Clinical Geropsychiatry

SECOND EDITION

ADRIAN VERWOERDT, M.D.

Professor of Psychiatry;
Duke University Medical Center,
Durham, North Carolina;
Director, Geropsychiatric Institute
John Umstead Hospital,
Butner, North Carolina

WILLIAMS & WILKINS
Baltimore/London

Made in the United States of America

First Edition, 1976

Library of Congress Cataloging in Publication Data

Verwoerdt, Adrian.
Clinical geropsychiatry.

Includes bibliographical references and index. 1. Geriatric psychiatry. I. Title.
[DNLM: 1. Geriatric psychiatry. WT150 V57c]
RC451.4.A5V47 1980 618.97'689 80-15759
ISBN 0-683-08592-1

Composed and printed at the
Waverly Press, Inc.
Mt. Royal and Guilford Aves.
Baltimore, Md. 21202, U.S.A.

To Christopher and Mark

PREFACE

To the Second Edition

In this second revised edition, the new nomenclature of DSM III (Diagnostic Statistical Manual of Mental Disorders) is being introduced in the text. Several chapters have been up-dated and a chapter on training has been added. Generally, the basic outline of the book and the sequence of the chapters is similar to that in the first edition.

PREFACE

To the First Edition

This book is intended for professionals involved in organizing or providing mental health services for the elderly. While the text is primarily aimed at psychiatrists and psychiatric nurse practitioners, an attempt has been made to reflect the multidisciplinary aspects of aging, and to make the book useful for gerontologic practitioners from other disciplines as well. Its purpose is to be of use to mental health professionals who practice in a variety of clinical settings, including private practice, community mental health centers, general hospitals, geriatric units of mental hospitals, and nursing homes.

Geropsychiatry is the psychiatry of late life. It encompasses the behavioral sciences, psychodynamic concepts, and psychiatric practices with reference to the aging personality and to the mental disorders of late life. This book is written within a medical-psychological frame of reference, in keeping with the concepts of modern ego psychology, and is based on consideration of three levels of human activity: biological, psychological, and social. Since the primary focus of the book is clinical, the presentation of theoretical concepts serves to facilitate a better understanding of the psychopathology of senescence and of an etiologically based treatment approach. Any theoretical construct stands or falls depending on its power to broaden the scope of scientific understanding and to facilitate effective clinical intervention.

Anyone who has done clinical work in the field of aging is confronted with arduous tasks, including the necessity to relinquish one's rescue fantasies, to be faced with death or despair, to struggle for value and meaning, and to keep the humanitarian and the scientist within one's self in dynamic equilibrium. If some measure of personal and professional maturation results from this, a proper sense of humility will be part of it. Surprisingly many can be our rewards: the challenge of work in what still is very much a terra incognita, the excitement of the team effort, and the therapeutic response of our patients.

ACKNOWLEDGMENTS

It has been my good fortune to have been associated with the Duke Center for the Study of Aging and Human Development for many years. Founded by Dr. Ewald W. Busse, who was director from its inception in 1957 until 1970, the Center was subsequently headed by Dr. Carl Eisdorfer (1970 until 1972) and Dr. George Maddox (1972 until the present). I am indebted to them in two ways: first, because of their remarkable success in bringing together a superb team of investigators, educators and clinicians in the field of aging, and providing unique opportunities for multidisciplinary work; and also, because my personal associations with them were a source of rich learning experiences.

The Center for the Study of Aging and Human Development and the Department of Psychiatry at Duke made it possible to develop a formal Geropsychiatry Training Program in 1966. Funded in part by grants of the National Institute of Mental Health, it has provided training in geriatric psychiatry, primarily for psychiatrists, but also for professionals of other disciplines. Throughout the years, it also has provided numerous contacts with the training faculty, including Dr. Dan G. Blazer, Dr. Daniel T. Gianturco, Dr. Daniel T. Peak, Dr. Eric Pfeiffer, Dr. H. S. Wang, and Dr. Alan D. Whanger. I have profited from our collaboration; to each of them I am indebted in a special way. The work we did was an exciting mix of research, teaching, clinical practice, and program planning. Their enthusiastic participation and individual creativity ensured the success of the Duke Geropsychiatry Training Program, and provided the impetus for other innovative programs, in the university itself, in the community, and statewide.

There are many others to whom I wish to express my appreciation. Dr. H. Keith H. Brodie, Professor and Chairman of the Duke Department of Psychiatry, Mr. Thomas J. Peters, III, Director of John Umstead Hospital, and Dr. Khalil S. Tanas, Director of Clinical Services, John Umstead Hospital, have given me enthusiastic support and encouragement. Dr. Pamela J. Trent has read the manuscript and given useful suggestions. Dr. Robert D. Miller, Dr. William M. Taylor, Dr. Alan D. Whanger, and Dr. Martha S. Wingfield contributed to the second edition of the book by up-dating the text in several chapters.

Most of the case material presented in this book became accessible to me through my participation in the Geropsychiatry Unit at John Umstead Hospital, Butner, directed by Dr. Gildegardo Alidon; and the OARS Geriatric Evaluation and Treatment Clinic and the Duke Geriatric Psychiatric Inpatient Service, both directed by Dr. Alan D. Whanger. Other clinical case material became available through contact with the Geropsychiatry Units of Cherry Hospital (Goldsboro) and Dorothea Dix Hospital (Raleigh). I wish to express my appreciation to the directors and the clinical staff of these programs for the many case conferences I had the privilege to attend.

I wish to thank Mrs. Mary Frances Ingold, Mrs. Pamela Smoak, and Mrs. Ruth Wortman for their excellent work in typing and preparing the manuscript.

CONTRIBUTORS

R. D. Miller, M.D., Ph.D.
Clinical Assistant Professor of Psychiatry
Duke University Medical Center, Durham, North Carolina
Director, Psychiatric Residency Training
John Umstead Hospital, Butner, North Carolina

W. M. Taylor, M.D.
Clinical Assistant Professor of Psychiatry
Duke University Medical Center, Durham, North Carolina
Staff Psychiatrist, John Umstead Hospital,
Butner, North Carolina

A. D. Whanger, M.D.
Professor of Psychiatry
Chief, Duke Geriatric Psychiatry Service
Director, OARS Geriatric Evaluation and
Treatment Clinic
Duke University Medical Center, Durham, North Carolina

M. S. Wingfield, M.D.
Clinical Associate Professor of Neurology
University of North Carolina School of Medicine
Chapel Hill, North Carolina
Director of Neurology
John Umstead Hospital, Butner, North Carolina

CONTENTS

1 aging and human development

BIOLOGICAL AGING

THE CONCEPT OF AGING

Role of Theories of Aging

The purpose and role of a *theory* is to systematize diverse phenomena into a single conceptual pattern and to explain how or why these phenomena occur. Thus, theories of aging must take into account the fundamental nature of the aging process, the mechanisms by which it comes about, as well as its manifestations and effects on the organism's functions. Since aging involves many diverse phenomena, a spectrum of biological, psychological, and social theories is needed, rather than a single theory. What aging essentially is and why it occurs, no one knows; these issues are just as complex as those pertaining to the concept of life. Since we are unable to define "life," we are likewise incapable of drawing a sharp line between such concepts as development, becoming, and aging. Their common denominator, however, is the factor of time-dependent change.

Factor of Time. Definitions of biological aging share the common denominator of the *factor of time*. Thus, a distinction between primary and secondary aging has been made. Primary aging refers to time-dependent biological processes, rooted in heredity, that are independent of stress, trauma, and disease. It is a time-related process that results in a decline in the efficiency of the various functions of the organism, and this deterioration progressively increases the probability of death. Secondary aging pertains to the disabilities resulting from trauma and loss.[1]

The factor of time is also essential in the Gompertz equation,[2] a mathematical formula expressing the probability of death at any given age. The Gompertz formula expresses not only the fact that the prevalence of aging phenomena increases exponentially with advancing age, but also the age-related rate of loss of functional cells. Thus, it represents the rate of aging on a cellular level and of human mortality in relation to age.

Longevity. With regard to *longevity*, variations exist between members of a species, but there is a maximum beyond which no system has been known to survive. The life span of members of a species, by and large, shows a fairly narrow distribution. There seems to be an intrinsic time clock for each species, or a genetically determined program that regulates the phases of the life cycle. In this framework, the moment of death is determined by the same genetic programming that determines the onset of the organism. The functional decline intrinsic in the senescent process is related to a logarithmic function of time.

Human longevity is the outcome of several interacting factors, including genetic makeup and environmental and nutritional factors, as well as psychological, social, and economic influences. The increase in average life expectancy has been largely due to the decrease in deaths attributable to infectious diseases. However, it is highly likely that measures that succeed in improving health and reducing death risk in early life positively affect health in the adult years as well, thereby diminishing the death risk. Few individuals of any species actually reach their potential maximum longevity, so that senescence may not be the major cause of death.[1]

Biological Clocks. Several subsystems of the system-as-a-whole have been considered as possible *biological clocks*. One example is the brain. In contrast to certain epithelial cells (e.g., skin or white blood cells) which are capable of mitotic cell division, the neurons are postmitotic all through life. Since these postmitotic neurons have the vital role of regulating the entire organism, the central nervous system may be viewed as a time clock. The brain is the only organ whose size is correlated with the potential lifespan of several species. The *cephalization index* is the ratio between the weight of the brain and the body, and appears to be correlated with longevity in the case of mammals and birds.[3]

Another example of a proposed biological clock is the mitochondria.[4] This is based on the premise that longevity in mammalian species is largely an expression of genetic control over the rate of oxygen utilization. The latter determines the rate of accumulation of mitochondrial damage produced by free radical reactions, the rate increasing with the rate of oxygen consumption, which ultimately causes death.

Finally, it has been proposed that no single part or process of the living system contains a time clock but that the latter is represented by the sum total of the system parameters themselves. The fact that species have fixed longevities, which are probably genetically determined, implies that the factors present at the beginning of the biological system are the same as those that result in senescence. In a mathematical sense, the origin of senescence is at the beginning of the system's existence.[5]

System Theory. The phenomenon of aging can also be conceptualized in the framework of *system theory*. A system can be defined as a dynamic order of parts and processes standing in mutual relationship. Living organisms, whether unicellular or metazoa, are open systems which function through the transfer of energy.[6] The phenomena of senescence are encountered only in systems. Only energy systems, not things, grow old. In biological energy transfers, the efficiency of the system reflects its ability to exist in its environment. In any system undergoing senescence, there is a steady decrease in the energy yields and a negative change in the rate at which utilizable energy is produced. Power is defined as work per unit of time. Hence, a decline in the functional capacity of a system is a negative acceleration in power. Senescence may be conceptualized as a decline in free energy production with time, a decline in power arising from intrinsic changes in the system.[7]

MECHANISMS OF SENESCENCE

There are several biological theories of aging (see also Table 1.1) which represent attempts to understand and explain the manner, method, or mechanisms by which aging comes about. The various theories of aging are by no means mutually exclusive, but rather tend to complement each other. Some theories focus more on cellular phenomena, others on interstitial tissue (e.g., collagen), and again others on intracellular structures (e.g., mitochondria). The number of possible interactions between intracellular and intercellular activities is so great that it is not possible

Table 1.1

Biological Theories of Aging

1. Cellular (intracellular)
   a. Genetic Theories
      —Stochastic
      —DNA damage
      —Somatic mutation (by radiation)
      —Hit theory
      —Error theory
   b. Nongenetic
      —Loss of reserve capacities
      —Wear and tear
      —Rate of oxygen uptake (mitochondrial damage)
      —Accumulation (lipofuscin, etc.)
      —Deprivation (of essential nutrients)
      —Free radicals (intra- and intercellular)
      —Cross-linkage (intra- and intercellular)
2. Physiological (intercellular)
   a. Single organ theories
      —Cardiovascular
      —Endocrine: thyroid, gonads, pituitary
   b. Homeostasis
      —Failure of adaptive mechanisms
      —Stress theory
      —Immunological; autoimmune theory
      —Endocrine control
      —Central nervous system control (cephalization index)

to determine which action, reaction, or interaction represents the mechanism of aging. The intrinsic processes which bring the cell inevitably to its death are probably the same as those with which the cell begins.[5]

Cellular Theories

Genetic Theories. Genetic theories of aging are based on the assumption that the life span is determined by the information in the DNA molecules of the gene. The focus is on the way that information is transferred from DNA molecules through various steps to the formation of proteins necessary for the normal functioning of cells.[8]

Since there are marked differences in average life span between different species, it is clear that there is a genetic program which sets the upper limit of the life span. A long life is related to many different genes and a large gene pool is advantageous for long life.

Women live an average of about 8 years longer than men. The same sex difference in favor of females exists in other species such as rats, mice, and dogs. Since gender is determined by the XY chromosomes in males and XX chromosomes in females, the sex difference in longevity may be due to the greater amount of X chromatin in females. Humans with long-lived parents and grandparents live an average of about 6 years longer than those with parents who die before the age of 50.[9]

Theories of preprogrammed aging have also been supported by studies which indicate that certain cells can divide only a limited number of times (40–50), after which they age and die.[10] Furthermore, cells from old animals can undergo only 20–25 cell divisions in contrast to the 40–50 divisions possible in cells taken from young animals.

Thus, on the one hand, a genetic program sets the upper limits of the potential life span in a species, but on the other hand, several other factors (gender, ancestry, nutrition, and environment, as well as psychological and socioeconomic influences) play a significant role in determining the actual life span.

Stochastic. Stochastic theories focus on cell depletion through cell death or somatic mutations due to radiation or other "hits." In time, defects develop in all cells, but in organs that can replace cells, the process of mitosis can eliminate aberrant cells. However, organs consisting of postmitotic cells (e.g., neurons) cannot rejuvenate, and hence would appear to have major responsibility for the aging process. From this point of view, aging is fundamentally the progressive increase of nonfunctional cells in organs whose cells are postmitotic.[1]

DNA Damage. The information needed by the cells to make essential proteins depends on the precise molecular structure of different parts of the large DNA molecules. Breaks in the chain of the DNA molecule or exchange of positions of parts of the chain alter the message and result in the cell's inability to make essential enzymes and death of the cell.

Somatic Mutation. According to the *somatic mutation* theory of aging, exposure to radiation accelerates aging. Experiments with rats showed that the incidence of abnormal chromosomes increased remarkably in radiated animals and progressively with age in nonradiatad animals.[11]

Hit Theory. The *hit theory* of aging[12] is a variation of the somatic mutation theory. Over the animal's lifetime, random hits would make a gene or its DNA molecules incapable of providing the precise information for making essential cellular proteins. A cell would become ineffective when the two similar chromosomes of a pair each suffer a hit in the same place or when one of the pair has been hit and the other has an inherited fault in this location. A fault is regarded as a recessive gene which makes the cell inviable only if it occurs in both genes of a pair. Some adults of a species may have shorter lives than others due to the difference in the number of inherited faults.

Error Theory. The information stored in the genetic code depends on the structure of the DNA molecule and is transcribed and translated in various steps until the final proteins or enzyme molecules appear. The assembly of amino acids to form specific proteins occurs at another place in the cell, namely on the ribosome. For this to occur, information from DNA is transferred to the proper place on the ribosome. This transfer occurs by the assembly of RNA molecules at specific points on the DNA molecule which then migrate to the ribosomes. The type of protein formed depends on what part of the large DNA molecule is decoded with the formation of an appropriate mRNA. The error theory[13] postulates that cell death is due to *errors* which may occur anywhere along the way *in the information transfer*, resulting in a protein which is not an exact copy and is unable to function properly. The error may be the incorporation of the wrong animo acid in the protein or a slight error in the normal sequence. DNA molecules are stable throughout the cell's life span, but RNA molecules have a half-life of 8 or 9 days. Consequently, new RNA molecules continuously replace enzyme molecules.

The cell's ability to produce proteins depends not only on the correct genetic information in the DNA molecules, but also on the competence of the protein synthetic apparatus, *i.e.*, enzymes necessary for translation and transcription of the information from the DNA to the final protein product. Thus, aging may be due to errors in enzymes involved in translation and transcription. Although there may be only a few errors at first, in the absence of cell division, the number of errors would increase exponentially over time leading to an "error catastrophe" and cell death.[14]

The error theory is linked to the mutation theory. Apparently, the development of chromosomal abnormalities is an intrinsic aspect of cellular aging and suggests the occurrence of mutation.[15]

Chromosomal abnormalities occur progressively with increasing age. Radiation further facilitates this phenomenon. It proposes age-related changes in deoxyribonucleic acid (DNA); these errors are then transferred on to messenger RNA, resulting eventually in the production of defective enzymes.

Sinex[16] discusses the possibility that aging results when inappropriate information is provided for normal cell function from the cell nucleus. This approach is consistent with the view that aging is related to some form of mutagenesis. When DNA is replicated, histone and other regulatory molecules are arranged on newly synthesized DNA in such a way as to ensure that daughter cells reproduce the parent cell or are suitably modified for the next stage of differentiation. There are two models concerning somatic mutation as a cause of aging: (1) somatic mutation due to intrinsic mutagenesis at the time of division and (2) a time-dependent mutagenesis in resting cells.

Nongenetic Theories. *Nongenetic cellular* theories of aging emphasize time-related changes in cellular proteins after their formation. These theories presume that time-related changes in molecules and other structural elements of cells impair their effectiveness.[8]

Loss of Reserve Capacities. Progressive *loss of reserve capacities* may be due to cell death and depletion of functioning units, results of increasing impairment of energy utilization, tissue repair, and elimination. Since no physiological process functions with 100 percent efficiency, there would be a progressive accumulation of failure in the course of time. This view is related to the concept of "mean time to failure" which would view living systems as a sort of biological machine with built-in obsolescence.[10]

Wear and Tear. The *wear and tear* theory assumes that organisms behave like machines.[17] From repeated use, parts wear out, and the machinery finally comes to a halt. However, unlike machines, living organisms have mechanisms for self repair. In some tissues, such as skin, the lining of the gastrointestinal tract, and red blood cells, which no longer divide in the adult, repair mechanisms are present and there is a constant turnover among many molecules within a cell.

Rate of Oxygen Uptake. Rubner[18] reported a direct relationship between *oxygen uptake* in various animals and their life span and hypothesized that the rate of living as measured by oxygen consumption was an important determinant of life span. Small animals, e.g., rat and mouse, have higher oxygen uptakes than large animals, e.g., horse and man. In fact, there is a rough correlation between the oxygen uptake per unit of body weight and life span: the higher the oxygen uptake, the shorter the life span. However, since the rate of all chemical reactions is influenced by temperature changes, all effects of temperature on life span could support any aging theory which involves chemical reactions, e.g., the cross-linking or error theories.

Nutrient Deprivation. *Deprivation theories* assume that aging is due to inadequate delivery of essential nutrients and oxygen to cells. These theories point to the increasing prevalence of atherosclerosis with advancing age and its effects on cellular and tissue functions. By the same token, cellular aging has also been ascribed to *accumulation of deleterious substances,* e.g., insoluble lipofuscin in neurons and muscle fibers of the heart.[19] These age pigments consist of lipids and protein molecules, and may represent an accumulation of nonmetabolized molecules. At present, there is no evidence of impaired function associated with these age pigments.

Free Radical Theory. Free radicals contain highly activated oxygen, and react quickly with other molecules. As a result, enzymes and other proteins may be altered. The formation of free radicals is accelerated by radiation and inhibited by antioxidants.[20]

Cross-linkage. The *cross-linkage* (eversion) theory applies mostly to noncellular material, especially collagen. A cross-linkage between polypeptide strands changes the structure of the collagen molecule and results in functional deterioration. With the passage of time, many large molecules of biological importance develop intra- or intermolecular crosslinking which alter the properties of these molecules. Since these crosslinks are stable, they accumulate with the passage of time. The accumulation of these cross-link molecules may be a primary cause of aging.[21] Most evidence comes from studies on extracellular proteins, namely elastin and collagen. With aging, cross-links develop between the two intertwined strands of the collagen molecule and between adjacent strands, resulting in loss of elasticity in many tissues, e.g., skin and blood vessels. The body contains many substances, primarily aldehydes, which accelerate the formation of cross-links. From these observations on extracellular protein, it has been assumed that similar changes occur in intracellular proteins, e.g., the DNA molecule. Since collagen becomes stiffer with age and constitutes 25–30 percent of total body protein and surrounds blood vessels and cells, age changes in collagen may have far reaching effects on other physiological functions.[22]

Physiological Theories of Aging

These theories focus on the interaction between cells and organs, and try to explain aging on the basis of impaired performance of a single organ or of physiological control mechanisms.[8]

Single Organ Theories. *Cardiovascular.* Failure of the *cardiovascular* system has long been regarded as the primary cause of aging. Aging would result primarily from the progressive deterioration of blood vessels due to atherosclerosis. However, atherosclerosis does occur in the young, and furthermore, aging occurs in lower animal species with no blood vessels, e.g., fruit flies, rotifers, and nematodes. McFarland[23] hypothesized that aging is primarily the result of reduced delivery of oxygen to critical tissues such as the brain, but the oxygen content of arterial blood does not fall with advancing age and blood flow to the brain is only slightly diminished after maturity.

Thyroid. Another hypothesis assumed that aging was due primarily to slowing of metabolic processes caused by *thyroid failure*. However, the age-related decline in basal oxygen uptake reflects tissue loss with advancing age rather than diminished oxygen consumption of individual cells.[24]

Sex Gland. Failure of the *sex glands* has also been looked upon as a primary cause of aging. This hypothesis led to the administration of sex hormones and the transplantation of gonads to induce rejuvenation. The use of female sex hormones for postmenopausal women has been advocated to minimize aging effects, but the risk of cancer in the genital tract by prolonged administration has led most clinicians to utilize the treatment on a short term basis.

Pituitary. Since the *pituitary gland* plays a central role in regulating the adrenal gland, thyroid, and gonads, aging has been ascribed to a failure of this gland.[25]

While failure of any organ system in the mammal may result in death, these failures cannot be regarded as a primary cause of aging, since aging also occurs in lower organisms which may not possess the specific organ system. Thus, physiological theories of aging need to look beyond a single organ system.

Aging and Physiological Controls. *Failure of Adaptive Mechanisms.* The overall performance of an animal is closely related to the effectiveness of various control mechanisms which regulate the interplay of different organs and tissues. It has been hypothesized that aging is due to *failure of adaptive mechanisms.*[26] Since adaptation to stresses involves the intact functioning of control mechanisms, the adaptation hypothesis is a special case of the broader theory of control mechanism failure. With advancing age, many control mechanisms lose their effectiveness. Any control mechanism must have a system to detect changes and a mechanism to carry out the proper adjustment. Thus, sensing devices may activate processes to readjust body temperature, blood glucose, blood pressure, heart rate, etc. In developing theories of aging based on control mechanisms, it is necessary to distinguish between alterations in the sensitivity of detecting devices and the effectiveness of the effector system necessary to maintain homeostasis. The primary control mechanisms operate through the endocrine system or nervous system.

Stress. The *stress theory* of aging[27] holds that aging results from the accumulated effects of life stresses. Any stress would leave a residual impairment from which the animal does not completely recover. These residuals, each perhaps quite small, accumulate over the life span so that eventually the reserve capacities are depleted. However, the assumption of residual damage which persists and accumulates, is not supported by experimental data. Also, stresses often induce hypertrophy and may be beneficial.

Immunological Theories. The immune system protects the body against invading microorganisms and mutant cells which may form in the body. The immune system produces antibodies and special phagocytic cells which digest foreign cells and substances. Aging has a marked impact on these capabilities. The production of antibodies reaches a peak during adolescence and then declines. The basic impairment may be a declining ability to recognize slight deviations in molecular structure or cell characteristics, so that mutant cells that would ordinarily be destroyed are no longer recognized and are permitted to grow. By the same token, impaired capacity of cell recognition might result in the development of antibodies which inactivate normal cells. Even though recognition occurs, the aging immune system may be unable to produce antibodies or phagocytic cells.

Autoimmune. The *autoimmune theory* of aging[28, 29] proposes that aging results from the development of antibodies which react even with normal cells and destroy them. This might occur because of failure to recognize normal cells as normal or the development of errors in the formation of antibodies so that they now react with normal cells as well as the deviate ones which stimulated the immune cells to form antibodies in the first place. This hypothesis gains its support from the age-related increase of autoimmune antibodies in the blood and the similarity between many so-called immune diseases (some types of anemia, rheumatoid arthritis, arteritis, maturity onset diabetes, thyroiditis, and amyloidosis) and the phenomena of aging.

Endocrine Control System. Tissues of senescent animals show a reduced binding capacity for many steroid hormones;[30] thus, the site of breakdown of the regulatory mechanisms through endocrine control may well be at the cellular level. With advancing age, the rate at which excess sugar is removed from the blood is significantly reduced. This is due to the reduced sensitivity of the β cells of the pancreas to a slight rise in blood sugar level.[8]

Nervous Control Mechanisms. Performances which require coordinated movements mediated through the nervous system show greater decrements with age than component parts of the total performance. For example, the maximum breathing capacity shows a greater age decrement than vital capacity itself.[31] When environmental temperatures are increased or decreased, young subjects can maintain body temperature, while old subjects show a change.

The ability to perform muscular work is a function of the integrated activity of the cardiovascular, respiratory and neuromuscular systems. Perhaps the greatest age-related decrements are in the area of exercise and work performance. Although decrements exist within each organ system involved, they are less than the decrements in total performance. The slower response in many organ systems in the elderly may be a reflection of impaired integrative functions both at the neural and endocrine levels.

THE MANIFESTATIONS OF AGING

Pattern of Age Decrement

As a rule, biological characteristics show earlier maturation and decline than psychosocial capacities and functions. The *pattern of age decrement* is individual for each person, and the rate of decline varies from one function to another, and from one individual to another. There is no direct or simple cause and effect relationship between the degree of structural impairment on the one hand, and the presence of impaired function or manifest disease, on the other hand. At an autopsy, for example, it is not unusual to find rather extensive changes in the brain vessels while there was little clinical evidence of mental impairment prior to death.[32]

The Concept of Health and Illness

The hallmark of health is the ability to maintain a steady state within, and a dynamic equilibrium between oneself and the environment. A healthy individual can maintain himself, and remain inwardly stable, in spite of changing external circumstances. This ability is called homeostasis or constancy principle. However, there are definite limits to this capacity. This is true for living organisms at any age, but with advancing age, the capacity for homeostasis gradually declines. The range of adjustment and adaptation becomes smaller and narrower.

Aging versus Illness

Progressive Loss of Physiological Capacities. Aging is the *progressive loss of physiological capacities* and functions in the organism. Muscle, fibrous tissue, cartilage, and bone deteriorate with age. Elastic and muscular tissue is replaced by fibrous elements. Changes in the elastic properties of collagen (due to increased cross-linkages between polypeptide chains) cause it to be tougher. Calcification of the arterial system is a linear function of age. Hardening of the arteries begins at an early age and continues to progress slowly. In the skeletal system, resorption of bone and osteoporosis occur, the latter more frequently in women, due to postmenopausal reduction of estrogen secretion. Other examples of age-related deterioration are the decline in myocardial, pulmonary, hepatic, renal, endocrine, and behavioral capacities. These deteriorations have been attributed to an increasing loss in functional (parenchymal) cells with replacement by nonfunctional connective tissue.

Normal and Pathological Aging. The distinction between age-related biological decline and specific diseases prevalent in late life is not always easy. One characteristic of biological deterioration is that the resting level of a function may show no significant change with age, except that during stress, return to the base level is prolonged (for example, displacements in acid-base balance and in blood glucose levels). Diabetes is an example illustrating the difficulty of distinguishing clearly between *normal* and *pathological aging*. If values indicative of diabetes in young adults are indiscriminately applied to the aged, many of them would be diagnosed as diabetic. Older persons taking a glucose tolerance test often show a "diabetic" type of curve, but do not necessarily show clinical evidence of diabetes. It is only under the stress of glucose overload that the aged person manifests a decline in the capacity to keep the blood glucose level within certain narrow limits.

Unique Health Status Evaluation. Therefore, *health status* of the aged should not be evaluated in terms of the standards for young adults. If one takes the latter as criteria for health, then indeed most of the aged would have to be considered ill. The phrase "well" in the case of a 30-year-old person and an 80-year-old person has entirely different meanings. On the other hand, creative individuals, e.g., musicians, may still be productive and "young" in their sixties.

HUMAN DEVELOPMENT

Over the life span there exists a continuously ongoing change of goals and interests, and the awareness of these changes results in a sense of becoming. During each of the phases of the life span, there are specific opportunities and challenges. The notion of development includes phenomena that are both progressive and retrogressive in nature. The thymus gland, for example, shows retrogressive changes (involution) early in life. On the other hand, in late life, there may be considerable social growth and expansion in spite of age-related biological decline.

PHASES OF HUMAN DEVELOPMENT

Cycle of Life Phases

Human development has been described in terms of a *cycle of life phases*, each phase being characterized by its own specific opportunities, sources of satisfaction, and developmental goals.[33] Successful completion of one life phase is a prerequisite to meeting the demands, and obtaining the gratifications of a subsequent phase. Failure in one phase leads to psychological problems related to that phase, and serves as a predisposition for subsequent failures in later phases. Because there are increasingly more chances to fail as time goes on, the last phase of life ("integrity") is necessarily the most difficult one to attain. Erikson's life phases may be summarized as follows (See also Table 1.2).

Basic Trust. *Basic trust* is the period covering the first year of life and is more or less the equivalent of the oral phase in psychoanalytic terminology. Essentially, the infant learns through the experiences of the

Table 1.2*

Psychosocial crises	Radius of significant relations	Related elements of social order	Psychosocial modalities	Psychosexual stages
Trust vs. mistrust	Maternal person	Cosmic order	To get To give in return	Oral-respiratory, sensory-kinesthetic (incorporative modes)
Autonomy vs. shame, doubt	Parental persons	"Law and order"	To hold (on) To let (go)	Anal-urethral, muscular (retentive-eliminative)
Initiative vs. guilt	Basic family	Ideal prototypes	To make (=going after) To "make like" (=playing)	Infantile-genital, locomotor (intrusive, inclusive)
Industry vs. inferiority	"Neighborhood," school	Technological elements	To make things (=completing) To make things together	"Latency"
Identity and repudiation vs. identity diffusion	Peer groups and outgroups; models of leadership	Ideological perspectives	To be oneself (or not to be) To share being oneself	Puberty
Intimacy and solidarity vs. isolation	Partners in friendship, sex, competition, cooperation	Patterns of cooperation and competition	To lose and find oneself in another	Genitality
Generativity vs. self-absorption	Divided labor and shared household	Currents of education and tradition	To make be To take care of	
Integrity vs. despair	"Mankind," "my kind"	Wisdom	To be, through having been To face not being	

* Reproduced from *Identity and the Life Cycle* by Erik H. Erikson, with the permission of W. W. Norton & Company, Inc. Copyright © 1959 by International Universities Press, Inc.

mother-child relationship that the world is a "good place," and that others are trustworthy; included is a sense of trustworthiness as far as the self is concerned. In adults, the impairment of basic trust is expressed in a basic mistrust: a tendency toward withdrawal, alienation, and lack of affiliation.

Autonomy. *Autonomy* (age 1–3) is the equivalent of the anal phase. During this period the child learns to make use of his basic neuromuscular capacities such as walking, talking, and sphincter control. The child begins to "stand out" as an individual. From a sense of self-control, not associated with loss of self-esteem, comes a lasting sense of autonomy and pride. Failure to reach such autonomy results in a sense of doubt and shame, and a tenuous capacity for self-control. The sense of shame interferes with standing out as a separate individual, and is related to loss of face and loss of dignity.

Initiative. *Initiative* (age 4–6) is a period of venturing out, exploring (curiosity), thrusting forward, and discovering what it means to be a boy or a girl. Failure in this developmental stage leads to an undue sense of "doing wrong" and guilt. Feelings of guilt are now possible due to the maturation of the child's conscience (superego). The phase of initiative is comparable to the infantile-genital stage in psychoanalytic terminology.

Industry. *Industry* (age 6–12), equivalent to the latency period, is the period of learning specific skills and acquiring knowledge. Failure in this phase leads to a sense of inferiority.

Identity. *Identity* (age 12–20) is the phase of adolescence (puberty). The task of this difficult period of life is to discover "who one is": what kind of man or woman one is going to be, what career to pursue, and what one's individual outlook on society and the world is. Identity diffusion leads to uncertainty in one or all of these aspects.

Intimacy. *Intimacy* refers to the closeness and affiliation in adult relationships, particularly between man and woman. This phase corresponds with that of mature genitality. To find sexual, emotional, and spiritual satisfactions in a socially approved relationship is a major developmental task of intimacy. Failure leads to a sense of isolation and self-absorption.

Generativity. *Generativity* pertains primarily to the establishing and guiding of the next generation, although there are people who, for various reasons, do not apply this drive to offspring but to other forms of altruistic activity, or to creativity, which may absorb their kind of parental responsibility. Generativity literally refers to productivity. An individual can generate a great variety of "works," such as offspring, money, business, teaching, and good deeds. Self-absorption and a sense of stagnation are typical of failure in the area of generativity.

Integrity. *Integrity* refers to the final identity of a person. Erikson[33] describes it as the acceptance of one's life and the significant people in it as something that had to be and that, by necessity, permitted no substitutions; also, there is the need for accepting one's life and what happened in it, as one's own responsibility. (Note the apparent paradox between the inevitability of one's life and one's responsibility for it). The ideal characteristic of the last phase of life is integrity which, at the same time, is also the specific task of this life phase. Failure in accomplishing this aim is indicated by the term despair.

Understanding the Psychological Issues of Old Age

Integrity, the sense of identity in senescence, presupposes the more or less successful passing through of previous life phases. The successful completion of developmental challenges is not simply an isolated affair, on the part of the individual. He needs, besides his own resources, the cooperation of the social environment. Thus, an infant will not develop "trust" if the mother does not provide the infant with the sense that life is worthwhile living; and the adolescent develops his sense of identity, by way of consensual validation, in contact with his peers.

It is no exaggeration to say that the social environment up until now has been less than conducive toward successful completion of the ultimate task in life: the final integration of one's self and of all past selves in the present self. Biological and social-environmental hazards contribute to a great number of crises and failures.

In as much as intimacy, generativity, and integrity are developmental phases of the adult and late years, they have special significance for *understanding the psychological issues of old age.* The counterparts of these three phases, *i.e.*, distancing and isolation, stagnation and self-absorption, and despair, play a major role in the psychopathological formations of late life.

Comparatively speaking, the senium has remained "terra incognita." A fuller understanding of this phase of life is a necessary step toward a comprehensive theory of human behavior and can provide additional insights into earlier periods of growth and development and their impact on the total personality.

SENESCENCE AS A DEVELOPMENTAL PHASE

Psychological Experiences of the Last Phase

When speaking of psychological experiences of the last phase of life, the emphasis here is on the word "last." Although we usually think of aging in terms of decline, this decline is a movement toward a final end. It is this that distinguishes senescence from previous life phases. The latter have a beginning and an end which, at the same time, is a new commencement. Besides being a temporal determinant, the term "the end" also connotes the element of purpose, goal, or task. In previous developmental stages, the end of a phase coincides with the goal toward which development is aimed. Toward which end is the stage of senescence aimed? Can we speak of a goal of task in senescence, as we do in previous life phases?

Although death is a "fact of life," one's position vis-à-vis death is an intensely personal matter. It is here that we may speak of a *developmental task,* in the sense that a person comes to view his own death as the appropriate outcome of his life. Stern offers the thesis that adaptation to death is necessary for full personality maturation and that deficiency in this adaptation is an integral factor in neurosis. The neurotic uses regressive fixation to symbiotic dependency (which in infancy protected him against trauma) to ward off fears concerning the inevitable final trauma.[34] Since there is no previous experience of death (only the death of others) to serve as a model for death anxiety, the latter is a creative act. It involves the synthesis of earlier anxieties (those along one or more specific dimensions of human experience) into a new form of anxiety which overarches all of these.

Adaptation to Death

The statistical definition, that "aging is a process that increases the probability of death" introduces the phenomenon of death. The impersonal quality and intellectual detachment inherent in statistics and mathematics, however, are alien to the immediacy of human experience. Inasmuch as aging represents a progressive shortening of the distance to death, there are several corresponding *milestones* in human development: (a) a cognitive, intellectual comprehension; (b) a subjective, emotional experience; and (c) a final existential perspective.

Cognitive. What distinguishes human aging from biological aging, in general, is the fact that the human being *knows* he will grow old and eventually die. This knowledge is not always present and during the first few years of life, it is completely absent. An intellectual comprehension of the fact of death develops at about the same time that the young individual learns the facts of life, i.e., during early adolescence. A cognitive grasp of the concept of a personal death depends on the attainment of specific psychological capacities, including the completion of the body image, a mature time perspective, and the capacity for abstract thinking. Through the abstract capacity, it becomes possible to imagine one's own death, that is, to apply the fact of the death of the other to oneself. The mature time perspective enables one to place this end of the self at the horizon of one's existence. And finally, the concept of death of the self is meaningful only to the extent that there is a self-concept and body image to begin with.

Emotional-Experiential: Mid-life Crisis. That point in life when the sum total of an individual's biological, psychological, and social capacities are in an optimal configuration, constitutes the peak or prime of life (climacter: Greek term meaning rung of the ladder). Most people perceive the period of life before the climacter as one of evolution, growth, or ascendance; and the time following the prime of life as a period of involution, decline, or descendance. (Again, these are not simple distinctions or absolute contrasts, because growth and expansion remain possible during the second half of life. What matters, however, is the net effect of the sum total of all changes at a given time.) Following the peak there is a change in tempo and direction: a deceleration and descent which are dimensions of the "change of life." The perception of the onset of age-related phenomena, and the subjective experience associated with the awareness of aging (*i.e.*, shorter distance to death) are dimensions of the *mid-life crisis.*[35] The latter presumably is a depressive crisis, and is often lucidly apparent in the lives of persons with creative genius. As an example, the opening stanzas of Dante's "Divine Comedy," written at the age of 35, may be quoted.[36]

"Midway life's journey I was made aware
That I had strayed into a dark forest,
And the right path appeared not anywhere.
Ah, tongue cannot describe how it oppressed,
This wood, so harsh, dismal and wild, that fear
At thought of it strikes now into my breast.
So bitter it is, death is scarce bitterer."

According to Jacques,[35] who investigated the midlife crisis with regard to its effect on creativity, it occurs around the age 35. In a random sample of 310 artists, the death rate showed a sudden jump between age 35–39. Between age 40–44, there is a big drop below the normal death rate, while in the late 40's the death rate returns to normal. The content and mode of creative work before and after the midlife crisis are different. The content of the creativity changes from the lyrical, in early adulthood; to the more tragic and philosophical, after the crisis; and, eventually on to the serene (in the sixties).

Existential: Life Review. As the biological phenomena of life, aging, and death are inextricably intertwined, so are, on the existential level, the meaning of life and death inseparable. Hence, the final perspective vis-à-vis death comes about by way of a retrospective evaluation of one's life. The task of the *life review*[37, 38] is to integrate one's life as it has been lived in relation to how it might have been lived. The life review is not a passive process, but a constructive effort to achieve a purposeful form of *reminiscence*. These reminiscences serve not primarily to recall facts, but to weave them into a harmonious perspective and to achieve a sense of closure. The old person may want to write a revised autobiography, as it were, to be left with those who survive him.

The forms of life review may range from a nostalgic recall to severe depression with anxiety, guilt, and suicidal tendencies. In general, the life review should not be viewed as a psychopathological phenomenon, but as a common normal experience. The lifelong personality of each individual influences the way in which he handles the life review, and whether he feels he has much time or only a few days to get his psychological house in order. The person's characteristic patterns of coping with conflict may be used to resolve his terminal conflicts.[38]

Reminiscing and the life review may be carried out in the privacy of one's mind, or it may involve an audience. A certain degree of "audience participation" is desirable, because the issue "Who am I and what have I been?" is intimately related to the notion of what one is and has been for others. In the life review, there is concern with the image that an individual wishes to leave behind. This may lead to forgiveness and reconciliation, and sharing one's own interpretation of the meaning of life with others.

References

1. Busse, E. W.: Theories of aging. In: *Behavior and Adaptation in in Late Life,* edited by E. W. Busse and E. Pfeiffer, ed. 2, chap. 2, Little, Brown and Company, Boston, 1977. pp. 8–30.
2. Gompertz, B.: On the nature of the function expressive of the law of human mortality. *Philos. Trans. Roy. Soc. Lond. 115*:513, 1825.
3. Sacher, G. A.: Relation of lifespan to brain weight and body weight in mammals. In: *Lifespan of Animals, Ciba Foundation Colloquia on Aging,* edited by G. E. W. Wolstenholme and M. O'Connor, vol. 5, Little, Brown and Company, Boston, 1959. pp. 115–141.
4. Harman, D.: The biological clock: the mitochondria? *J. Am. Geriatr. Soc. 20*:145–147, 1972.
5. Calloway, N. O.: A general theory of senescence. *J. Am. Geriat. Soc. 12*:856, 1964.
6. von Bertalanffy, L.: General system theory and psychiatry. In: *American Handbook of Psychiatry,* edited by S. Arieti, vol. 3, chap. 43, Basic Books, New York, 1966. pp. 705–721.
7. Calloway, N. 0.: The role of entropy in biologic senescence. *J. Am. Geriatr. Soc. 14*:342, 1966.
8. Shock, N. W.: Biological theories of aging. In: *Handbook of the Psychology of Aging,* edited by J. E. Birren and K. W. Schaie, chap. 5, van Nostrand Reinhold Company, New York, 1977. pp. 103–115.
9. Dublin, L. L., Lotka, A. J., and Spiegelman, M.: *Length of Life: A Study of the Life Table,* Ronald, New York, 1949.
10. Hayflick, L.: Biomedical gerontology: current theories of biological aging. *Gerontologist 14*:454, 1974.
11. Curtis, H. J.: *Biological Mechanisms of Aging,* Charles C Thomas, Springfield, Ill., 1966.
12. Szilard, L.: On the nature of the aging process. *Proc. Natl. Acad. Sci. U. S. A. 45*:32, 1959.
13. Medvedev, Zh. A.: The nucleic acids in development and aging. In: *Advances in Gerontological Research,* edited by B. L. Strehler, vol. 1, Academic Press, New York, 1964. pp. 181–206.
14. Orgel, L. E.: The maintenance of the accuracy of protein synthesis and its relevance to aging. *Biochemistry 49*:517–521, 1963.
15. Jacobs, P. A., Court Brown, W. M., and Doll, R.: Distribution of human chromosome counts in relation to age. *Nature (Lond.) 191*:1178, 1961.
16. Sinex, F. M.: The molecular genetics of aging. In: *Handbook of the Biology of Aging,* edited by C. E. Finch and L. Hayflick, chap. 2, van Nostrand Reinhold Company, New York, 1977. pp. 37–62.
17. Sacher, G. A.: Abnutzungstheorie. In: *Perspectives in Experimental Gerontology,* edited by N. W. Shock, Charles C Thomas, Springfield, Ill., 1966. pp. 326–335.
18. Rubner, M.: *Das Problem der Lebensdauer and seine Beziehungen zu Wachstum und Ernahrung.* R. Oldenbourg, Munchen, 1908.
19. Strehler, B. L.: On the histochemistry and ultrastructure of age pigment. In: *Advances in Gerontological Research,* edited by D. B. Strehler, vol. 1, Academic Press, New York, 1964. pp. 343–384.
20. Harman, D.: Free radical theory of aging: effect of free radical reaction inhibitors on the mortality rate of male LAF mice. *J. Gerontol. 23*:476–482, 1968.
21. Bjorksten, J.: The crosslinkage theory of aging. *J. Am. Geriatr. Soc. 16*:408–427, 1968.
22. Kohn, R. R.: *Principles of Mammalian Aging.* Prentice-Hall, Englewood Cliffs, N. J., 1971.
23. McFarland, R. A.: Experimental evidence of the relationship between aging and oxygen wants in search of a theory of aging. *Ergonomics 6*:339–366, 1963.
24. Shock, N. W.: Metabolism and age. *J. Chronic Dis. 2*:687–703, 1955.

25. Dilman, V. M.: Age-associated elevation of hypothalamic threshold to feedback control, and its role in development, aging, and disease. *Lancet 7711*:1211–1219, 1971.
26. Frolkis, V. V.: Neuro-humoral regulations in the aging organism. *J. Gerontol. 21*:161–167, 1966.
27. Selye, H.: The future for aging research. In: *Perspectives in Experimental Gerontology*, edited by N. W. Shock, Charles C Thomas, Springfield, Ill., 1966. pp. 375–387.
28. Blumenthal, H. T., and Probstein, J. G.: The pathogenesis of diseases of senescence. In: *Surgery of the Aged and Debilitated Patient*, edited by J. D. Powers, W. B. Saunders Company, Philadelphia, 1968. pp. 44–81.
29. Wolford, R. L.: The immunologic theory of aging. *Gerontologist 4*:195–197, 1964.
30. Roth, G. S.: Age-related changes in specific glucocorticoid binding by steroid-responsive tissues of rats. *Endocrinology 94*:82–90, 1974.
31. Norris, A. H., Shock, N. W., Landowne, M., and Falzone, J. A., Jr.: Pulmonary function studies: age difference in lung volumes and bellows function. *J. Gerontol. 11*:379–387, 1956.
32. Zerbin-Ruedin, E.: Genetics. In: *Modern Perspectives in the Psychiatry of Old Age*, edited by J. G. Howells, chap. 1, Brunner/Mazel, New York, 1975. pp. 1–23.
33. Erikson, E. H.: Identity and the life cycle. In: *Psychological Issues*, International Universities Press, New York, 1959.
34. Stern, M. M.: Fear of death and neuroses. *J. Am. Psychoanal. Assoc. 16*:3–31, 1968.
35. Jacques, E.: Death and the mid-life-crisis. *Int. J. Psychoanal. 46*:502–514, 1965.
36. Alighieri, D.: The divine comedy: inferno, canto I. In: *The Portable Dante*, translated by L. Binyon, The Viking Press, New York, 1947. p. 3.
37. Butler, R. N.: The life review: an interpretation of reminiscence in the aged. *Psychiatry 26*:109–114, 1963.
38. Birren, J. E.: Life review, reconciliation and termination. In: *The Psychology of Aging*, chap. 12, Prentice-Hall, Inc., Englewood Cliffs, N. J., 1964.

2

psychodynamic aspects

CHANGES IN THE MENTAL APPARATUS

Considerations of mental phenomena include several dimensions: the time factor, aspects of energy, the concept of structure, and the factor of dynamic interaction. The time factor is reflected in the developmental aspects of human behavior, in processes of becoming, and in the time-related changes of aging. Aspects of energy (the so-called economic point of view in psychoanalytic theory) refer to such phenomena as motivation, activity, drives, needs; to surplus energy for productivity, creativity, or recreation; to energy required for adaptational or defensive purposes; and so on. Structural considerations pertain to concepts such as ego and superego, which represent organization, order, or information. Finally, the term psychodynamic refers to the interaction of intrapsychic forces, on the one hand, and interpersonal-environmental influences on the other hand.

Simple as these definitions may sound, they pertain to complex mental phenomena. With regard to their existence and characteristics, we can only make inferences, not direct observations. In addition, since there are no separate compartments in the mind, they are closely inter-related and cannot be viewed as being independent. The sum total of the attributes of the mental apparatus makes up the individual's *character* (from the Greek verb which means "to groove," e.g., in stone, as a hieroglyph; hence, our use of the term character for a printed or engraved symbol). Thus, one's character is the indelible imprint of life's experiences on one's self. Implied here is the notion that personalities can change over a lifetime. These changes can be described in terms of intrapsychic and social changes as well as their dynamic inter-relationships.[1] Such considerations about the effects of aging on the mental apparatus will be metapsychological on the one hand, and must be in conformance with clinical observations on the other hand.[2, 3]

ENERGY, DRIVES, AND NEEDS

The organism is an intrinsically active system. A stimulus does not cause a reaction in an otherwise inert system, but rather modifies processes in an autonomously active system. Since the organism is able to maintain a disequilibrium (i.e., the steady state of an open system), it can dispose of tension in spontaneous activity or through responses to stimuli.[4]

Characteristics of Drives

Characteristic of drives is the tendency to seek gratification through activities of consummation. *Drives represent "bits of energy"*; this energy can be estimated in terms of the amount of work performed in the process of satisfying the drive. The term "id" (Latin for the English "it") connotes something impersonal. What is impersonal about the drives of the id is that all humans (and animals) possess similar sets of biological drives. Therefore, what makes a human being distinctive, i.e., a personality, is not his id, but how he handles himself in a complex world in which he has to maintain relationships with others.

With regard to the drives, it must be kept in mind that these can be categorized in several ways. Traditionally, a distinction has been made between libidinal and aggressive drives. It is clear, however, that the distinction between drives involving the discharge of surplus energy and those involving the need for replenishment is also important. The former type includes active impulses, catabolic in nature, or aimed at discharge of tension. The latter can be thought of as (more or less) passive needs, e.g., fatigue, hunger, sleep, thirst, cold, which involves anabolic processes, and eventually aim at building up of tension or surplus energy.

General Characteristics of Biological Aging

Typical of the biological senescence of living systems is the progressive decline in ability to produce energy. A young organism can produce more energy per unit of time than an old one. From the standpoint of energy, an old organism has less power. Applying this concept of biological drives, it appears plausible that with aging, the strength of the active drives declines, and would become less powerful (e.g., genital sexuality, generativity in the areas of work and parenthood, mastery of novel situations, etc.).

Another general characteristic of biological aging is that the resting level of a function may show no significant change with age, but that during or after stress, *return to the baseline level is prolonged* (e.g., displacements in electrolytes, blood glucose levels, heart rate). Thus, there is an increase in the amount of time needed to restore and replenish the organism, with advancing age. On the psychological level, this can be expressed in terms of an increase in needs. With advancing age, it takes increasingly more time for anabolic processes of restoration and replenishment to take place, even though the absolute quantity (intensity) of the passive, anabolic needs may actually decrease with age. For example, an older person may need fewer calories, but the metabolic processes of intake and assimilation of food, as well as production of utilizable energy, may require more time. Such a constellation amounts to an *increase in passive needs*. The intensity of such needs, then, becomes progressively stronger since more time is required to fulfill them. With increasing age, then, the needs for stability, shelter, rest, etc. will become relatively more important. These biologically oriented needs, whose quantity or intensity increases with age, have a quality of being relatively more "narcissistic," self-oriented, passive, and aimed at self-preservation. Important in this context is the fact that, because of declining strength and resources, the aged person does not have the same power he used to have to bring about the fulfillment of his particular needs and wishes.

STRUCTURAL ASPECTS

The Ego

Order and Information. While the energy of drives lacks structure, in the case of ego, energy is utilized in an organized manner. This corresponds, respectively, to the difference between primary and secondary process. Thus, "ego" is, in a sense, equivalent to *order and information*. The ego is a set of regulatory principles whose main task is to maintain a balance between pressures from different directions: inner needs and drives, the opportunities and constraints of the external world, and the guidelines of one's conscience and aspirations (see Table 2.1).

The achievement of adaptation is a creative process, involving continuous problem solving and being facilitated by the *synthetic* and the *autonomous* ego functions. Hartmann developed the concept of autonomous ego apparatuses which, in rudimentary nature, are present at birth and develop outside the area of psychic conflict.[5] This area of conflict-free ego functioning presumably includes perception, intuition, comprehension, thinking, language, certain phases of motor development, learning, and intelligence. However, in the course of development, these functions may become involved in psychic conflict; e.g., when unduly aggressive impulses impinge on the function of intelligence, thinking, and memory, a learning inhibition may result.

The human organism, being an open system, is capable of maintaining a *steady state*. This is not a simple condition of harmony or of static equilibrium, but involves the maintenance of a constant ratio between input (sensory-afferent stimuli, etc.) and output (motor-efferent responses, etc.). This steady state is further characterized by *equifinality*. While the equilibria in closed systems depend on initial conditions, an open system can attain a time-independent state, which depends on the parameters of the system rather than its initial condition.[4] On the psychological level, this principle corresponds with the phenomenon of personal identity. Thus, the functions of the ego include, but also go beyond, the traditional concept of homeostasis.

Table 2.1
Ego Functions and Their Components*

1. *Reality testing:* distinction between inner and outer stimuli; accuracy of perception of external and internal events.
2. *Judgment:* anticipation of consequences of intended behavior; appropriateness of behavior to external events.
3. *Sense of reality:* extent of derealization and depersonalization; self- identity and self-esteem; clarity of boundaries between self and world.
4. *Regulation of affects and impulses:* directness of impulse expression; effectiveness of delay mechanisms.
5. *Object relations:* degree and kind of relatedness (narcissistic attachment or symbiotic object choices); primitivity versus maturity; degree to which others are perceived independently of self; object constancy.
6. *Thought processes:* memory and attention; ability to conceptualize; primary versus secondary process as reflected in language.
7. *Regression in the service of the ego:* ability to regressively relax cognitive acuity and to allow new configurations to emerge in thinking.
8. *Defensive functioning:* success or failure of defenses.
9. *Stimulus barrier:* threshold for stimuli; management of excessive stimulus input.
10. *Autonomous functioning:* intactness of primary and secondary autonomy apparatuses.
11. *Synthetic-integrative functioning:* degree of reconciliation of incongruities and relating together of events.
12. *Mastery-competence:* actual competence (capacity to master and affect environment); feeling of competence as measured by person's expectations of success on actual performance; discrepancy between actual competence and feeling of competence.

* Reprinted with permission from Bellak, L., and Sheehy, M.: The broad role of ego functions assessment. *Am. J. Psychiatry 133:*1259–1264, 1976.

The basic model of cybernetics is the feedback schema which, in the case of the living organism, is called *homeostasis.* The homeostatic feedback mechanism involves an ensemble of regulations that maintain variables constant, and direct the organism toward a goal, with the result of the reaction being monitored back to the receptor side so that the system is held stable or led toward a target. However, the homeostatic schema does not explain several types of specifically human behavior, such as exploring and curiosity; activities aimed at building up, rather than reducing, of tension; creativity; etc. In psychopathology, on the other hand, the homeostatic model is more suitable because nonhomeostatic functions usually decline in mental illness. Thus, mental disease may be described as a series of defense mechanisms, settling down at ever lower homeostatic levels until more preservation of physiological life is left (e.g., in senile regression).[6] The concept of progressive teleological regression in schizophrenia is similar.[7]

The accurate perception and interpretation of reality is an ego function, called the *reality principle*; it is based on an integration of several part functions: perception, apperception, thought, and memory. Characteristic of all living systems is the property of boundary. The boundary of the personality (the self) is not simply concrete and spatial such as the skin.

Rather, the *ego boundary* is a dynamic structure that functions *like* a membrane. It is the subjective line of demarcation between self and not-self, me and not-me, inside and outside. The concept of ego boundary is related to other ego functions, such as the reality principle, the self-image, and the body image. In states of depersonalization, there is both a blurring of the ego boundary and impaired reality testing.

The body occupies a unique position with regard to inner and outer reality. In one sense, the body is part of myself so that what occurs to it, occurs inside of me. But, one can also take some distance from one's body, look at it, touch it, perceive sensations coming from within, and so on. In this sense, the body is external to the perceiving self and comparable to other external objects. We may even feel that we "own" our body, a possession to be proud or ashamed of, to be concerned about it, or to be taken for granted. The term *body image* refers to an individual's subjective image of his own body. In addition to this inner mental picture, the body image includes a set of personal values, assigned to parts of the body, and to the body as a whole (pride in physical prowess; shame about physical shortcomings, etc.). The role of the body and the body image is particularly relevant with regard to somatic expressions of psychiatric illness (e.g., conversion, hypochondriasis).

The ego matures in a gradual way and this involves a great deal of learning, first in the family, and later in school and work, through friendships, marriage, parenthood, and so on. In fact, the ego has the opportunity for a lifetime of continuing education. By the same token, life, through its corrective emotional experiences, may act as a therapist. The autodidact may learn from life's experiences without the formalized instructions of school or interventions typical of therapy.

Age-related Changes. *Age-related changes* may affect the autonomous ego functions or the ego's defense mechanisms, both of which require the expenditure of energy.

Autonomous Ego Functions. The *autonomous* ego functions (perception, thought, etc.) may be affected when insufficient energy is available to them, or when there is a withdrawal (decathexis) of the energy normally invested in the operation of these capacities. This can be seen in various psychopathological conditions; decathexis of perception may lead to hysterical conversion symptoms, e.g., hysterical blindness, and decathexis of memory may cause amnesia. It is possible that in schizophrenia and in certain cases of senile regression, the loss of abstract intelligence is based on a withdrawal of energy from the autonomous ego function of thought.

Delay of Gratification. One of the earliest functions of the ego is to interpose a time lag between stimulus and response. Thus, motor responses are no longer necessarily automatic. During this *delay of gratification,* there is opportunity for selecting those behavioral responses which are likely to be maximally effective and for creative problem solving. Thus, the mature ego (secondary process) stands in opposition to the pleasure principle (the urge toward immediate gratification, typical of primary process). Regression of this ego function may result in "the geriatric delinquent," dominated by the pleasure principle, and oriented toward immediate gratification, often at the expense of long-range plans.[8]

Time Perspective. The decline in the ability to delay gratification in some old individuals is probably related to an *altered time perspective*: the sense that time is running out, and there is no point in continuing to delay gratification. Such a trend is not necessarily pathological; it may be healthy, depending on many factors. In some old persons, however, this ego change may result in the acting out of socially undesirable behavior.

Defense Mechanisms. As is true for ego functions in general, *defense mechanisms* require energy to function effectively. Repression, the ego's (unconscious) attempt to prevent certain thoughts or feelings from entering conscious awareness requires a continuous expenditure of energy (countercathexis). With less energy being available to the ego, it may become difficult to maintain repression. In such a case, there are two possible developments. Some of that which was repressed may begin to emerge into conscious awareness; and, if this repressed mental content is threatening or unacceptable to the individual, anxiety will be the result. Or, with repression itself being unable to do the job, auxiliary defenses are called into action, e.g., denial or projection.

High-Energy Defenses. Some individuals, throughout life, habitually use defenses that may require large amounts of energy. As a result, they have little energy left over for work, social contacts, leisure activities; etc. *High-energy* defense patterns (the "fight" patterns of response) include: reaction formation, counterphobic defenses, overcompensation, obsessive-compulsive defenses, the "manic" cluster (denial, hyperactivity, and suppression through diversion), and the "paranoid" cluster (projection, hostile aggression against the externalized problem, or repeatedly fleeing away from the externalized threat).

Regressive Defenses. On the other hand, defenses that are basically *regressive* (e.g., withdrawal and increased dependency) require less energy. The high-energy defensive patterns become more vulnerable as the years go by, due to physical illness or age-related decline in energy production.

The Superego

The *superego* is more or less equivalent to conscience. Like the ego, it develops over a period of years, through assimilation of standards and guidelines from significant people, especially the parents. The mental processes that play an important role in superego development are introjection and identification. The superego may be involved in intrapsychic changes that are favorable or unfavorable.

Mellowing. Favorable, adaptive changes are probably related to the phenomenon of "mellowing with age." There may be two ways in which *mellowing* can come about. First, when the instinctual drives are less strong and urgent, the superego may no longer have to be as alert or on guard. As a result, less energy is taken up by the censorship function of the superego. A relaxed superego may be inwardly perceived as a sense of freedom. Whatever energy has been freed may now become available for other, possibly creative, purposes. Secondly, an individual who has been "on good behavior" for most of his life may come to feel that it is now time for a reward. He may allow himself to reap the benefits of a lifetime of work through the experience of leisure during retirement.

Unfavorable Developments. *Unfavorable developments* occur, when in the course of aging, needs or impulses emerge which are unacceptable to the superego. For example, an individual who is physically disabled and faced with the need to accept help from others, may consider such dependency gratifications unacceptable, or inconsistent with his self-concept, so that feelings of shame and guilt develop, or an attitude of rebellious protest.

Ego Ideal

Part of the superego is the idealized self concept, the *ego ideal,* which refers to one's aspirations and life goals. At some point in life, frequently in the middle years, an individual begins to wonder if he will reach the goals he has set for himself. Some people will feel that they have arrived; others, that they have fallen short of their aspirations. The phrases "having arrived," and "having it made," are commonly used to refer to a sense of status in life, or the attainment of a plateau on which success comes in one's grasp. A sense of satisfaction arises from perceiving the merger of the actual self with the idealized self. The success is the sense of succeeding into the ego ideal. Once attained, this succession into the ego ideal will serve as insurance against the risks of loss of self-esteem that would result from "being over the hill."

In contrast to despair, the coming into one's own, the succeeding into the ego ideal, is a moment of integration, of integrity.

PSYCHODYNAMICS OF ADAPTATION

THE ROLE OF LOSS

Apperception

For any loss or stress to become meaningful, it has to be perceived, registered in the mind, and evaluated through the process of *apperception.* The latter refers to a mental scanning process of comparing incoming stimuli and images with those already stored in memory. The fact of a loss cannot be undone by the ego, but it is possible for the ego, through its defense mechanisms, to try to prevent the loss from reaching conscious awareness. The situation may become rather complex, when the ego itself is changing as well, e.g., in organic brain syndrome (compare case on p. 132). In these instances, the ego's ability to perceive reality is impaired and the impact of these losses may be blunted. Reality perception may also be diminished through a process of withdrawal which prevents the individual from feeling the pain that would have come with clear awareness of having suffered a loss, a factor that may play a role in the development of senile regression.

The Quality of Stress and Loss

Specific clusters of social events requiring change in ongoing life adjustment are significantly associated with the onset of an illness.[9] The relationship between life stress and object loss, on the one hand, and illness onset, on the other hand, has been demonstrated by several investigators.[10] The etiological significance of stresses and losses is that they represent a necessary, but not sufficient, cause of illness, and that they account in part for the time of onset of illness. In addition to determining the number and type of stressful factors, it is also necessary to be able to assess them in terms of their qualitative aspects, e.g., the subjective meaning of an event or its personal value. Holmes and Rahe developed a rating scale listing a series of life events, the qualitative significance of the latter being numerically expressed.[11] It must be remembered that such a rating scale is based on data obtained from a cross-sectional study of a large number of subjects. Therefore, the rating scale cannot simply be applied to one particular person. In addition, it is very likely that, in a given individual, the qualitative stress aspects of some of the life events would change in the course of time.

According to Levin,[12] loss represents a deficiency of external supplies needed to satisfy drives and needs. Loss of an object into which much narcissistic libido was invested is a precipitating factor for depression. In addition, there are other precipitating factors: attack, restraint, threat, and "loss equivalents." Attack refers to any external force producing pain or injury. Restraint is any external force which restricts those actions needed for satisfaction of drives. Freedom from restraint therefore represents freedom to find satisfactory outlets for one's drives. Older people are restrained by physical infirmities, fears of "overdoing it," and cautionary attitudes on the part of family and society (e.g., in the area of sex). Threat is a warning of possible future loss, attack, or restraint. Threats may contribute to depression and conversely depression may increase one's feeling of being threatened. "Loss equivalents" occur when somebody else's gain is experienced as a loss for oneself (as in envy). Or, there may be exposure to a seductive situation which leads to increased desire which cannot be satisfied.

Object, Aim, Source of Drives

For further understanding of the effects of loss, it is necessary to keep in mind the distinction between losses pertaining to the non-self (e.g., material possessions, love objects) as compared to the self (e.g., the body). Again, a few definitions may be in order. An *object* refers to the instrument that brings about satisfaction of a need or drive (food, sexual partner, etc.). The *aim* of a drive is the specific activity required for satisfying the drive (in case of hunger: biting, chewing, swallowing, etc.; in case of the sex drive: sexual intercourse, masturbation, etc.). The *source* of a drive refers to the body area where the excitation arises, e.g., the upper gastrointestinal tract or the genital organs.

The *object*, the "instrument" bringing about drive satisfaction or need fulfillment, may be lost through death, or may be less accessible due to illness. Thus, because of a specific object loss, the quality of the sexual drive, for example, may change from a heterosexual to an autoerotic orientation. The loss of an external object may be resolved by a process of *substitution*: directing the drive or interest toward a new object. The economy of the mind is then only temporarily upset.

The situation, however, is different in the case of an *"internal" loss.* When an important part of the body is lost (or declines in effectiveness), psychic economy may be considerably disturbed. For example, due to the loss of teeth or a gastrectomy, the aim of the hunger drive can be significantly altered: the activity normally required for satisfying the drive can no longer be performed. Likewise, an arthritic or cardiac patient can be incapable of performing activities required for certain sexual gratifications.

It is also possible that the decline in the overall amount of available energy may affect the *aim* of the drive or need. This may involve a shift from being active to being passive. A physically infirm man, for example, may change from active sexual performance to being a more or less passive participant.

Again another consideration pertains to possible changes in the *source* of the drives. Anatomical and physiological alterations in specific organs may diminish the intensity of excitations, a shift which may involve a simultaneous increase in the urgency of another need. The source (erogenous zone) where the genital-sexual drive is considered to originate, for example, is the genital apparatus. If there should be a major anatomical loss involving these organs, or a physiological change affecting the endocrine glands providing sex hormones, the biological basis of the sex drive itself may be altered. And, the psychological effect will be different, compared with the loss of an external object. Likewise, the source of the hunger drive is altered in conditions such as diabetes or hyperthyroidism.

Under certain circumstances, *special problems* may develop. For example, any acute sudden change in the drive, its objects, aim, or source, usually represents a major stress resulting in profound psychological reactions. Also, any discrepancy between the rates of change in the aim and the source of the drive sets the stage for conflict. Thus, a young man with a disabling skeletomuscular condition may be unable to consummate the sexual act while his sex drive is relatively normal. Optimally, losses in the realm of the object, aim, and source would be in keeping with each other so that no discrepancy between wish, capability, and opportunity takes place.

> Some of the above is illustrated by the case of a 68-year-old man hospitalized because of chronic depression. The psychodynamics involved a dependent premorbid personality, with regression and hypochondriacal concerns being quite prominent in the clinical picture. What actually had brought the patient to the hospital was his sexual behavior toward his wife: he insisted on being held at her bosom and her nursing him, 2 hours every day. The wife had become increasingly indignant about this, especially in view of the fact that "he cannot raise a hard one." Thus, in the context of his depression (and some age-related infirmities), the following changes in drive and drive satisfaction had occurred. The source of the sexual drive had changed from being genital to pregenital (oral and skin eroticism); the aim of the drive changed from active consummation to being passive and receptive (being held). The object of the drive shifted from vagina to breasts. The area of sexuality, however, in which these regressive changes occurred, represented a displacement of other, nonsexual concerns (need for security, self-esteem, etc.). The fact that the patient tried to solve a nonsexual problem by way of sexual means was responsible for his insatiable demands, no amount of breast feeding would have been sufficient. This point was vividly demonstrated following admission to the hospital. As the result of various therapeutic measures, his spirits improved and the regressive and hypochondriacal features disappeared, along with the insatiable oral tension.

THE ROLE OF SUBLIMATION

While a psychologically healthy person is flexible enough to revise his mental economy, such a readjustment is difficult or impossible for a person with long-standing psychological problems. One reason for this is the often rigid and limited repertoire of defenses; also, the very magnitude of the underlying conflict may be sufficiently frightening that the individual feels he has to be constantly on guard and that he can't afford a period of relative defenselessness during which he could experiment with new coping techniques. In such a situation, then, marked anxiety or depression may develop. The failure to establish new patterns to deal with conflict or stress tends to be resolved finally by resorting to the way of least resistance, i.e., regression or withdrawal. These defensive maneuvers, in fact, may take the person away from the conflict area, but since he has never adequately developed the habit of optimal regression (e.g., regression in the service of the ego), the newly adopted defense tends to overshoot. Examples of this can be seen when an individual, who used to be compulsively active or excessively self-reliant, experiences an illness or a stressful change, following which he remains unduly passive and dependent.

All important for mental health is the capacity to sublimate. Sublimation is the optimal way of handling drives that, in their original form, are not permitted free expression by society. Many such impulses belong to the domain of infantile sexuality; they are drives which, later in adult life, ordinarily find their appropriate niche in the realm of genital sexuality. They are called component drives because they are to become subsidiary to adult genital drives. Normally, these infantile drives come under the hegemony of adult sexuality, and being more temperate under the auspices of love and intimacy they become useful and permissible. Another possibility, however, is for one or more of the pregenital drives to be sublimated which involves the following. The drive changes in quality so that it now becomes socially acceptable. The energy involved in the original infantile drive is fully expressed; this is different from repression, where the drive energy is wasted due to its confinement in the unconscious. In contrast to repression, there is no need for a continuous countercathexis in the case of sublimation. The id and the ego join forces, as it were, and are not at cross-purposes; hence, energy is freely available for constructive purposes. Finally, sublimation involves a process of neutralization: the sexual or aggressive-destructive aspects of a particular drive is removed and neutralized.

What is the significance of this for the psychodynamics of senescence? The notion of changing a need, interest, or drive into socially acceptable channels implies an orientation on the part of the individual toward society, its members, and values. An *outward orientation* toward others and toward external resources can be an extremely useful coping device when the aging person's inner resources are dwindling and provide less intense gratification.[13] Thus, an aging individual may shift his interests and values away from himself, toward external objects: his children, business, church, community, etc. Individuals with a high degree of abstraction may shift their interest to society, the world, science, or art. In the previous chapter, we had raised the question of whether it is possible to speak of development in old age. In view of the continued possibility for intrapsychic changes, including the opportunities for sublimation, it is certainly appropriate to speak of continued psychological development in late life.

References

1. Neugarten, B. L.: Time, age, and the life cycle. *Am. J. Psychiatry 136*:887–894, 1979.
2. Baltes, P. B., and Willis, S. L.: Toward psychological theories of aging and development. In: *Handbook of the Psycholog of Aging,* edited by J. E. Birren and K. W. Schaie, chap. 7, von Nostrand Reinhold Company, New York, 1977. pp. 128–154.
3. Zetzel, E. R.: Dynamics of the metapsychology of the aging process. In: *Geriatric Psychiatry,* edited by M. A. Berezin and S. H. Cath, International University Press, New York, 1965. pp. 109–119.
4. von Bertalanffy, L.: General system theory and psychiatry. In: *American Handbook of Psychiatry,* edited by S. Arieti, vol. 3, chap. 43, Basic Books, Inc., New York, 1966. pp. 705–721.
5. Hartmann, H.: *Essays in Ego Psychology,* International Universities Press, New York, 1967.
6. Menninger, K., Mayman, M., and Pruyser, P.: *The Vital Balance,* The Viking Press, New York, 1963.
7. Arieti, S.: Schizophrenia. In: *American Handbook of Psychiatry,* edited by S. Arieti, vol. 1, chap. 23, Basic Books, Inc., New York, 1959.
8. Wolk, R. L., Rustin, S. L., and Scotti, J.: The geriatric delinquent. *J. Am. Geriatr. Soc., 11*:653–659, 1963.
9. Rahe, R. H., Meyer, M., Kjeer, G., and Holmes, T. H.: Social stress and illness onset. *J. Psychosom. Res. 8*:35 1964.
10. Eisdorfer, C., and Wilkie, F.: Stress, disease, aging and behavior. In: *Handbook of the Psychology of Aging,* edited by J. E. Birren and K. W. Schaie, chap. 12, van Nostrand Reinhold Company, New York, 1977. pp. 251–275.
11. Holmes, T. H. and Rahe, R. H.: The social readjustment rating scale. *J. Psychosom. Res. 11*:213–218, 1967.
12. Levin, S.: Depression in the aged. In: *Geriatric Psychiatry,* edited by M. A. Berezin and S. H. Cath, International Universities Press, New York, 1965. pp. 203–225.
13. Cath, S. H.: Some dynamics of middle and later years: a study in depletion and restitution. In: *Geriatric Psychiatry,* edited by M. A. Berezin and S. H. Cath, International Universities Press, New York, 1965. pp. 21–72.

3 dynamic psychopathology

STRESS AND COPING IN LATE LIFE

The aged person's environment is characterized by changes which are stressful in varying degrees. Stresses in the external environment include loss of occupation, income, and prestige. In the internal milieu, decline in all biological systems is obvious.

In living organisms, the response to a stressful event is a reaction aimed at removing or neutralizing the stress and repairing the damage. On the cellular level there is, for example, the formation of antibodies and other immune mechanisms. Specific cells or organs play a major role in physiological defenses: white blood cells, spleen, adrenal glands, etc. The same principles apply to phenomena on the psychological level. A mental stress or psychotrauma leads to a psychological defense or a behavioral coping pattern.[1-3]

In dynamic psychopathology, we need to differentiate between the stress itself; the immediate emotional distress caused by it (e.g., loss of a spouse resulting in immediate distress of grief); the defense mechanisms employed to deal with the stress and its associated distress (e.g., denial); and the psychological and behavioral phenomena associated with, or resulting from the defense mechanisms (e.g., denial leading to patterns of manic hyperactivity).[4, 5]

EMOTIONAL DISTRESS

Emotional distress includes various negative feelings such as fear and anxiety, grief and depression, shame and guilt, anger and hostility, and so forth. It is important to keep in mind that there is no such thing as an abnormal feeling per se. What makes feelings abnormal is not so much their quality, but the extent of their duration and intensity, and their appropriateness in the context. Thus, sadness and grief are an essential aspect of the experience of living; it would be "abnormal" not ever to feel sadness and grief. These same feelings, however, if more prolonged and severe, become pathological, i.e., a depression.

Fear of Loss

Fear is the normal emotional reaction in response to impending injury or loss. *Primary anxiety* (or traumatic anxiety) concerns the response of the organism to maximal internal and external stimulation. *Signal anxiety* is the warning signal in response to impulses and fantasies that might result in disaster. This type of anxiety is the signal of an internal danger situation relevant to ego-alien impulses. In old age, signal anxiety becomes less important. Also, traumatic anxiety as a response to overwhelming stress is relatively unusual, although it does occur. Thus, the nature of anxiety in the aged does not correspond to primary (traumatic) anxiety, nor to signal anxiety. According to Zetzel, anxiety in the aged resembles the type of anxiety stimulated by fear of *loss and separation.*[6] A danger anticipated may be actual (real) or imagined (existing in fantasy only). The more a person reacts to imagined dangers and losses, the more the psychological capacity of reality evaluation is impaired. In a neurosis there is only a mild to moderate impairment of reality testing, while in a psychosis, the impairment of contact with reality is severe or total. Thus, a psychotic patient may live entirely in a fantasy world. Some aged individuals, for example, withdraw from reality and retreat into their inner self in order to "live off" their memories.

Grief Reaction

The normal emotional response to a loss which actually took place is a *grief reaction* (simple bereavement). This should be distinguished from depression which, although difficult to define in exact terms, is generally considered as a pathological emotional reaction. A grief reaction involves a clear and conscious recognition, on the individual's part, of an actual loss. Following the initial emotional shock on the part of the bereaved person, there is an increasing realization of the significance of the loss and all its ramifications in every day life.[7] During this period, there are recurring episodes of specific physiological distress, such as waves of sadness. The feelings of bereavement and sadness are expressed verbally and nonverbally, e.g., crying. Toward the end of the grief reaction, which may last for several months, there is a resolution which involves a redirecting of energies and interests toward new people, goals, or activities.[8–10]

When a close person is lost, the psychic energy invested in that person first has "no place to go," but eventually, the resolution of the grief reaction results in a reinvestment of this psychic energy in new objects, in the direction of other people. When, however, part of the self is lost (e.g., amputation), resolution of the grief reaction is more complex and involves a form of inner realignment and reappraisal of the self and one's relations with others. Adjustment of the latter type is characterized by continuation of self-esteem, rooted in a religious or philosophical frame-

3

work that views personal worth on the basis of one's intrinsic value as a unique person; by accepting and integrating the limitation into a new self concept; and by finding new ways of maintaining closeness to others and realizing remaining potentials.[10, 11]

PSYCHODYNAMIC ASPECTS OF COPING BEHAVIOR

The aged individual has to cope with a multitude of losses that often interact and accumulate in the manner of a vicious circle, at a time when the physical and mental energy needed for effective coping is decreasing.[12] This has two implications. First, the usual ways of coping, especially the "high energy" defenses, may have to be replaced by new techniques of adaptation. Active or aggressive mastery, for example, may be replaced by acceptance and the capacity to resign oneself to the inevitable without self-reproach, bitterness, or cynicism.[6]

Capacity for Coping

The *capacity for coping* with stress (the range of capacity, and the types of defenses chosen) is a function of the ego. Ego strength determines, to a large extent, the degree of success in coping. When a person overextends himself in his attempts toward mastery, we can speak of a crisis. Whether or not a crisis will be resolved depends, by and large, on the ego's potential for growth; crisis resolution, in turn, results in further ego growth. We can try to assess ego strength by exploring the individual's manner of coping with stress in the past, his mastery of novel situations, as well as the objective signs of achievement and subjective sense of satisfaction with regard to previous life phases (marriage, parenthood, work, etc.) (see Table 2.1).

Range of Coping Mechanisms

The *range* of coping mechanisms is based on a repertoire determined largely by past experiences and relationships to significant people in childhood and young adult life. A person, whose earlier life was relatively wholesome and free from major intrapsychic conflicts, possesses more flexibility and a greater range of effective behavioral responses to stress since less effort is expended in dealing with internal (neurotic) pressures. On the other hand, an individual who has always had limited psychological resources and resilience, and who has managed only a precarious adjustment, is more likely to respond maladaptively to stress.[13] The overly independent person, for example, who has always resisted any appearance of weakness may perceive a disabling disease as catastrophic, responding to it in a disorganized fashion; while another individual with fewer conflicts may be able to adjust to the same disability more gracefully.

The individual's capacity to adapt successfully is also influenced by *organic problems* such as mental retardation, congenital or required deformities, organic brain damage, etc. The person who cannot fully comprehend a problem or who lacks the physical capacity to respond efficiently is clearly limited in his attempts at adaptation.

The aged person's *external environment* is a very influential factor in the ability to adapt successfully. The ability of a spouse or other family member to move in supportively when greater physical dependence is unavoidable, will enable the aged person to remain in his environment for a longer time.

Adaptive versus Maladaptive

Whether coping or defense mechanisms are adaptive or maladaptive depends upon the type and intensity of the defense as well as upon its appropriateness to the situation.[14] *Adaptive* coping techniques imply a re-establishment of an equilibrium that was disturbed due to the loss. In the case of coping with physical illness, for example, adaptive devices presuppose some amount of cognitive awareness regarding the illness, a willingness to seek medical help and a realistic adjustment to the sick role. *Maladaptive* defenses aggravate the patient's suffering, deplete his resources and weaken his resistance. Maladaptive coping behavior typically leads to a vicious circle which aggravates the very problem against which it is directed. In the language of cybernetics: adaptive coping represents a "negative feedback" leading to corrective intervention, while maladaptive coping involves a "positive feedback" leading to a vicious circle. In the latter case, unpleasant emotions and painful tension do not abate, but accumulate in the individual.

Selection of Specific Defenses

The *selection* of a particular defense frequently results in certain characteristic behaviors. This has definite implications, not only for the individual's adjustment, or lack thereof, but also for clinical management.[15] The various defense techniques and the behavioral patterns commonly associated with them can be grouped into three main categories, i.e., those aimed at retreat from the threat and conservation of energy, exclusion of the threat or loss from awareness, and mastery and control.

TYPES OF DEFENSES AND COPING (see Table 3.1)

RETREAT AND CONSERVATION

Defenses aimed at *retreat from the threat* and at *conservation of energy* include regression, giving up, and withdrawal.

Regression

Regression is the retreat into earlier, more primitive modes of adap-

Table 3.1
Types of Defenses

A. *Retreat from threat and conservation of energy* ("low energy" defenses)
regression
withdrawal
giving up
B. *Exclusion from awareness*
repression
suppression
denial
rationalization
externalization (projection)
internalization (introjection)
C. *Mastery and control* ("high energy" defenses)
intellectualization
isolation of feelings from thoughts
obsessive-compulsive mechanisms
reaction formation
overcompensation
counterphobic

tation and relating to others. Its chief features are restriction of interest in the external world, self-centeredness, bodily overconcern, and increased dependency on others. Regression commensurate with the severity of a disability or illness is useful since it enables the patient to accept appropriate help in a dependent relationship. Excessive regression tends to backfire because others (relatives, medical personnel) will view the patient as "bad and uncooperative."

In some cases, the patient is apprehensive about "letting go" and fights against the regressive pull tugging inside of him. Although this may seem convenient for the environment (the patient is not "demanding"), it does present a problem to the person who clings to an independence which may have been appropriate but now has lost its usefulness. Moreover, once the facade of independence crumbles, the regressive manifestations of the underlying dependency now coming to the fore, may be exceptionally severe, and all the more difficult to manage.

The egocentricity and bodily overconcern of the regressed patient are closely related. Being engrossed in his own self, little interest is left over for others and the world around. Due to the reduced scope of the patient's world, his reality testing is hampered and he is less able to form reliable judgments about what happens around him. Consequently, he feels insecure and the need for continuous reality testing arises. Some of the resulting disturbing behavior represents attempts to find out where he stands with other people.

The patient is often uncomfortably aware of his dependent state; the guilt feelings generated by it make him easily suspicious of the goodwill of those attending him. He may imagine that they do not come to his aid quickly enough because they resent waiting on him or get exhausted by his demands. The patient also feels ambivalence toward those who care for him. While he may be grateful for the support, he is resentful because of what seems to him his inferior position. Some patients express this ambivalence by becoming more demanding.

The individual who accepts dependency eagerly causes other problems. He may develop excessive dependency on one person, so that he feels no one else can satisfy his needs. Such patients need to have their relationships with the medical personnel carefully structured to prevent overdependence on any one individual.

> A 69-year-old man of national prominence, hospitalized for a myocardial infarct, irritated and alienated nurses with his demanding, hostile behavior. In contrast to his responsible preillness behavior, characterized by precision in his work and conscientiousness in his relations with other people, the patient's illness behavior was marked by extreme dependence upon his wife, and obnoxiousness toward everyone else. He frequently passed flatus in the presence of nurses and other medical personnel without any appearance of embarrassment.

As regression deepens, dependence upon the familiar, and upon the established order extends to routines and to inanimate objects. Patients find small disruptions of daily routine upsetting; they need to have their activities fall into a stable, predictable pattern. One feature of regression, relevant in this context, is the alteration of the time sense and time perspective. While normal, healthy adults look ahead months or years, the regressed patient, like the child, views life in a time scale composed of smaller units, such as days or weeks. One of the consequences of this is the patient's inability to wait, and a frustrating sense of impatience.

The existence of organic problems, e.g., Organic Brain Syndrome, predisposes to regressive phenomena of psychotic nature. An 85-year-old woman with senile dementia would fill her shoes with bath powder and shredded paper; then she would tear up her clothes. She expressed the delusion that she had just given birth to a baby, even mentioning the baby's father by name, but the baby had died, and now she did not know what to do with the clothing. The themes of conception, birth, and death are represented through archaic, primary process symbols. Her own impending death was no longer in sight since she had regressed to a point where she still could give birth (a psychotic restitution fantasy). At the same time, her own death was represented by the young baby who already had died. The baby's death was concretely dramatized by tearing up her clothes. The delusional and hallucinatory phenomena in patients who are psychotic or profoundly regressed (e.g., schizophrenia, senile regression) are comparable to the manifest contents of a dream. The mental mechanisms causing the distortion of the underlying, latent thoughts and feelings are frequently rather naive and unsophisticated.

Hence, it may be relatively easy to arrive at an understanding of the psychotic manifestations. (see also pp. 250 through 252).

Giving Up

The orderly retreat inherent in adaptive regression is a sort of flexible "giving in." If, however, the retreat is carried to its extreme, it may end in surrender and capitulation to the threat. In this *giving up* there is a sense of complete loss of control and intactness of the self. In such a state of hopelessness and helplessness, the entire homeostatic machinery may collapse. The organism may lose its capacity for maintaining order in the internal (psychophysiological) environment. Giving up the will to live may well have psychophysiological repercussions which lower the individual's resistance, aggravate existing symptoms, and perhaps even hasten the moment of death.[16]

> A 59-year-old divorced woman expressed the desire to go to sleep and never wake up. Her present condition of giving up was the outcome of a long process of decompensation. Early in her marriage, her husband "committed adultery" but she stayed with him, and even supported him, "because he was close to being an alcoholic." She worked as a personnel director, an illustration of her strong sense of duty. Since they were unable to have children of their own, she wanted to adopt a child, but he refused. The patient continued to function responsibly in her work until she had a depression following her father's death, 8 years ago. This depression lasted 6 months. Since then, however, she began to drink, and this increased to the point of her being hospitalized several times because of alcohol abuse. Meanwhile, her husband left her which resulted in a divorce 2 years ago. After this, he began to do remarkably well as a salesman, and even stopped drinking. Having lost her husband, the patient next lost her job, and then her home. Being on welfare, she had to move into a rooming house. Thus, at the age of 58, she felt that nothing was left: no parents, no child, no husband, no job, no home, no meaning, no future. Living alone, she let herself deteriorate: drinking by herself and keeping others away by locking herself in her room which became more and more filthy. Eventually, she started to wander about aimlessly at night, was told to pack up and leave, and lost this last shelter.

Withdrawal

While regression is moving away from adult role responsibilities, *withdrawal* is a moving away from people. As such, it is a more serious development than regression. The response of withdrawal is often based on feelings of inadequacy or shame. For example, disfigurements resulting from illness or surgery may cause a person to expect disgust from others. To protect himself from this mortification, he withdraws from the contact with others. The loss of youthful attractiveness also can prompt a protective withdrawal. The "ravages of time" may be experienced as a narcissistic injury that is particularly painful. As a result, there may be attempts to cover oneself from the exposure to the eyes of others. In intimate relations, withdrawal sets up a vicious circle. The attitude of lowered esteem for oneself is contagious: others are likely to end up feeling embarrassed, too. Thus, withdrawal as a means to maintain self-esteem and avoid shame becomes a self-fulfilling prophecy; and, the price of maintaining dignity through withdrawal is isolation and loneliness.

A woman in her early 60's had been in psychotherapy because of multiple somatic complaints, most of which had a psychogenic origin. As her physical symptoms began to abate, she became more depressed. With embarrassment, she began to relate concerns about her marriage. She accused her husband of not being interested in her, and ruminated that, many years ago, he might have had a fleeting interest in another woman. Now, she and her husband were estranged, no longer intimate. At this point she confided, with visible shame, that her body was like a battlefield. In the course of many years, multiple surgical procedures had been performed on her abdomen and breasts, leaving scars all over. She hated the sight of it and kept herself "under cover." Her embarrassment, however, was communicated to her husband; he too began to feel a sense of shame. By participating in the cover up, he confirmed her doubts about herself and consolidated a pattern of mutual withdrawal.

EXCLUSION FROM AWARENESS

Defenses aimed at *excluding the threat or its significance from awareness* include suppression, denial, rationalization, depersonalization, externalization (projection), internalization (introjection).

Suppression

Suppression is a conscious attempt to dismiss certain ideas or feelings from awareness. Typically, the individual tries to push unpleasant thoughts to the back of his mind by getting busy with something else. Such diversionary activities become more difficult, when a person becomes weaker due to progressive disability or illness. Also, suppression may be put out of commission by the increased idleness inherent in being sick, disabled, or isolated. Nighttime may be especially difficult because of the additional lack of sensory input. Unable to sleep, the patient may find himself increasingly preoccupied with anxiety-provoking concerns.

A 63-year-old man was hospitalized because of addiction to glutethimide (Doriden). He had taken this for several years, gradually requiring more and more. The patient had been a prominent and successful person in his small community. He viewed his personal identity almost exclusively in terms of his work (director of a community agency) which involved much strain and irregular hours. The thought of retirement in the nearby future was a threat because this loss of social role was equated by him with a loss of identity. During daytime or working hours, he could suppress awareness of this threat by keeping busy, but at nighttime the "ghosts came out of the closet." Hence, the insomnia which in turn led to the addiction pattern.

Denial

Denial is a mental mechanism by which an observation, fact, or its significance, is denied or not recognized. Denial is frequently manifested by a person's spontaneous negation ("Now, don't get me wrong, what we have talked about doesn't worry me one bit"). Denial may be aimed at the factual existence of a loss, at the implications of the loss, or at one's emotional reactions resulting from the loss. Complete denial of the *fact* of an illness or loss suggests serious psychopathology of psychotic proportions. Denial of *feelings* or *problems* associated with an illness or loss is much more common. Mild forms of denial are often conducive to good adjustment, but extreme denial, frequently coupled with rebellious protest, is self-destructive, since the person tends to neglect appropriate counsel and assistance.

A 66-year-old man was hospitalized repeatedly because of recurrent cardiac decompensation. A psychiatric consultation was requested. During the interview, the patient was in a jovial, expansive mood (denial of feelings of concern about his illness). He did acknowledge the fact that he had a heart disease, but denied its importance. At one point, he leaned over and whispered with a mischievous look on his face: "Every so often, I get away from here, go downtown, and treat myself to a hearty, salty steak." He opened the drawer of his nightstand and pointed with a chuckle at a hidden salt shaker.

Rationalization

Closely related to denial is *rationalization*, a type of reasoning whereby true causal relationships are not recognized, minor aspects of a situation are emphasized out of proportion, or major aspects minimized. Facts, conditions, or symptoms are ascribed to causes that are less threatening than the real ones.

A male patient, in his early 60's, had undergone a prostatectomy and bilateral orchiectomy because of cancer. When asked about his condition, he stated that "my testicles are not gone—they just pull up in here—or maybe they pool in here" (pointing to his groin).

The ineffectiveness of denial mechanisms may become apparent in several ways: worsening of physical illness, inability to rationalize away traumatic changes in the body, and so on. One interesting example showing the ineffectiveness of denial is the emergence of the denied phenomenon in dreams.

> A woman, widowed for more than a year, said, "I never look at my husband's pictures, or I would think of him all the time." She had been quite ambivalent about her husband. Since his death, she had a repetitive dream: "I see his casket in the ground—there is no soil on it, no dirt on it yet—the top of the casket is lifted up." The tenuous intrapsychic equilibrium also showed up in nightmares: "I am falling off the top of a building." Rather than heeding these warnings from within, she resorted to sleeping pills to bolster the denial attempts. When this failed, an agitated depression developed, requiring hospitalization.

Depersonalization

Depersonalization is a mechanism that involves a protective blurring or ego boundaries. The usual distinction between self and not-self becomes less clear and the result is a sense of estrangement from reality. The protective quality of depersonalization lies in the individual's feeling that "this experience is not really happening to me—it is just like a dream." If the emphasis is on external reality being different, the term *derealization* can be used.

> A 64-year-old woman, with several physical illnesses of a serious nature, developed an acute trance-like confusion. After the confusion had cleared up, she described her experience as follows: "I felt like I was plumb gone, as if I was facing the end—I looked at my watch and saw that the face of my watch was black." This episode of unreality represented a dying experience: she was facing the end of herself ("being plumb gone") and the end of time ("the black face of the watch").

Externalization and Internalization

Externalization and *internalization* involve a displacement and a blurring of boundary between the self and the not-self. The former is the mechanism by which one ascribes one's own undesirable condition, thoughts, or feelings to other people; the latter being the reverse process. By way of internalization a person may attribute to himself something that actually came from without.

> A patient with lung cancer, told by his physician about the existence of metastases, said later: "I am not sure what I was told—I think the idea of malignant spread was, after all, my own idea."

In externalization (or projection), the *fact* of a loss or illness cannot be ascribed to others unless mental disorganization is of psychotic proportion. Its occurrence suggests massive ego breakdown due to terminal processes.

> A woman with terminal uremia thought it was not she herself,

but the nurse and her husband who were going to die. A patient, terminally ill with leukemia, had the delusion that she was spreading a bad odor throughout the entire hospital.

Much more common is the projection of the *cause* of one's condition onto somebody or something external. It is as though the person says: "It is nothing about me that makes me weak or less valuable, but you outsiders are responsible." Projection of *feelings* (e.g., anger, envy) is very common; it causes a person to think that the people around him do not like him, not recognizing that the source of this hostility is inside of himself.

An 86-year-old man, living with his 84-year-old wife in a rest home, had been preoccupied with his "loss of manhood." Contributing to his general sense of loss were his children's lack of interest, the sale of his home, and the loss of other belongings due to a fire. He resented his financial dependency and required his wife to "pin their spending money to her underwear"; all expenditures needed his authorization. All the losses, however, appeared to converge into the overriding concern of losing his manhood and sexual potency. He then used projection to deal with this specific concern: he accused his 84-year-old wife of having an affair with the rest home operator.

Externalization may also be accomplished by displacement onto objects and situations which can serve as an external symbol of inner concerns, feelings, or drives. Thus, a *phobia* originates. Once the internal problem has become an external threat, i.e., a phobia, the patient may feel in a position to cope, either by flight from the external threat, or, as in the case of counterphobic defenses, by fighting the external enemy.

MASTERY AND CONTROL

Defenses aimed at *mastery and control* include intellectualization, isolation of feelings from thoughts, certain obsessive-compulsive mechanisms, overcompensation and counterphobic defenses.

Intellectualization (Isolation)

Intellectualization and the separation of ideas from painful feelings associated with them (i.e., *isolation*) represent attempt at mastery by reliance on a cognitive, intellectual approach. While obsessions usually refer to ideational phenomena, compulsions pertain to behavioral-motor manifestations.

Obsessive-Compulsive

Obsessive-compulsive phenomena involve the mental mechanisms of reaction formation, undoing, and isolation. The following case illustrates some of these mechanisms.

A 62-year-old widow had been living with her married daughter for several years. The 9-year-old granddaughter who had problems in school, was being seen by a counsellor who allegedly recommended that the grandmother would do well to leave the home. Shortly after this, the elderly woman became progressively withdrawn. She stopped taking baths, so that the adult daughter had to bathe her mother. The latter, however, refused to take her clothes off or be touched. She also refused to sit down for a meal, but would eat standing in a corner; she was picky about the food. She began holding her purse in her hand, at all times. Finally, she started compulsive handwashing. In trying to understand this behavior, it appeared that the idea of being-in-the-way was a core theme. The patient saw herself as somebody who did not belong, an untouchable. Hence she tried to be inconspicuous, taking up minimal space by withdrawing, ready to go at a moment's notice (standing up to eat, not taking her clothes off, having her purse with her). By staying out of touch with others, she intended to stay out of their way and be allowed to stay. But her standing up during mealtime served as an ominous symbol of nemesis; and her complaints about the food also expressed her resentment about being mistreated. The compulsive handwashing represented her self image as being untouchable; it was a subtle, but vindictive demonstration that she was given a dirty deal; and, it symbolized that she was taking her hands off them, and washing them in innocence.

Not infrequently, obsessive-compulsive phenomena occur in the context of major depressive disorders. Their psychodynamic significance depends on the individual case, but, not uncommonly, this involves attempts to maintain control over unacceptable aggressive or sexual impulses.

A 55-year-old woman complained of depression, a compelling urge to walk, a handwashing compulsion, and a "crazy feeling of wanting to rip off my clothes and go naked on the street." Her husband had gradually become disabled due to cardiac illness. He was now staying at home, doing housekeeping chores, and no longer sexually interested in her. She was not aware of conscious anger at her husband. Instead, she was preoccupied with "these crazy ideas intruding in my mind like a foreign body—this is not like me—this urge to walk, rip off my clothes, getting irritated when my husband rhythmically pets—I mean taps—his foot."

Obsessive doubting and indecision, as well as *compulsive rituals* and ceremonies, may serve the ulterior motive of avoiding decisive action, and of stalling and temporizing.

A 74-year-old woman had spent most of her life in a mental hospital. She was released when her schizophrenic symptomatology had become minimal and placed in a boarding home. The patient was still remarkably capable of grasping the intellectual, emotional, and social nuances inherent in her new existence. She verbalized regret that so much of her life had passed her by— would it not be wonderful if she could do some catching up? Soon after this, she began to spend hours in the toilet, refusing to come out even though others were waiting in line. She would also go shopping, spending all her time and energy in trying to decide what to buy, but coming home empty-handed. In this patient, both the toilet and the shopping behavior reflected her wish to temporize; if she could only make time stand still, her wish to make up for lost time in the past would come true.

Obsessive-compulsive mechanisms also may occur in aged persons caught in a regressive drift. With the ebbing away of their energy or resources, their life span and personal hygiene may progressively deteriorate. Compulsive rituals may emerge in a last effort to prevent the life space from decaying into a micro-slum. In such cases we see the evidence of breakdown scattered all over the place, with the individual concentrating on keeping one tiny detail straightened out.

Overcompensation and Reaction Formation

Overcompensation refers to behavioral patterns aimed at repairing deficiencies or overcoming shortcomings, real or imagined. The notion of overcompensation implies a surplus effort. This reminds us of *reaction formation.* In the latter, however, the aim is not repairing a deficiency, but sealing off repressed feelings or thoughts. Overcompensation and reaction formation do have in common the fact that they require the expenditure of considerable psychic energy; and for this reason they become increasingly inappropriate and maladaptive in the course of aging.

A 73-year-old woman had been married for 32 years to a man, 10 years her junior. She herself had 2 years of college education, while her husband never went beyond the 4th grade. At the age of 8, he had lost his left leg due to an accident. Throughout their married life, she had supported him and kept their age difference and his alcoholism a secret. At the age of 65, she refused to apply for financial assistance because of the lien law and wanting to keep her age a secret. Her pattern of excessive self-reliance was based on overcompensating for a self-image of being a "weakling." (This "negative identity" had developed in early adolescence. During a routine physical examination, a heart murmur was discovered and she had been advised to get as much rest as possible, and to avoid dating, dances, etc. Her classmates had made fun of her handicap. After 6 years of a regimen of getting as much rest as possible, it turned out that the heart murmur was a functional one.) The patient was able to maintain an illusion of strength and dignity by means of this high energy defense, until a series of traumatic events pulled the rug from underneath her. At the age of 68, because of cancer, she got a permanent colostomy. This also forced her into requesting financial aid for herself. One year later, she had a mastectomy. Her sense of having lost strength was reflected by an ever increasing fear that her husband would leave her. Feelings of shame were revealed by her daily dress: a bedsheet. She refused to wear anything that might be insufficient for a complete coverup of her deformities. This idiosyncratic coverup turned her into a caricature (a reactivation of the negative identity during adolescence), and the patient, aware of failure all around, fell back on the next line of defense: projection. She accused her husband of stealing her money.

Counterphobic

While in overcompensation the source of the deficiency and the challenge posed by it is perceived to be inside, in the case of *counterphobic* mechanisms, the behavioral pattern is in response to a challenge outside. Thus, counterphobic behavior tends to be aimed at the mastery of a situational, external challenge. When the individual's resources are equal to the challenge, the stage is set for the possible accomplishment of unusual, impressive feats. But, when his resources decline due to the aging process, the counterphobic mechanisms become highly maladaptive, or self-destructive. These mechanisms also may play role in the psychodynamics of certain paranoid states (see p. 94).

References

1. Dohrenwend B. S., and Dohrenwend, B. P. (eds.): *Stressful Life Events: Their Nature and Effects*, John Wiley and Sons, Inc., New York, 1973.
2. Rahe, R. H.: Life change events and mental illness: an overview. *J. Human Stress* 5:2–10, 1979.
3. Hinkle, L. E., Jr.: The concept of "stress" in the biological and social sciences. *Int. J. Psychiat. Med.* 15:335–357, 1974.
4. Hurst, M. W., Jenkins, C. D., and Rose, R. M.: The assessment of life change stress: a comparative and methodological inquiry. *Psychosom. Med.* 40:126–141, 1978.
5. Rabkin, J. G., and Streuning, E. L.: Life events, stress, and illness. *Science* 194:1013–1030, 1976.
6. Zetzel, E. R.: Metapsychology of aging. In: *Geriatric Psychiatry*, edited by M. A. Berezin and S. H. Cath, International Universities Press, New York, 1965. pp, 109–119.
7. Parkes, C. M.: *Bereavement: A Study of Grief in Adult Life*, Tavistock, London, 1972.
8. Lindemann, E.: Symptomatology and management of acute grief. *Am. J. Pyschiat.* 101: 141, 1944.
9. Clayton, P. J.: Mortality and morbidity in the first year of widowhood. *Arch. Gen. Psychiatry* 30:747-750, 1974.
10. Cath, S.: Depletion and restitution. In: *Geriatric Psychiatry*, edited by M. A. Berezin and S. H. Cath, International Universities Press, New York, 1965. pp. 21–72.
11. Neugarten, B. L.: Personality and aging. In: *Handbook of Psychology of Aging*, edited by J. E. Birren and K. W. Schaie, chap. 26, van Nostrand Reinhold Company, New York, 1977. pp. 626–649.
12. Andrews, G., Tennant, C., Hewson, D. M., and Vaillant, G. E.: Life event stress, social support, coping style , and risk of psychological impairment. *J. Nerv. Ment. Dis.* 166: 307–316, 1978.

13. Tennant, C., and Andrews, G.: The pathogenic quality of life event stress in neurotic impairment. *Arch. Gen. Psychiatry 35*: 859–863, 1978.
14. Coelho, G. V., Hamburg, D. A., and Adams, J. E.: *Coping and Adaptation*, Basic Books, New York, 1974.
15. Verwoerdt, A.: Psychopathological responses to the stress of physical illness. In: *Advances in Psychosomatic Medicine* vol. 8, Karger, Basel, 1972. pp. 92–114
16. Verwoerdt, A.: *Communication with the Fatally Ill.* Charles C Thomas, Springfield, Ill. 1966. pp. 59–60.

4

organic mental disorders*

PHENOMENOLOGY

There are certain typical syndromes (symptom clusters) which represent the clinical manifestations of disturbed brain function. The essential feature of organic mental disorders is transient or permanent dysfunction of the brain, due to specific organic factors. Associated features include emotional, motivational, and behavioral reactions to the awareness, subjective meaning, and socioeconomic consequences of cognitive deficits. Each organic mental disorder reflects the localization, rate of onset, progression, and duration of the underlying brain pathology. The presence of one or more of these syndromes suggests brain pathology, to be confirmed by laboratory testing.

Organic mental disorders can be grouped in the following categories: delirium, dementia, amnestic syndrome, organic hallucinosis, organic delusional syndrome, organic affective syndrome, organic personality syndrome.

The organic mental disorders are no longer categorized as psychotic versus nonpsychotic, or acute (reversible) versus chronic (irreversible). However, delirium, dementia, amnestic syndrome, organic hallucinosis, and organic delusional syndrome are roughly equivalent to organic *psychotic* disorders. Delirium is usually equivalent to an *acute* organic brain syndrome, while dementia, amnestic syndrome, and organic personality syndrome tend to correspond to *chronic* brain syndrome.[1]

The clinical course of organic mental disorders is quite variable, both cross-sectionally between different patients and longitudinally in the same patient over time. More than one brain syndrome can occur simultaneously (e.g., delirium superimposed on dementia), and one syndrome may follow another (e.g., a delirium followed by an organic personality syndrome). The onset may be sudden (e.g., trauma, vascular, infection) or insidious (e.g., degenerative disease). The clinical course may be steady or irregular, progressive or remittent, static or resolving.

* In collaboration with W. M. Taylor, M.D. and M. S. Wingfield, M.D.

A key determinant of the course is the type of etiology. A transient metabolical disorder, for example, usually causes a delirium of short duration with full recovery. Acute brain edema tends to precipitate sudden reduction of the level of awareness (clouded sensorium). Significant loss of neurons causes some degree of permanent psychological impairment.

The prognosis, by and large, depends on the type of etiology and diagnosis. In one study, patients with chronic organic brain syndrome had a median duration of pre-hospital illness of about 3 years; one-half of these patients died within 2 years of hospitalization. This suggests that the duration of chronic brain syndrome is about 5 years. In contrast, acute brain syndromes developed, on the average, 1 week before hospitalization; and these patients tended to die within 1 month or recover.[2]

DELIRIUM

Symptomatology

Disorder of Attention. This syndrome includes a great variety of clinical pictures, of different organic etiologies, whose basic feature is a *disorder of attention.* Goal-directed thinking and behavior cannot be sustained because attention wanders. Thinking is disorganized and speech may be incoherent because the patient loses his train of thought. Since reasoning and goal-directed behavior (secondary process) are impossible, there may be perseveration of speech or behavior and other regressive phenomena.[1]

Memory Deficit. Due to the difficulty in registering new information, there is a short-term *memory deficit.* Thus, the patient may be unable to remember, after a few minutes, the names of three objects presented to him. Since there is difficulty focusing attention on past events, there may also be a deficit in long-term memory. The amnesia is retrograde (impaired recall of memories formed before onset of delirium) as well as anterograde (impaired information registration after onset of delirium).

Clouded Sensorium. Usually there is a *clouded sensorium* ranging from drowsiness to stupor or coma. Some patients, however, may be hyperalert and have insomnia. Often there are fluctuations from reduced wakefulness to insomnia with lucid intervals.

Perceptual Disturbances. *Perceptual disturbances* result in illusions or hallucinations. Although perceptual disturbances are usually visual in nature, they may occur in other sensory modalities. Psychomotor behavior is frequently disturbed, and may shift from agitation to sluggishness.

Associated Features. Emotional disturbances, such as anxiety, depression, anger, irritability, euphoria, or apathy are often present and these may change unpredictably. Threatening hallucinations may cause profound fear and can lead to attempts to escape without regard to injury. Delusions may lead to attacks on others who are perceived as threatening. Autonomic arousal is manifested by tachycardia, sweating, dilated pupils, and elevated systolic blood pressure. Neurological signs are uncommon, except for coarse tremors. Other disorders of cortical function include impairment in naming objects (dysnomia) and in writing ability (dysgraphia).

Course

The onset is rapid. Prodromal symptoms include nocturnal restlessness alternating with somnolence during the day, hypersensitivity to stimuli, and difficulty in thinking. The duration is usually brief, an average of 1 week. The tendency is either full recovery or death, but if the underlying cause persists, dementia may develop.

Differential Diagnosis

Schizophrenia. It may be marked by hallucinations, delusions, and disordered thinking, but in a delirium these symptoms are shifting and poorly systematized. Impaired memory and orientation and clouded sensorium are usually absent in nonorganic disorders. Finally, in delirium there often is a generalized slowing of the background activity in the electroencephalogram.

Sometimes it may be impossible to tell how much cognitive impairment is due to delirium and how much is due to dementia, e.g., in case of delirium superimposed on dementia. It is best to defer judgment for a few weeks; the delirium will then subside and any remaining deficits are probably due to a concomitant dementia.

Factitious Illness with Psychological Symptoms. This illness sometimes simulates an organic brain syndrome (pseudodementia). The differential diagnosis is based on the inconsistent mental status findings in factitious illness. A normal electroencephalogram also helps rule out delirium.

Dissociative States and Hysterical Psychosis. In the *Diagnostic and Statistical Manual of Mental Disorders* (DSM III),[1] the dissociative disorders (hysterical neuroses, dissociative type) include psychogenic amnesia, psychogenic fugue, and depersonalization disorder. In a dissociative state, psychological conflicts may result in apparent personality disorganization. Repressed unacceptable impulses, wishes, or fantasies may find expression, or are acted out, during a state of altered consciousness. Clinical manifestations of the dissociative state include depersonalization, stupor, trance states, and hysterical fugues. Typically, there is amnesia for the dissociative episode. The differential diagnosis of hysterical dissociation includes temporal lobe epilepsy and other types of organic brain syndrome which involve an alteration of consciousness. The following case illustrates the difficulties in differentiating between delirium, dissociative disorder, and depression.

A man in his 60's was hospitalized in a state of stupor. He would not respond to questions and was, in fact, mute. Although there was extreme restriction in psychomotor activity, the few movements which he did perform were not remarkably slowed. The behavioral response to any question was stereotypical: he would lie down on his bed, cross his hands over his chest, and close his eyes. It was obvious, from occasional eye contact, that the patient was aware of what went on around him. But his consciousness and attention seemed to be focused exclusively on one point. The nature of these ideas could be inferred from his ritual behavior: acting out a fantasy of being dead. The patient's trance-like behavior, the narrowing of his consciousness onto one exclusive thought, and the enactment of the fantasy of being dead suggested the diagnosis of dissociative reaction (hysterical psychosis). It would not have been incorrect to make the diagnosis of a psychotic depression, but the point is that the depression presented itself in the form of an hysterical psychosis (i.e., profound personality disorganization, an altered state of consciousness, and the acting out of a dominant fantasy). Electric shock treatment in this case resulted in immediate improvement.

DEMENTIA

General Features

Chronic, Diffuse Cerebral Dysfunction. This syndrome is associated with *chronic, diffuse cerebral dysfunction* and is characterized by insidious onset, chronicity, and progressive course. Specific pathological changes are usually demonstrable in the cerebral tissue, but in some reversible disorders causing dementia (e.g., vitamin deficiencies, metabolic disorders), the neuropathological changes may not be demonstrable unless treatment is delayed too long.[3]

Basic Symptoms. The *basic symptoms* are intellectual deterioration interfering with social and occupational functioning, impairment of memory, abstract thinking, judgment, and impulse control; as well as personality change. Most prominent is the *memory impairment,* which is anterograde (an ongoing inability to learn new things) as well as retrograde (difficulty with recalling past events). Remote past events are better preserved than recent ones, but at the advanced stages remote memory is also impaired.[1]

Impairment in abstract thinking is manifested by reduced capacity for generalizing, synthesizing, logical reasoning, and concept formation. This basic deficit results in difficulty in coping with new tasks, which in turn prompts the patient to avoid situations that involve processing of new information, or responding to such situations with profound anxiety and irritability (catastrophic reaction).

Language may be normal in the early stages, but later becomes vague, stereotyped, and imprecise with frequent naming errors, and finally incomprehensible or absent (mutism). Difficulties in performing complex motor tasks (apraxia) may lead to inability to dress, use utensils, and other impairments in activities of daily living.

Impaired judgment and impulse control is manifested by coarse language and jokes, neglect of personal hygiene, and disregard for conventional rules of social conduct without regard for the consequences ("geriatric delinquency"). Impaired judgment and impulse control is especially characteristic in dementias due to frontal lobe damage.

> A 75-year-old male patient used comraderie as a way to get out of the predicament of not knowing certain answers. He would playfully slap the interviewer on the shoulder, arm, or knee. But while doing so, he would begin to perseverate in this activity, probably also on the basis of short term memory impairment. That is, he had forgotten what this bonhommie was all about. At this point, additional trouble developed on the basis of the combination of impaired impulse control and the psychological phenomenon of regression, specifically the so-called aggressivization of libidinal impulses. In everyday language, he no longer knew the difference between a friendly slap and a hostile one. In the interview setting, this was apparent by the increasing amplitude and force of his slapping movements. As this went on, the patient's face revealed outwardly the extent of his inner chaos; he looked puzzled and his eyes filled with tears although he kept up his smile. Finally, he stopped the activity, his arm being extended straight up, poised for a blow, in utter bewilderment. Before hospitalization, this patient had been beating up his wife to whom he had been happily married for 40 years.

Personality changes may involve accentuation of premorbid personality traits, e.g., increased compulsivity, impulsiveness, suspiciousness, dependency, vindictiveness, etc. Patients with a premorbid active personality, however, may become apathetic and withdrawn. The patient's spectrum of interests becomes impoverished and is reduced to a narrow range of preoccupation with personal comfort and hypochondriacal concerns.

Course of Illness. Dementia may be progressive, static, or reversible. The mode of onset and course of illness depend on the etiology. Alzheimer's dementia is usually insidious and slowly progressive to death over a period of several years. Dementia from brain tumors, subdural hematomas, and metabolical disorders may also have a gradual onset. When due to specific neurological disease, e.g., brain hypoxia, encephalitis, or head trauma, dementia may begin suddenly but then remain stationary for a long time. When the underlying pathology can be treated, such as hypothyroidism, dementia may be arrested or even reversed.

Primary Idiopathic Dementia

Prevalence. Senile dementia is one of the major causes of morbidity and mortality. Alzheimer's dementia is the fourth most common cause of death in the United States. In the future, with more people surviving into advanced old age, the number of patients with senile dementia will certainly increase. It is now estimated that about 3 percent of the population age 65 and over suffers from progressive idiopathic dementia. The prevalence is approximately 4 times as great among family members as in the general population; and the disorder is more common in women.[1, 5] Among hospitalized aged individuals, the incidence is much higher. One survey showed that among old patients first admitted to a psychiatrical institution, almost 80 percent received a diagnosis of organic brain syndrome; and less than 10 percent, the diagnosis of a functional psychosis.[6]

Symptomatology. Dementias in the senium and presenium are associated with Alzheimer's and Pick's diseases, or with vascular disease. Senile dementia has been arbitrarily distinguished from presenile dementia by the age at onset being over 65. Because dementias are usually associated with Alzheimer's disease and the differentiation of Alzheimer's and Pick's disease depends on histopathological data, they are now grouped together as primary idiopathic dementia. The latter is subtyped according to the age of onset for the sake of historical continuity, but the clinician will rarely be able to identify the specific underlying neuropathology. The usual age at onset for primary idiopathic dementia is in the 70's, rarely before 65 (presenile onset). When it does, the average age at onset is 58. The essential feature is the insidious onset of a dementia with a progressive deteriorating course for which all other specific causes have been excluded by history, neurological examination, and laboratory investigation. There are disturbances in memory, abstract thinking, judgment, impulse control, and personality (see above).

A superimposed delirium may occur with an associated infection or following emotional stress. Delusions, usually paranoid, may occur and warrant a designation: with delusional features. Depressive symptoms are common, and if associated with many features of the depressive syndrome, warrant the designation: with depressive features.[1]

Course. In the early stage of Alzheimer's disease, only the memory deficit may be apparent, with mild personality changes. In the middle stage, various cognitive disturbances are more obvious, and behavior may be disturbed. The patient may be increasingly querulous, slovenly, irritable, and agitated. In the late stage,[5] the patient may be mute, inattentive, and grossly uncooperative. The average duration of illness is about 5 years.

Differential Diagnosis. Mild intellectual impairment, particularly memory difficulty, is common in *normal aging,* but usually this does not significantly interfere with social and occupational functioning. In primary idiopathic dementia, there is clear evidence of progressive deterioration of function.

An important differential diagnosis is with *treatable dementias,* such as those associated with subdural hematomas, normal-pressure hydro cephalus, brain tumors, substance intoxication, infections, and other medical diseases (e.g., pernicious anemia and hypothyroidism). The diagnosis requires a complete medical and neurological evaluation.

In *multi-infarct dementia,* the course of the illness is more variable and progresses in stepwise fashion, and there are more frequent focal neurological signs.

Superimposed *delirium* is a frequent complication. In delirium, there is a disturbed level of awareness, while in an uncomplicated dementia this is not the case. The severity of symptoms in delirium fluctuates, while in dementia it is relatively stable unless there is a reaction to a stressor or progression of brain pathology.

In *chronic schizophrenia* there may be some intellectual deterioration, but no identifiable brain pathology.

In *depression,* the difficulty in thinking, concentration, and memory are secondary to the disturbed affect. If there is no specific organic factor, and if the symptoms of depression are as prominent as those of dementia, it is best to diagnose a depressive episode with a pseudodementia secondary to depression. A therapeutic trial with antidepressant drugs or electroconvulsive therapy (ECT) may clarify the situation. In a depressive episode, the "cognitive impairment" may resolve as the mood improves.[1, 7, 8]

Factitious illness with psychological symptoms may rarely mimic a dementia (Ganser syndrome). This is also one of the causes of pseudodementia.

Multi-infarct Dementia

Symptomatology. The basic symptoms are a stepwise intellectual deterioration which, in the early phases of the illness, may leave some cognitive functions relatively intact (patchy deterioration), as well as focal neurological signs. This entity was called organic brain syndrome with cerebral arteriosclerosis in DSM II. However, this disorder is related to repeated infarcts of the brain rather than the extent of cerebral arteriosclerosis. The diagnosis multi-infarct dementia is restricted to patients in whom a clear-cut succession of strokes has destroyed enough brain tissue to cause the syndrome of dementia. The age at onset is often earlier than in primary idiopathic dementia. Predisposing factors include arterial hypertension, extracranial vascular disease, and valvular or other diseases of the heart that may cause emboli.[9] Multi-infarct dementia is less common than primary idiopathic dementia.[10]

Common focal neurological signs are monopareses or hemiparesis, reflex asymmetries, extensor plantar responses, dysarthria, and small-stepped gait. Evidence of vascular disease such as hypertension is usually present. There may be pseudobulbar palsy with dysarthria, dysphagia, and fleeting episodes of laughing and crying. Fluctuation in mental status with clear-cut episodes of confusion may be present, probably because of further vascular insults. Early treatment of hypertension may prevent progression.[11]

Course. The onset is usually abrupt and the course is stepwise and fluctuating with rapid changes, rather than uniformly progressive. The pattern of deficits is patchy, depending upon which regions of the brain have been destroyed.

Differential Diagnosis. Multi-infarct dementia must be distinguished from a single stroke which causes a circumscribed neuropsychiatric impairment, such as an aphasia or an amnestic syndrome from infarction of the posterior cerebral arteries. In multi-infarct dementia there are several strokes, at different times, producing the full syndrome of dementia. Multi-infarct dementia is differentiated from primary idiopathic dementia by the step-like course, focal neurological abnormalities, and evidence of cerebrovascular disease.[12, 13] When primary idiopathic dementia is followed by the typical course of multi-infarct dementia, both diagnoses are made (see p. 259).

AMNESTIC SYNDROME

Symptomatology

The basic symptoms of the amnestic syndrome (Korsakoff's syndrome) is a *short-term memory disturbance.* Since the patient cannot integrate memory into permanent memory storage, nor retrieve memory from storage, he cannot form new memories (anterograde amnesia). Because the exact time needed to transfer information from immediate into permanent storage is not known, 25 minutes is taken as an arbitrary criterion. Most patients cannot remember events that occurred prior to this time, but do remember events immediately after they happen. Thus, a patient has a short-term (but not immediate) memory disturbance if he has normal digit span but cannot recall three objects presented to him 25 minutes earlier. Usually there is some impaired memory for events that occurred before the illness (retrograde amnesia). Remote events are better preserved than recent past events.[14]

A significant amount of short-term memory deficit has the consequence of producing some degree of *disorientation.* Because such patients do not remember the immediate past, they tend to become quite *suggestible.* Clinically, this is explored by following a certain line of questions. For example, the interviewer, who has just met the patient for the first time, may ask: "Did I not meet you last week?" The suggestible patient will answer in the affirmative. One can measure the extent of suggestibility (and thus, indirectly, the memory deficit) by adding more questions. (For example: "Did we not meet at your home?," and "Were we having something to drink?").

Confabulation, i.e., filling the memory gaps with invented stories, is common, but not pathognomonic.[13] The patient may actively deny his obvious memory deficits. Awareness of self and environment is usually intact. Patients are often friendly and agreeable, but with shallow affect. Confabulations, a form of paramnesia, are products of fantasy being substituted for memory gaps. These accounts of past experiences may be rather fantastic, like a fable; hence the name confabulations.

> A 74-year-old man had suffered a stroke when he was 55 years old. Since then he had been disabled due to hemiplegia, and more recently due to a slowly progressive dementia. He had been able to walk with a cane until recently, when he had become so infirm that he was confined to bed or wheelchair. All these years, his wife had taken care of him, accepting their fate with courage and matter-of-factness. But her matter-of-factness, which had served both of them so well and so long, became a focal point for periodic friction. Whenever the patient would boast that he "had gone for a walk around the block" (a reassuring confabulation), she would correct him by pointing out the facts of the matter. There upon the patient, usually a mild-mannered man, would angrily repeat his boastful assertion.

Course

The onset depends on the etiology and usually is fairly sudden. About one-third of these patients show good improvement with adequate therapy; one-third show some improvement, while the remainder does not improve. The confabulations generally decrease in the course of time. This is also true for those patients who show no overall clinical improvement; in them the confabulations make room for increasing deterioration through withdrawal.

Differential Diagnosis

In dementia there are, in addition to impaired short-term memory, signs of other cognitive and behavioral abnormalities. In delirium there is impaired attention and sensorium. In factitious illness with psychological symptoms (pseudodementia), memory testing yields inconsistent results and there is no organic etiology. When the amnestic syndrome is the result of alcoholism and vitamin deficiency, other neurological complications (e.g., peripheral neuropathy, cerebellar ataxia) may occur.

ORGANIC DELUSIONAL SYNDROME

Symptomatology

Delusions in a state of clear sensorium are the predominant symptoms. The delusions vary depending on the particular organic etiology, but frequently are poorly formed paranoid ideas. Almost any psychiatric symptoms may be an associated feature, including mild cognitive deficits, language disorders such as incoherence or tangentiality, psychomotor disturbances (pacing, rocking, or apathy), ritualistic or stereotyped behavior with magical thinking, and dysphoric mood.[1] (See also "Paranoid Reactions in Organic Brain Syndrome" in Chapter 5.)

> An 80-year-old widow was hospitalized because of delusions and marked agitation. Three weeks previously, the patient began to think that somebody was trying to get in her house through the window. She first said there were six people outside looking at her and that this scared her to death. She then began to have pain in her lower abdomen and stated that the people outside were trying to kill her. The patient's daughter reported that her mother had the idea that there was an 18-year-old girl living in the house, and that this girl tried to do everything that the patient did. For example, if the patient changes her dress, so would this girl. Also, the girl had a room which is attached to the patient's house, and she has furniture similar to that of the patient. So it appeared that this girl was trying to imitate her. At first, the girl was good, but recently she has become nasty. She is stealing the patient's belongings, and she does not respond when the patient talks to her. By this time, the group of six people outside had swelled to a crowd of fifty.

Differential Diagnosis

Organic delusional syndrome must be differentiated from nonorganic psychotic disorders by the evidence of a specific organic factor. The hallucinations of a nonorganic psychosis are usually auditory and in organic delusional syndrome, visual or tactile. In organic hallucinosis, hallucinations are predominant and delusions are secondarily related to the hallucinations.

ORGANIC HALLUCINOSIS

Symptomatology

The basic symptoms are persistent or recurrent hallucinations in clear sensorium. Any delusional content is in keeping with the content of the hallucinations. Elaboration of delusional material beyond this (for example, systematized persecutory delusions to account for the hallucinations) suggests an organic delusional syndrome. The hallucinations usually are auditory, but specific organic etiologies tend to manifest themselves in a specific sensory modality. For example, cataracts often cause visual hallucinosis, while the organic hallucinosis caused by alcohol is usually auditory.[1]

In some cases, one can observe the following pathogenesis of a hallucinatory experience. The patient may have certain age-related changes in perception and alterations in sensory modality, such as paresthesias.

For example, a dry skin may cause itching—"as if ants are crawling over my skin." When the patient undergoes regression, the abstract capacity may be replaced by concrete thinking. As a result, the metaphor becomes the real thing; what was figurative, becomes literal. Thus, the sensory experience is expressed in a literal, concrete form: "ants are crawling over my skin."

Course

The *course* depends upon the underlying etiology. Alcohol hallucinosis lasts from weeks to years. Bilateral cataracts or otosclerosis may cause a permanent organic hallucinosis. When due to sensory deprivation, the course may be brief.

Differential Diagnosis

In delirium, hallucinations are accompanied by disturbed attention and impaired sensorium. In dementia, the intellectual deficits are more striking and prominent than any hallucinations that occur. In organic delusional syndrome, the delusions are more prominent than the hallucinations. In nonorganic psychotic disorders, hallucinations may occur but no organic factor can be demonstrated.

ORGANIC AFFECTIVE SYNDROME

Symptomatology

The predominant symptoms are disturbances in mood similar to those of a depressive or manic episode. Any associated features of the affective disorders can be seen with an organic affective syndrome. Delusions of persecution and worthlessness may be present. Hallucinations are rare, usually auditory, and related to the emotional state. Hallucinations and delusions are more common in the manic than in the depressive form.[1]

The case example of the patient with a psychotic manic disorder, described on p. 111 also can be used to illustrate an organic affective syndrome.

Differential Diagnosis

Organic affective syndrome must be differentiated from affective disorders; a specific organic factor is necessary for the diagnosis. In organic personality syndrome, there may be a mood disturbance, but this is less prominent than the other symptoms.

ORGANIC PERSONALITY SYNDROME

Symptomatology

The basic symptom is a marked personality change. The syndrome depends mainly on the nature and localization of the pathological process. A common cluster of symptoms is emotional lability, impaired impulse control, temper outbursts, and socially inappropriate behavior. Another pattern is marked apathy, and lack of interest in one's usual hobbies and environment. Both patterns are associated with frontal lobe damage, and used to be called "frontal lobe syndrome." Irritability and mild cognitive impairment are often present. Impairment is variable. Despite relatively intact cognitive function, poor social judgment may lead to marked impairment requiring close supervision or custodial care. Socially unacceptable behavior may result in social or legal difficulties. Impulsive or explosive behavior may be dangerous to the patient or others.[1]

Course

The *course* depends on the etiology and may range from a transient disturbance (e.g., drug-induced personality disturbances), to stable changes (e.g., pseudobulbar palsy). The disease may also be the first sign of a subclinical dementia.

Differential Diagnosis

In dementia and organic affective syndrome, there frequently are personality changes. The diagnosis of an organic personality syndrome needs to be changed to dementia when intellectual impairment becomes the predominant feature. In schizophrenia, paranoid disorders, affective disorders, adjustment disorders, and disorders of impulse control, no specific organic factor can be demonstrated.

ETIOLOGY AND PATHOGENESIS

PHYSICAL FACTORS

Pathogenesis includes consideration of two sets of factors: primary etiological factors and secondary effects. The etiological agent may impinge directly on the brain causing a primary organic brain syndrome (e.g., trauma) or indirectly, by way of extracerebral pathology, leading to a secondary organic brain syndrome (e.g., uremia). Furthermore, the etiologic factor may be a known organic agent; or unknown (idiopathic) as in Alzheimer's disease.

Structural damage to the brain tends to be irreversible, because neurons have limited recuperative capacity and do not reproduce. Structural alterations include a loss of neurons, and an increase in senile plaques and the amount of neurofibrillary degeneration. Physiologically, there is a reduction in the metabolic activity of brain.

Although brain impairment is usually accompanied by deficits of those cognitive functions which depend on the intactness of the tissue involved, the pathogenic role of other factors should not be overlooked. Usually, multiple factors (physical, psychological, social, and environmental) are operating, either simultaneously or as successive links in a cause-and-effect chain. The outcome of such interactions is the formation of one or more vicious circles: one pathogenic process exerting a positive feedback effect on another. Hence, it is useful to consider the pathogenesis of organic brain syndrome in a sociopsychosomatic framework.[15]

Physical factors which may cause organic brain damage can be grouped in two major categories: cerebral-organic and extracerebral-somatic factors.

Organic-Cerebral Factors

Organic-cerebral factors may be of known or unknown origin. Organic etiological factors of *known origin* include the following.

Trauma, e.g., concussion, contusion, subarachnoid hemorrhage.

Infection, e.g., neurosyphilis, Jakob-Creutzfeldt disease (slow virus), acute viral encephalitis (herpes simplex), meningitis, postencephalitic syndromes.

Neoplasm.

Chemical, e.g., toxins such as CO, lead, alcohol.

Drug-related, e.g., CNS side effects of psychotropic drugs; the central anticholinergic syndrome.

Cerebrovascular, e.g., atherosclerosis of cerebral arteries, cerebral thrombosis, multi-infarct dementia.

Heredodegenerative, e.g., Huntington's chorea.[16]

Other: pseudobulbar palsy, normal pressure hydrocephalus, progressive supranuclear palsy (Steele-Richardson-Olszewski syndrome).

Organic-cerebral factors whose etiological nature is *unknown* are involved in the senile and presenile dementias. These are global neurodegenerative processes of unknown origin producing the clinical syndrome of Alzheimer's disease.

Extracerebral-Somatic Factors

Many diseases frequently occurring in old age can have an adverse effect on the brain, causing a secondary organic brain syndrome. Physical illnesses which may interfere with brain function include cardiovascular and pulmonary disease. For example, elderly persons with cardiovascular disease have a high incidence of EEG abnormality, and a greater decline in intellectual function.[17, 18] In any patient with sudden and unexpected mental change, possible physical causes must be considered. A brain syndrome may be the first sign of a major disease outside the central nervous system. The syndrome may be an indication of myocardial infarction which in the elderly often is without chest pain; of pneumonia in which there may be little or no temperature rise or leukocytosis; or pulmonary embolism in which there may not be dyspnea, or chest pain.[2]

Metabolic Factors

Physical factors that interfere with brain metabolism can cause *delirium,* and these can be classified as follows:

Decreased Supply of Oxygen. Hypoxic hypoxia: low ambient oxygen, respiratory depression, pulmonary diseases; anemic hypoxia: various anemias; ischemic hypoxia: hypotension, insufficient pulse pressure, myocardial infarction, arteriosclerosis of vessels supplying blood to the brain, especially carotid arteries.

Decreased Supply of Glucose. Essential hypoglycemia; due to insulin.

Decreased Utilization of Essential Brain Nutrients. Due to drugs: barbiturates interfere with the cerebral metabolism of oxygen and glucose; vitamin deficiencies: e.g., vitamin B_{12}, thiamine (B_1); metabolic disorders: e.g., hypothyroidism, diabetes, alcoholism, hyperthyroidism; electrolyte disturbances: dehydration, acidosis, alkalosis, uremia, hyponatremia, hypernatremia.

The metabolic disturbances in the brain may, in turn, lead to anatomical-structural brain damage. It is because of the latter that it is so important to diagnose as quickly as possible, any physical factors which could interfere with brain function. By treating such physical diseases, one may prevent the development of permanent brain damage.

Dementia

Etiology of *dementia*: there appears to be no consistent relationship between intellectual deterioration and organic brain changes, (especially in the milder cases). In one study, 20 percent of the patients with a diagnosis of senile psychosis had little or no senile plaque formation on autopsy examination, while moderate or severe senile plaque formation occurred in 9 percent of patients with a functional psychosis.[19] In another investigation, no evidence of dementia was found in almost one-fourth of individuals who turned out to have severe brain atrophy. Although all patients with severe intellectual impairment did have demonstrable cerebral atrophy, in some cases the extent of atrophy was less than what had been anticipated on the basis of neuropsychological test data.[20]

Obrist et al.[21] found that, in a group of patients with presenile or senile dementia, cerebral blood flow was normal in about one-third of the cases. Furthermore, demented patients may have a normal EEG, while aged individuals in apparently good psychological condition can have gross abnormalities in their EEG.[22] These discrepancies can be taken as evidence that multiple factors play an etiological role in dementia and other organic brain syndromes.

Organic Amnestic Syndrome

Etiology of *organic amnestic syndrome*: several exogenous agents may cause the syndrome. Bilateral damage to certain limbic structures in the diencephalon and temporal lobe (e.g., mammillary bodies, fornix, hippocampal formation) produces the amnestic syndrome; it can be caused by head trauma, anoxia, infarction of the posterior cerebral arteries, and herpes simplex encephalitis. The most common form is associated with thiamine deficiency and chronic alcohol use, commonly referred to as Wernicke-Korsakoff syndrome.

Organic Hallucinosis

Etiology of *organic hallucinosis*: the most common causes are alcohol, sensory deprivation, and seizure foci in the temporal lobes.

Organic Affective Syndrome

Etiology of *organic affective syndrome*: this syndrome is usually caused by toxic or metabolical factors, including drugs (for example, reserpine, and methyldopa); hormonal disorders, e.g. hyperadrenalcorticalism (Cushing's disease or excessive steroid medication); hyper and hypothyroidism; malignancies; viral illnesses; brain trauma or tumor.

Organic Personality Syndrome

Etiology of *organic personality syndrome*: organic personality syndrome may be due to structural brain damage such as tumors, trauma (e.g., postconcussion syndrome), or vascular accidents (e.g., psuedobulbar palsy); drugs (e.g., steroids); or an endocrine disorder (e.g., thyroid disease). Usually, the lesion involves the frontal lobes; less often the temporal lobes, as in temporal lobe epilepsy.

PSYCHOLOGICAL FACTORS

Premorbid Personality

The possible existence of a link between certain premorbid personality traits (compulsiveness, aggressiveness, rigidity) and an increased vulnerability to dementia is mentioned by several authors. Patients whose premorbid personality is characterized by versatility in adaptation tend to have relatively less intellectual impairment in association with a certain amount of cerebral neuronal loss.[23, 24] It is, indeed, reasonable to expect that any premorbid behavioral style involving aggressive and "high energy" defenses is especially vulnerable to the psychotrauma of loss of mastery (resulting from organic brain changes); and that compulsive, rigid individuals are prone to react with profound anxiety, when faced with the necessity to change their habitual style, and accommodate themselves to ego-alien constraints.

Psychodynamic Aspects

The stress of intellectual decline produces the immediate response of anxiety, and mobilizes specific defenses. The latter are often precisely those defenses whose continued operation is being threatened (compare organic personality syndrome). Thus, the aggressive, ambitious person may try to defend against the threat of loss of control by becoming even more aggressive and controlling; likewise, the compulsive person may become more rigid and set in his usual ways. Inasmuch as the patient tries to meet the threat head-on, there will be more opportunities to experience failure. The emotional distress is compounded by more anxiety, frustrating helplessness, as well as feelings of shame and anger.

A second vicious circle is set in motion when auxiliary defenses, such as projection, are called into action (as in many cases of organic delusional syndrome). When this entails accusatory behavior, the patient may alienate the very persons whose support is vital. If, on the other hand, he tries to cope by withdrawal, the net effect will be similar: again the loss of external support, this time due to being out of reach. Still other vicious circles may be set in motion, linking up with those already there, and adding to their momentum. The combination of persisting high energy defenses, intensifying negative emotions, and weakening environmental support, sets the stage for another systems breakdown, e.g., a new physical illness, accidents.

In other individuals, the course of events is less stormy, because they use defenses that are less harmful, such as mild or moderate degrees of regression or denial. Some patients are almost naive in their attempts to deny; for example, they may respond to a question from the interviewer by saying, "I never learned that in school." (offering an alibi). Others are somewhat more sophisticated, e.g., "Let's see now, what was it you asked me—Oh, yes, well I often ask myself the same thing.—What do you think yourself, doctor?" (turning the tables). A third type tries to cover up the deficit by "beating around the bush," by circumlocution, stalling, and temporizing. Or, a patient may smile and wave with his hand—a waiver of the question—"This is not important, I already answered that yesterday." Thus, the ways and means of denial are legion, and they often strike the observers as funny, prompting giggles or laughter. The patient may then join in and feel off the hook: he is learning that being funny is one way to escape disaster.

The disaster dreaded is that particular situation of failure referred to as the "catastrophic condition." This tends to occur especially in patients with impairment of abstract capacity. The catastrophic condition is not a conscious awareness of, and reaction to, the failure, but rather belongs intrinsically to the overall situation of the organism-in-failure.[25] In this disintegration of the personality as an intact organism, the anxiety experienced is in the nature of nameless terror (the primary anxiety, or traumatic anxiety in psychoanalytical terminology). Because of the risk of this devastating experience, the patient's defenses should be handled gingerly (see pp. 252 and 258).

SOCIAL AND ECONOMIC FACTORS

Dementia is related to many social factors including family organization, housing conditions, type of household, social outlets, etc. The common denominators for most of these are economic status and level of education. Elderly persons of low socioeconomic status tend to have more physical illness which is associated with inadequate housing, nutrition, and medical care, as well as lack of social contacts. Social isolation, commonly associated with chronic illness, facilitates regression and withdrawal which, in turn, contribute to the development of intellectual deterioration. Consequently, the low socioeconomic status frequently predisposes to an early onset and a rapid rate of intellectual decline.[6, 22, 26]

ENVIRONMENTAL AND SITUATIONAL FACTORS

Because of difficulties in perception, comprehension, memory, as well as slowness in psychomotor skills, aged persons become more sensitive to environmental changes. Relatively minor alterations, such as a shift in household arrangements or family relationships, can cause severe psychological upsets. The brain is the "organ of adaptation," and whether it is in a state of compensation or decompensation, depends on the demands made on it. Cardiac status, by way of analogy, may decompensate, when the input presented or the output demanded, exceeds the heart's potential for work. Likewise, the brittle brain status of an old person may decompensate because of changes in the input or the output.

Abnormal Sensory Input

Abnormal sensory input may be quantitative or qualitative in nature.

Quantitative Changes. Quantitative input changes include: sensory *overload*, e.g., chronic overcrowding of a three- generational family in a small dwelling; another example is the acute sensory overload experienced by an old person, hospitalized for the first time in his life, undergoing a battery (sic!) of examinations and tests by many specialists, then is operated on, all within a few days; as well as sensory *underload*, i.e., an undue decrease in the number of stimuli (exteroceptive, proprioceptive, kinesthetic, etc.)

These quantitative changes can be chronic or acute; abrupt or insidious; or of minor or major proportions. Sensory deprivation or social isolation may be imposed on the individual (e.g., being alone in the hospital room; having the eyes covered following cataract surgery); they may be the outcome of life-long ego-syntonic character traits (e.g., the isolation which the schizoid prefers); or, they may be the consequence of major psychopathology (e.g., self-absorption in severe depression).

Qualitative Changes. These changes in the input pertain to exposure to unfamiliar stimuli, e.g., sudden transfer of elderly persons from their homes to an institution.

Changes in the Output

In addition, the brain may decompensate because of *changes in the output*. These include quantitative or qualitative changes pertaining to the individual's behavior activities or motor patterns; changes in the demands of performance and work, and modifications in coping techniques (e.g., exhaustion due to manic hyperactivity).

Disturbances in the Through-put

Inasmuch as the brain, in our cybernetic schema, is interposed between the sensory input and the motor output, the phrase *through-put* can be used to refer to the "black box" function of the central nervous system. Disturbances in the through-put (apart from structural brain changes) may develop on the basis of progressive accumulation of disturbing emotions. Accumulating anxiety and tension may produce a neuronal turmoil, which reduces the homeostatic and information-processing capacity of the brain. When the status of the brain is already borderline, any further decrease of its efficiency is enough to tip the balance toward decompensation.

EVALUATION

The *recognition of the syndrome* of dementia is the first step in the diagnostic process. The second step is to identify the specific organic etiological factor.

In dementia, there is usually cortical atrophy, widened cortical sulci, and enlarged ventricles. This may be demonstrated in the live patient by computed tomography. There are three characteristic histopathological changes: senile plaques, neurofibrillary tangles, and granulovacuolar degeneration of neurons. These changes are the same as in Alzheimer's disease, the most common form of primary idiopathic dementia.

Dementia of unknown cause constitutes the largest single diagnostic category, accounting for roughly half of all cases of dementia. Alzheimer's disease is the basic pathological process in most demented patients in whom no other specific cause can be found.[10] Many other types of disorders, however, requiring specific therapy, may cause dementia. The following *potentially reversible* disorders are responsible for the dementia in l0 to l5 percent of the cases: reversible normal pressure hydrocephalus, benign intracranial masses, drug toxicity, epilepsy, pernicious anemia, hypothyroidism, hyperthyroidism, liver disease, and pseudodementia. However, if diagnosis and treatment are delayed too long, irreversible brain damage may develop.[3, 13, 27]

The second step in the diagnostic process is the *identification of the specific etiological organic factor*. Although a number of diseases may cause dementia, we are interested mostly in the identification of treatable dementias. Most of these diagnoses can be established through information from the history, the physical and neurological examination, and certain auxiliary diagnostic procedures.[27, 28]

Although fully developed dementia is easily recognized on clinical examination, early symptoms may suggest a functional disorder. In the initial evaluation, one should suspect the possibility of dementia, particularly if the patient complains of various physical symptoms that fit no discernible pattern of physical disease, and manifests psychological symptoms that fit no specific functional diagnostic category (especially if there is no past history of psychiatric disease); and if the patient's history and complaints remain unclear and vague after lengthy and sympathetic listening.[29] The findings on the mental status examination may be far from characteristic in early stages of dementia.[30]

Another possibility for diagnostic error arises in the patient who has *pseudodementia,* the syndrome in which dementia is mimicked or caricatured by functional psychiatric disorders.[31–33]

The following case illustrates some of the difficulties in diagnosis and the need for early therapy of treatable dementias.

> A professional woman in her mid-50's was admitted to the mental hospital with the diagnosis of presenile dementia. Prior to this admission, she had spent several weeks in a university-affiliated hospital, where she had undergone numerous tests and examinations. The primary symptomatology which had prompted hospitalization consisted of a profound inability to concentrate and shortening of her attention span. As a result, she began to make more and more mistakes in her work, which involved a great deal of abstract thought and delicate judgment. Since the patient was clearly not depressed, organicity was suspected right from the beginning. Having undergone a "thorough check-up" in the university-affiliated hospital, the patient was finally told that her condition was "irreversible, and it was a case of premature aging." She was then transferred to a nearby state mental hospital, with the diagnosis of presenile dementia. It so happened that the alert internist of the state hospital began to pursue some leads along a pathway which eventually established the diagnosis of myxedema. Immediately after the patient began to receive thyroid replacement therapy, her "senility" cleared up. Commenting, in retrospect, on her initial symptoms of impaired concentration and attention, the patient stated: "It was not like me to be that way—that problem in concentrating came over me, as something foreign, that was not part of me—I was too weak to resist it." Such a discrepancy between an intact observing ego on the one hand, and a specific severe mental impairment on the other hand, would suggest an organic brain syndrome other than Alzheimer's dementia.

PHYSICAL ASSESSMENT

Organic-Cerebral Factors

Histopathological. A brain biopsy is the only procedure which permits direct examination of brain tissue in vivo. Yet, even such *histopathological* techniques do not always provide conclusive information.[34]

Pneumoencephalography. A definitive diagnosis of cerebral atrophy formerly depended on *pneumoencephalographic* evidence. This procedure which involves injection of air into the subarachnoid space to obtain a clear outline of the ventricular system, thus providing information about the extent or cortical atrophy, has been replaced by the use of the cranial tomography scan.

Computed Cranial Tomography. The *computed cranial tomography* (CT scan) offers more information than the pneumoencephalogram with less morbidity. The CT scan can be used for the detection of focal or diffuse cerebral atrophy, intracranial masses, hydrocephalus, and cerebral infarction.[35] The CT scan is especially useful in ruling out intracranial masses. Similar to pathological specimens, the CT scan data are not always closely correlated with the clinical picture. A mild to moderate degree of atrophy is not unusual in the normal elderly and does not indicate atrophic brain disease when the clinical symptoms are incompatible. Conversely, one may find little or no evidence of atrophy by CT scan in patients who are demented clinically. There are several possible explanations for such discrepancies. The clinical symptoms could simply precede the development of gross atrophic changes, and a later CT scan may reveal the progression of the process so that by then the atrophy is not incongruent with the cognitive and behavioral changes. On the other hand, when significant dementia is seen without significant atrophy, a reversible cause for the dementia should be suspected. In these instances, the possibility of pseudodementia should be considered.

Echoencephalography. In the past, *echoencephalography*, which employs high-frequency, ultrasound waves has been used to demonstrate a midline shift (due to a space-occupying lesion, or unilateral cerebral edema), and to measure the size of the ventricles. The width of the third ventricle is greater in persons aged 70 or older, than in young adults (a mean of 7.0 versus 5.0 mm). This technique is no longer in common use.

Nuclear Diagnostic Techniques. These techniques, e.g., the radioactive iodinated serum albumen (RISA) scan, make it possible to measure the rate of supracortical absorption of radioactive substances injected into the cerebrospinal fluid of the lumbar subarachnoid space. This is of special value in detecting so-called normal pressure hydrocephalus. In the case of a true hydrocephalus, a ventriculoperitoneal shunt may be helpful. However, poor absorption is not a clear indication for such operations, especially when the brain syndrome is of long duration.

Static brain scanning involving the use of radioactive materials (e.g., technetium 99) has some value as a screening test; it is indicated when a localized lesion such as a metastatic tumor, subdural hematoma, or decreased blood flow is suspected. The *dynamic brain scan* involves the intravenous injection of a radioactive substance. Uptake and flow of patterns of radioactive dye are recorded on tape and played back through programmed computers. Dynamic brain scanning makes it possible to pick up gross deficiencies in blood flow of major arteries.

Cerebral Metabolism and Blood Flow. Since the brain obtains its energy mostly from aerobic oxidation of glucose, cerebral metabolism is reflected by the rate of oxygen and glucose utilization. In healthy old persons, the values of cerebral oxygen consumption and blood flow are similar to those in younger persons.[36]

The *cerebral uptake of oxygen* (represented by the difference between the amount of oxygen in arterial blood and that in the internal jugular vein) is a reliable indicator of oxygen utilization only when the cerebral blood flow is constant.

Methods for measuring *cerebral blood flow* depend on a diffusible indicator, usually an inert gas administered by inhalation. Its uptake by, or clearance from, the brain is determined by monitoring intracranially in the case of a radioactive indicator. The inhalation method using xenon 133 is not traumatic but less reliable than other techniques.[37]

Regional cerebral blood flow can be measured by inhalation of a radioactive inert gas, and provides specific information about different areas of the brain. Metabolism and blood flow in specific regions of the brain may differ greatly under normal circumstances, and likewise, in pathological conditions.

Cerebral angiograms make it possible to determine the location and blood supply of space-occupying lesions. Cerebral angiography, by way of injecting radio-opaque compounds in the brachial or carotid artery, permits the visualization of the entire cerebrovascular network.

Electroencephalography (EEG). The incidence of abnormal EEG's is higher in elderly persons with brain disorders than those with psychogenic disorders. Among hospitalized elderly patients, EEG abnormalities are very common; patients with diffuse slowing in the EEG are more likely to remain hospitalized and have shorter life expectancy than those with a normal EEG. These abnormalities consist of *diffuse slow activity* in the θ or δ range and are probably due to reduced metabolic activity. Usually, the EEG abnormalities correlate well with the severity of intellectual and clinical deterioration. However, the EEG may be normal in patients with definite organic brain syndrome; and, old persons apparently in good psychological health may show abnormalities in their EEG.[22, 38]

Other common EEG abnormalities are *focal disturbances* which seem to appear first during middle age. With advancing age, their incidence increases. They usually consist of slow wave activity, mostly over the left anterior temporal region. Although such focal disturbances are not uncommon in organic brain syndromes (e.g., due to arteriosclerosis or neoplasm), they may persist for several years without manifest symptomatology. But there is some evidence that aged persons with such foci do undergo a faster rate of decline in verbal intelligence than those without such foci. Decline in performance abilities tends to be associated with diffuse slowing in the occipital rhythm or decreased blood flow in the left parietal cortex. Decline in verbal abilities tends to be related to focal EEG disturbances in the left anterior temporal region.[22, 38]

Because the EEG changes are not pathognomonic and because of the wide variations among old persons of comparable age and health, a single EEG tracing has limited value. On the other hand, serial EEG's are quite useful, especially to follow up patients suspected of having a brain syndrome. Healthy old persons with consistently normal EEG's do not show an intellectual decline over a period of several years.

Somatic-Extracerebral Aspects

These include all the physical factors and somatic illnesses which secondarily affect brain function, and in the course of time may produce brain damage. They include disorders which may be endocrine, metabolical, or nutritional; systemic infection; intoxication with drugs, alcohol; and so on. The prompt diagnosis and treatment of these somatic conditions is important, as was already emphasized, and often requires consultation with the internist, neurologist, or other specialists.

NEUROPSYCHOLOGICAL ASPECTS

Neuropsychological testing may be more sensitive than clinical examination in demonstrating intellectual or perceptual impairment. While these impairments usually indicate the presence of brain damage, they cannot be directly related to the location or extent of the pathological process. An impaired intellectual function may result from any one of a number of anatomical or physiological abnormalities in the brain.[39] The efficacy of neuropsychological test procedures is limited by the level of the patient's motivation, the consistency and scope of his attention span, the degree of his anxiety and various defensive responses vis-à-vis the test situation. Thus, the psychological test data must be interpreted in a framework that takes into consideration the clinical history, psychiatric examination, laboratory data, and so on.

Among the aged, intellectual decline is so common, that intelligence tests must be evaluated with a corrective factor for age. An old person is expected to have a verbal ability of 7–27 percent below, and a performance ability of 26–50 percent below that of a young adult. Most intellectual abilities seem to reach a peak in early adulthood and then gradually decline. Verbal abilities and stored information show relatively little deficit, in contrast to psychomotor skills, especially those involving speed and perceptual-integrative abilities. This increasing discrepancy between verbal and performance abilities can be used to indicate the degree of intellectual deterioration.[40–44]

BEHAVIORAL MANIFESTATIONS

On the basis of psychiatric history and mental status examination, it may be feasible to differentiate types of organic brain syndrome, especially in cases of rather severe brain damage.

Dementia is usually diagnosed by mental status examination which shows defects in several functions suggesting diffuse cerebral impairment. The findings on mental status examination must be such that they cannot be explained satisfactorily by loss of a specific cerebral function due to a focal brain lesion, e.g., pure aphasia (caused by a left hemisphere lesion) or memory loss alone (as in the amnestic syndrome).

In patients with brain impairment of mild to moderate degree, the anamnesis and the mental status may not be sufficient to make a certain diagnosis, and auxiliary diagnostic techniques will be required. Specific refinements of, and additions for, the psychiatric examination of elderly patients have been developed.[45] The issue of reliable behavioral rating scales has particular relevance for clinical research projects aimed at evaluating responses to psychotropic drugs.[46]

Sensorium

Sensorium refers to the extent that a person is capable of utilizing data from his sense organs. If the sensorium is intact, the individual is attentive and alert to his environment. If the sensorium is not intact, consciousness may be clouded and the person confused; in severe cases, there is stupor and coma. In delirium, the sensorium may be clouded ranging from drowsiness to stupor or coma; but some patients may be hyperalert.

Attention

The ability to focus in an alert way on a particular phenomenon depends, among other things, on the state of consciousness. A disturbed sensorium leads to a disturbance in attention, e.g., inability to concentrate, distractibility. Attention may also be affected by intense emotional states. In severe depression, for example, there may be intense preoccupation with depressive thought content.

In delirium, there is a basic disorder of attention, manifested by inability to sustain attention to external stimuli and to maintain goal-directed thinking. As a result, thought processes, memory, and orientation are impaired.

Orientation

Orientation is the process by which a person uses sense data (from internal and external origins) to gain information about the spatiotemporal characteristics of his whereabouts, the position he occupies in his milieu, and how and why he came to be there. For orientation to be intact, the sense organs must provide a minimum of sensory input, to be integrated centrally in an intact brain (apperception). Thus, disorientation can be caused by peripheral or central factors, or by a combination of both.

Perceptual Abnormalities

These include illusions and hallucinations. An *illusion* is a misinterpretation of an actual stimulus; such perceptual distortions frequently occur in delirium, and other psychiatric disorders, but also occasionally in normal individuals. *Hallucinations* are perceptual experiences in the apparent absence of external stimuli, and usually indicate the existence of a psychosis. When examining the patient in this respect, it is not wise to simply conclude that a patient is hallucinating when he reports that he "sees or hears things." One should also ascertain to what extent imagination or perceptual imagery play a role. This can be done by inquiring whether the visions or voices are "inside the patient's head—inside of him," or whether he perceives them as coming from outside of himself. In the case of visual and auditory imagery, the perceptual experiences are felt to be "inside"; they can be evoked and dismissed at will. Hallucinations, on the other hand, are not evoked and dismissed voluntarily.

Persistent and recurrent hallucinations are the essential features of organic hallucinosis; they may occur as associated features in delirium, dementia, organic affective syndrome, and organic delusional syndrome.

Memory

The capacity of *memory* includes the ability to register, store, and retrieve information. Learning, the storing of new information, requires intact memory. Memory disturbances may be due to impaired registration, retention, or retrieval of stored information. For the purpose of mental status examination, there appear to be four types of memory deficits: immediate, short-term, recent, and remote. *Immediate* recall refers to retrieval of stimuli presented to the patient a few minutes earlier; this memory function is impaired in delirium. *Short-term* memory has been defined, for clinical purposes, to cover events that occurred within the last 25 minutes; its impairment is the essential feature of the amnestic syndrome. *Recent* memory refers to events that occurred anywhere from ½ hour up to one or more weeks ago. This is impaired in several disorders, including delirium, amnestic syndrome, and dementia. *Remote* memory pertains to events that occurred earlier than a few weeks ago, or to so-called overlearned information (name, birthday, address, etc.). It is impaired in delirium (secondary to the attention deficit) and in dementia (one of the essential features).

Immediate and short-term recall is tested by asking the patient to remember something (a word, number, or name). After a while, e.g., 1–5

Table 4.1
Mental Status Questionnaire (MSQ)*

1. Where are we now?	Orientation for place
2. Where is this place located?	Orientation for place
3. What is the day of month?	Orientation for time
4. What month is it?	Orientation for time
5. What year is it?	Orientation for time
6. How old are you?	Memory, recent or remote
7. When is your birthday?	Memory, recent or remote
8. What year were you born?	Memory, recent or remote
9. Who is president of the U. S.?	General information, memory
10. Who was president before him?	General information, memory

Rating of MSQ

Number of errors	Chronic brain syndrome
0–2	Absent–mild
3–5	Mild–moderate
6–8	Moderate–severe
9–10	Severe

* Modified from: Kahn, R. L., Goldfarb, A. I., Pollack, M., and Peck, A.: Brief objective measure for the determination of mental status in the aged. *Am. J. Psychiatry 117*:326, 1960.

minutes (up to 25 minutes), the patient is asked to reproduce the item.

Recent memory can be tested by asking questions, such as: Where do you live? How long have you lived there? How long have you been here? Where were you one week ago? How many meals did you have today? What did you have for breakfast? What is my name? When did you see me for the first time? Have you been in this room before?

Remote memory can be tested by asking the following type of questions: Where were you born? Where did you go to school? Highest grade completed? How old were you when you finished school? How old were you when you began working? Name of first employer? Who was U. S. President when you began your first job?

Kahn and Goldfarb and co-workers[45] introduced a Mental Status Questionnaire (MSQ) consisting of 10 questions that pertain to orientation for time, place, and person; recent and remote memory; and general information. The patient's performance is scored in terms of the number of wrong answers. The error scores appear to be a reliable indicator of the degree of organicity (see Table 4.1).

Face-Hand Test

Another approach is the *Face-Hand Test* (FHT), a series of double simultaneous stimulations of the face and hand.[47] Failure to correctly report touch on the back of the hand is presumptive of cortical neuronal loss. The patient sits facing the examiner, hands resting on his knees. He is touched simultaneously on one cheek and the dorsum of one hand, in a specific order. The Face-Hand Test is done first with the patient's eyes closed, then repeated with eyes open. Anxious persons may make more errors with eyes open than with eyes closed. In 80 percent of persons who make errors with the eyes closed there is no improvement with eyes open. In the four initial trials, the patient gets used to the procedure. In the teaching trials 5 and 6, the examiner informs him where he is touched, or reinforces a correct response by saying "that's right." A person who learns to report correctly where he is touched after trials 5 and 6 is presumed free of brain damage. Only errors on steps 7 and 10 (which are a repeat of 1 to 4) are considered presumptive of brain damage. Major changes in score upon repeat testing are rare when chronic brain syndrome is present. However, in acute brain syndrome, the score may vary over a short period of time.

Errors include not reporting the touch to the hand (extinction); localizing the hand touch to the cheek, the knee, or elsewhere (displacement); pointing to the examiner's hand (projection); or pointing outside in space (exsomesthesia). The testresults correlate with the degree of brain syndrome as measured by the MSQ or psychiatric evaluation. Extinction of the touch to the face is rare and suggests a functional disorder (see Table 4.2).

Table 4.2
Sequence of Stimulation in Face-Hand Test

Stimulation	Comment
1. Right cheek-left hand 2. Left cheek-right hand 3. Right cheek-right hand 4. Left cheek-left hand	Initial trials. Response evaluated in context of further trials.
5. Right cheek-left cheek 6. Right hand-left hand	Teaching trials. Usually reported correctly. Examiner informs, or reinforces, response that there were two touches.
7. Right cheek-left hand 8. Left cheek-right hand 9. Right cheek-right hand 10. Left cheek-left hand	Brain damage suggested by: —incorrect response and stimulation not reported; —felt but displaced; —projected or located in space.

* As modified from Bender, Fink and Green by Kahn and Pollack, in Goldfarb, A. I.: The evaluation of geriatric patients following treatment. In: *Evaluation of Psychiatric Treatment*, edited by P. H. Hoch and J. Zubin, Grune & Stratton, New York, 1964, p. 291.

Table 4.3

Factors	Differential diagnosis of organic brain syndromes				
	Depressive disorders	Multi-infarct dementia	Alzheimer's disease senile onset	Alzheimer's disease presenile onset	Pick's disease
Usual age of onset	Any age	55–70 average: 65	70+ average: 75	50–60 average: 56	45–55 average: 50
Sex distribution	Early life: more women Late life: more men	Men:women = 3:1	Men:women = 2:3	Men:women = 2:3	Men:women = 2:3
Duration	Varies from weeks to years	Varies from days to many years average: 4 years	Varies from months to years average: 5 years	Average: 4 years	Average: 4 years
Mode of onset	Gradual or sudden; precipitating stress often apparent	Gradual or acute	Insidious	More sudden and less gradual than S. D.	Slow and insidious
Course	Self-limited, but tendency to recur	Intermittent, fluctuating	Slowly or rapidly progressive	Rapidly progressive	Progressive and fatal
Prognosis	Responsive to drugs or ECT	Varies depending on multiple factors	Poor (in moderate or severe cases)	Very poor	Very poor
Outcome	Usually recovery; sometimes suicide or regression to paranoid level	Death from CVA, heart disease, or infection	Death from general organismic failure; infection		
Hereditary and precipitating factors	Involution; previous history of depression	Some familial tendency	Multiple genetically determined factors	Multifactorical inheritance, genetic factors causing premature aging	Heredodegenerative process

Table 4.4

Factors	Differential diagnosis of organic brain syndromes				
	Depressive disorders	Multi-infarct dementia	Alzheimer's disease senile onset	Alzheimer's disease presenile onset	Pick's disease
Signs of brain damage	None	Diffuse or focal	Diffuse, generalized	Diffuse, generalized more severe than in senile onset	Circumscribed atrophy; frontal, temporal or parietal lobes
Impairment of higher cortical functions	No structural impairment	Some isolated impairments: e.g., aphasia, apraxia, agnosia	Progressive dementia	Involvement of cerebral associative areas; transcortical aphasia, apraxia, agnosia, etc.	Focal cortical impairments; e.g., motor or sensory aphasia
Neuromuscular	Psychomotor retardation or agitation	Paralyses; minor extrapyramidal signs	Tremors, uncertain gait, variable muscular rigidity, incontinence	Transient or progressive paresis; unsteady gait; increased muscle tone; occasional tremors, incontinence	Primitive reflexes; extrapyramidal signs; attacks of muscular hypotonia, incontinence
Seizures	None	Epileptiform attacks	Rare	Occasional	Rare
Medical	Physiological concomitants of depression (sleep, appetite, weight, energy)	Common history of CVA; headaches, dizziness & syncope (in 50%); "little strokes"; arteriosclerosis in heart, kidney, legs etc.	Infections, contractures, fractures, decubitus	Infections, contractures, fractures, decubitus	Infections, contractures, fractures, decubitus

Table 4.5

Neuropathology	Differential diagnosis of organic brain syndromes				
	Depressive disorders	Multi-infarct dementia	Alzheimer's disease senile onset	Alzheimer's disease presenile onset	Pick's disease
Macroscopic	None characteristic	Large or small areas of softening and hemorrhage	Diffuse generalized shrinkage of brain, especially gray matter; dilated ventricles; internal hydrocephalus	General cerebral atrophy; dilated ventricles; internal hydrocephalus	Circumscribed lobar atrophy, mostly —orbitofrontal —temporal
Microscopic	None characteristic	Granular atrophy of cortex diffusely with hypertensive cardiovascular disease; destruction of neurons, nerve fibers and glia; focal neuronal & selective cortical degeneration Secondary gliosis Senile plaques not typical	Neuronal degeneration and shrinking; most damage in upper layers of cortex; deposition of lipofuscin & intracellular fibrils Moderate gliosis, especially in outer layer of cortex Senile plaques	Diffuse loss of neurons, especially in cortex layers 3 & 5; disturbed cortical layers Neuron degeneration: pyknosis; granulovacuolar; Alzheimer's neurofibrillary change Gliosis more severe than in senile onset Senile plaques throughout cortex	Progressive atrophy of neurons; no predilection for cortical layers; neuron degeneration; increased pigment pyknosis; swollen cells; argyrophilic cytoplasmic; inclusions Gliosis prominent Senile plaques rare
Vascular	None characteristic	Vascular *Large arteries:* —atherosclerosis *small* vessels: —endothelial —proliferation —medial hypertrophy —intima hyalinization	Endothelial degeneration; media fibrosis; adventitial proliferation; vascular loops	Degenerative changes of endothelial and adventitial cells	Endothelial proliferation; hyaline degeneration

Table 4.6

Psychiatric symptomatology	Differential diagnosis of organic brain symdromes				
	Depressive disorders	Multi-infarct dementia	Alzheimer's disease senile onset	Alzheimer's disease presenile onset	Pick's disease
Orientation	Intact, except in depressive stupor	Episodes of acute confusion; lucid intervals	Progressive disorientation in all spheres Loss of time perspective		
Perception	Occasional auditory hallucinations	Auditory and visual during acute exacerbations	Various types of hallucinations in advanced stages	Occasional hallucinations	
Intellect and thought	No mental impairment; Delusions consistent with affect Insight varies	Lacunar types of intellectual deficit; Delusions: rare Insight present in early stages	Progressive, generalized dementia; Delusions depend on degree of regression and premorbid personality No insight	Progressive dementia & loss of abstraction; Aphasia, alexia, agnosia, asymbolia, agraphia, apraxia No insight	*Frontal lobe* syndrome: progressive loss of abstraction; *Aphasic* syndrome: aphasia, alexia, etc. *Alogic* syndrome: agnosia, apraxia, etc. No insight
Memory	Transient memory problems due to CNS slowing	Varying deficits of recent & remote memory, of retention & recall Confabulations: rare	Progressive impairment of all memory functions Confabulations in presbyophrenic type	Progressive impairment of all memory functions Confabulations: rare	Progressive impairment of all memory functions Confabulations: common

Table 4.7

Psychiatric symptomatology	Differential diagnosis of organic brain symdromes				
	Depressive disorders	Multi-infarct dementia	Alzheimer's disease senile onset	Alzheimer's disease presenile onset	Pick's disease
Affect	Depressed; guilt; low self-esteem	Emotional lability; anxiety & depression Later: blunting of affect	Depends on subtype simple:apathy depressed:agitated delirious:anxious paranoid:hostile presbyophrenic:shallow euphoria	Variable at first; later: apathy	Apathy and indifference
Psychomotor	Retardation sometimes: agitation	Hypoactive or hyperactive or restless agitation	Hyperactive or hypoactive, or restless agitation	Hyperactive; repetitive, primitive motor behavior; extrapyramidal signs	Hypo- or hyperkinetic; primitive reflexes; stereotyped activity; preseveration; echolalia; logoclony
Personality changes	Transient regressive changes	Regressive changes are intermittent or slowly progressive	Progressive deterioration of social behavior and personal habits		

References

1. Task Force on Nomenclature and Statistics of the American Psychiatric Association: *Diagnostic and Statistical Manual of Mental Disorders,* ed. 3, American Psychiatric Association, Washington, D. C., 1978.
2. Reichel, W.: Organic brain syndromes. In: *The Geriatric Patient,* edited by W. Reichel, chap. 5, HP Publishing Company, New York, 1978.
3. Wells, C. E.: Diagnosis of dementia. *Psychosomatics 20:* 517–522, 1979.
4. Katzman, R., and Karasu, T. B.: Differential diagnosis in dementia. In: *Neurological and Sensory Disorders in the Elderly,* edited by W. S. Fields, Stratton Intercontinental, New York, 1975. pp. 103–134.
5. Heston, L. L., and Mastri, A. R.: The genetics of Alzheimer's disease, associations with hematologic malignancy and Down's syndrome. *Arch. Gen. Psychiatry 34:*976–981, 1977.
6. Wang, H. S., and Busse, E. W.: Dementia in old age. In: *Contemporary Neurology,* edited by C. E. Wells, chap. 9, F. A. Davis Co., Philadelphia, 1971.
7. Cavenar, J. O., Maltbie, A. A., and Austin, L.: Depression simulating organic brain disease. *Am. J. Psychiatry 136:*521–523, 1979.
8. Post, F.: Dementia, depression, and pseudodementia. In: *Psychiatric Aspects of Neurologic Disease,* edited by D. F. Benson and D. Blumer, Grune and Stratton, New York, 1975.
9. Hontela, S., and Schwartz, G.: Myocardial infarction in the differential diagnosis of dementias in the elderly. *J. Am. Geriatr. Soc. 27:*104–106, 1979.
10. Tomlinson, B. E., Blessed, G., and Roth, M.: Observations on the brains of demented old people. *J. Neurol. Sci. 11:*205–242, 1970.
11. Robbins, S.: Stroke in the geriatric patient. In: *The Geriatric Patient,* edited by W. Reichel, chap. 8, HP Publishing Company, New York, 1978.
12. Hachinski, V. C., Iliff, L. D., Zelhka, E., et al: Cerebral blood flow in dementia. *Arch. Neurol. 32:*632–637, 1975.
13. Seltzer, B., and Sherwin, I.: Organic brain syndrome: an empirical study and critical review. *Am. J. Psychiatry 135:*13–21, 1978.
14. Victor, M., Adams, R. D., and Collins, G. H.: *The Wernicke-Korsakoff Syndrome,* F. A. Davis, Philadelphia, 1971.
15. Wang, H. S.: Organic brain syndrome. In: *Behavior and Adaptation in Late Life,* edited by E. W. Busse and E. Pfeiffer, chap. 13, Little, Brown and Company, Inc., New York, 1969.
16. Caine, E. D., Hunt, R. D., Weingartner, H., and Ebert, M. H.: Huntington's dementia: clinical and neuropsychological features. *Arch. Gen. Psychiatry 35:*377–384, 1978.
17. Obrist, W. D., and Bissell, L. F.: The electroencephalogram of aged patients with cardiac and cerebral vascular disease. *J. Gerontol. 10:*315–330, 1955.
18. Eisdorfer, C.: Psychologic reaction to cardiovascular change in the aged. *Mayo Clinic Proc. 42:*620–636, 1967.
19. Corsellis, J. A. N.: *Mental Illness and the Aging Brain.* Oxford University Press, London, 1962.
20. Willanger, R., Thygesen, P., Nielsen, R., and Peterson, O.: Intellectual impairment and cerebral atrophy—a psychological, neurological and radiological investigation. *Dan. Med. Bull. 15:*65–93, 1968.
21. Obrist, W. D., Chivian, E., Cronqvist, S., and Ingvar, D. H.: Regional cerebral blood flow in senile and presenile dementia. *Neurology 20:*315–322, 1970.
22. Busse, E. W., and Wang, H. S.: The value of electroencephalography in geriatrics. *Geriatrics 20:*906–924, 1965.
23. Gianturco, D. T., Breslin, M. S., Heyman, A., Gentry, W. D., Jenkins, C. D., and Kaplan, B.: Personality patterns and life stress in ischemic cerebrovascular disease: I. Psychiatric findings. *Stroke 5:*453–460, 1974.
24. Kiev, A., Chapman, L. F., Guthrie, T. C., and Wolff, G.: The highest integrative functions and diffuse cerebral atrophy. *Neurology 12:*363–385, 1962.
25. Goldstein, K.: Functional disturbances in brain damage. In: *American Handbook of Psychiatry,* edited by S. Arieti, chap. 39, Basic Books, New York, 1959. pp. 770–793.
26. Kaszniak, A. W., Garron, D. C., Fox, J. H., Bergen, D., and Huckman, M.: Cerebral

atrophy, EEG slowing, age, education, and cognitive functioning in suspected dementia. *Neurology 29*:1273–1279, 1979.
27. Wells, C. E.: Chronic brain disease: an overview. *Am. J. Psychiatry 135*:1–12, 1978.
28. Haase, G. R.: Disease presenting as dementia. In: *Dementia*, ed. 2, edited by C. E. Wells, F. A. Davis Company, Philadelphia, 1977. pp. 27–67.
29. Wells, C. E.: Diagnostic evaluation and treatment in dementia. In: *Dementia*, ed. 2, edited by C. E. Wells, F. A. Davis Company, Philadelphia, 1977. pp. 247–276.
30. Nott, P. N., and Fleminger, J. J.: Presenile dementia: the difficulties of early diagnosis. *Acta Psychiatr. Scand. 51*:210–217, 1975.
31. Kiloh, L. G.: Pseudo-dementia. *Acta Psychiatr. Scand. 37*:336–351, 1961.
32. Wells, C. E.: Pseudodementia. *Am. J. Psychiatry 136*:895–900, 1979.
33. Wells, C. E.: Dementia, pseudodementia, and dementia praecox. In: *Phenomenology and Treatment of Schizophrenia*, edited by W. E. Fann, I. Karacan, A. D. Pokorny, et al., Spectrum Publications, 1977.
34. Smith, W. T., Turner, E., and Sim, M.: Cerebral biopsy in the investigation of presenile dementia: II. *Br. J. Psychiatry 112*:127–133, 1966.
35. Fox, J. H., Topel, J. L., and Huckman, M. S.: Use of computerized tomography in senile dementia. *J. Neurol. Neurosurg. Psychiatry 38*:948–953, 1975.
36. Dastur, D. K., Lane, M. H., Hansen, D. B., Kety, S. S., Perlin, S., Butler, R., and Sokoloff, L.: Effects of aging on cerebral circulation and metabolism in man. In: *Human Aging: A Biological and Behavioral Study*, edited by J. E. Birren, R. N. Butler, S. W. Greenhouse, L. Sokoloff, and M. R. Yarrow, U. S. Government Printing Office, Washington, D. C., 1963.
37. Obrist, W. D., Thompson, H. K., Jr., King, C. H., and Wang, H. S.: Determination of regional cerebral blood flow by inhalation by 133-Xenon. *Circ. Res. 20*:124–135, 1967.
38. Obrist, W. D., Sokoloff, L., Lassen, N. A., Lane, M. H., Butler, R. N., and Feinberg, I.: Relation of EEG to cerebral blood flow and metabolism in old age. *Electroencephalogr. Clin. Neurophysiol. 15*:610–619, 1963.
39. Benton, A. L.: Psychological tests for brain damage. In: *Comprehensive Textbook of Psychiatry*, edited by A. M. Freedman, H. I. Kaplan, and B. J. Sadock, ed. 2, vol. 2, chap. 12.4, The Williams and Wilkins Company, Baltimore, 1975.
40. Wechsler, D.: *The Measurement and Appraisal of Adult Intelligence*, ed. 4, The Williams and Wilkins Company, Baltimore, 1958.
41. Botwinick, J.: *Cognitive Processes in Maturity and Old Age*. Springer Publishing Co., Inc., New York, 1967.
42. Craik, F. I. M.: Age differences in human memory. In: *Handbook of the Psychology of Aging*, edited by J. E. Birren and K. Warner Schaie, chap. 17, van Nostrand Reinhold Company, New York, 1977.
43. Birren, J. E.: Increments and decrements in the intellectual status of the aged. In: *Aging in Modern Society: Psychiatric Research Report 23*, edited by A. Simon and L. J. Epstein, American Psychiatric Association, Washington, D. C., 1968.
44. Botwinick, J.: Intellectual abilities. In: *Handbook of the Psychology of Aging*, edited by J. E. Birren and K. W. Schaie, chap. 24, van Nostrand Reinhold Company, New York, 1977.
45. Kahn, R. L., Goldfarb, A. I., Pollack, M., and Peck, A.: Brief objective measures for the determination of mental status in the aged. *Am. J. Psychiatry 117*:326–328, 1960.
46. Salzman, C., Shader, R. I., Kochansky, G. E., and Cronin, D. M.: Rating scales for psychotropic drug research with geriatric patients. *J. Am. Geriatr. Soc. 20*:209–221, 1972.
47. Goldfarb, A. I.: The evaluation of geriatric patients following treatment. In: *Evaluation of Psychiatric Treatment*, edited by P. H. Hoch and J. Zubin, Grune and Stratton, New York, 1964.

5

thought disorders and paranoid phenomena*

Primary thought disorders in late life occur as a major feature in dementia, schizophrenia, and paranoid disorders. The latter two categories of illnesses may be carried over from earlier years into old age, or they may appear to arise for the first time in the senium.

THE NATURE OF THOUGHT DISORDERS AND PARANOID PHENOMENA

The term dementia praecox was coined in 1857 by Morel, to designate psychoses which would end in deterioration. Some approaches to the concept of schizophrenia have emphasized the tendency toward deterioration (Kraepelin), the presence of a specific underlying disturbance in psychological processes (Bleuler), or pathognomonic symptom complexes (Schneider). The phrase praecox (= precocious) implied that this process started in early life, in contrast to the mental deterioration in old age. In 1896, Kraepelin delineated dementia praecox as a group of mental disorders; and, in 1911 Bleuler introduced the term schizophrenia, because in his view, the illness did not necessarily lead to dementia. The term dementia nowadays is reserved for thought disorders which have an organic basis. Schizophrenia, however, is considered to involve a primary disorder in thinking, which is not secondary to brain damage.

According to the *Diagnostic and Statistical Manual of Mental Disorders* (DSM-III),[1] the basic features of schizophrenia are disorganization of a previous level of psychosocial functioning, as well as psychotic features in the areas of thought and language, perception, affect, personal identity and object relations (autism). The diagnosis is not made unless the illness has persisted for at least 6 months. Illnesses of shorter duration (schizophreniform) probably have different pathogenesis and course. The premorbid personality may meet the criteria for paranoid, introverted, schizotypal, or borderline personality disorder.[1]

Bleuler's[2] four primary symptoms of schizophrenia include the following.

* In collaboration with W. M. Taylor, M.D.

1. Defect in association (characterized by loosening of associations and by other evidence of a thinking disturbance).

2. Defect in affect (characterized by being flat or blunted or inappropriate to the ideation or situation).

3. Autism (characterized by a detachment from external reality and a proclivity to withdraw into one's fantasies and inner life).

4. Ambivalence (characterized by the existence of opposite feelings and thoughts simultaneously).

Schneider's[3] first-rank symptoms include six symptoms, any one of which is thought to be pathognomonic.

1. Auditorization of thought (the patient hearing his own thoughts).

2. Auditory hallucinations that occur in the form of a running commentary on the patient's current thoughts and activities or experienced in the form of a conversation between two or more people who refer to the patient in the third person.

3. Thought withdrawal, thought insertion, and thought broadcasting.

4. Somatic hallucinations that the patient attributes to the will, influence, or motive of outside agencies.

5. Delusional perceptions (delusions based on perceptions).

6. All events in the sphere of feeling, drive, and volition that are experienced as made or influenced by others.

EVALUATION OF THOUGHT PROCESSES

The only satisfactory method to examine a person's thoughts is through the medium of words, spoken or written. The communicative framework in which thoughts are transmitted to the receiver includes verbal messages and the metacommunicative signals accompanying them.

Quantitative

Quantitative changes in thought may be reflected by changes in the tempo of speech, e.g., pressure of speech in mania; or slowing of speech in depression. But there is not always a close correlation between thought and speech; for example, a hostile, fearful, or withdrawn patient may be tight-lipped, while his thoughts are racing at high speed. Quantitative abnormalities are not essential features of a primary thought disorder. In fact, these are more typical of affective disorders.

Qualitative

The types of words selected, the configuration of speech patterns, and other formal aspects of speech, may be an indicator of *qualitative* disturbances in thought. In true thought disorders, there is a qualitative abnormality, affecting the *formal* aspects of thought.

> A 63-year-old chronic schizophrenic woman, when asked if she was the head of the household, answered: "My is a residential

president." When asked about her health, she responded: "The united crusaders of the medical sciences have some gifts to give each individual as to prosperity." The inappropriateness and incoherence of this speech pattern reflects the patient's thought disorder. To other questions, she would respond by whispering telephone numbers. The patient had with her many scraps of paper on which she had written numerous telephone numbers; throughout these numbers, a few words were scattered adding up to a cryptic message of reassurance from God. Each phone number represented a person considered helpful and friendly (illustrating the typical features of autism, magical thinking, telecommunication with supernatural powers, etc.).

A thought disorder can be defined as the intrusion of a primary process into secondary process thinking. Secondary process thinking is the goal-directed logical thinking typically used by most adults. Primary process thinking is typical of the thinking of small children and of dreams. Oppenheimer[4] describes seven types of formal thought disorders. Four (desymbolization of the word, semantic shift, metonymic distortion, and neologism) are based on word use, and three (asyndesis, system shifting, and sham language) are based on sentence use. All of these are based on the intrusion of primary process thinking into the secondary process, and most rely heavily on the concept of predicative identification (see below).

The Concept of Association. The relatively unencumbered flow of thought that occurs in the stream of consciousness is called "free associations." When examining a series of thoughts, we may discover that each thought in the sequence expresses the same underlying theme. The associative links between the thoughts represent a "red thread" tying them together into a cohesive statement. A single thought is not an association; an association can only exist between two or more thoughts. A pattern of thought processes is evaluated by examining the associative *links* between thoughts. The nature of these links can be predominantly logical and orderly (secondary process), or illogical and irrational (primary process).

Primary process corresponds with the pleasure principle and is characterized by a tendency to immediate discharge of drive energy, and extreme mobility of cathexes, so that substitute ways of discharge are easily achieved. The secondary process refers to the reality principle and involves the delay of immediate discharge or gratification, the use of logic, the presence of the time sense, the awareness of alternative modes of action, and the ability of decision-making. Primary process thinking is characterized by the absence of negatives and conditionals; by absence of time sense; and by the use of allusions, analogies, displacements, condensation, and symbolic representation. The primary process quality of psychotic thought processes is illustrated by the following case.

An 82-year-old schizophrenic woman who had been preoccupied for years with sex and being pregnant, stated that "When I put my hand on the red knob of the railing, my thumb becomes swollen." Such a delusion can be viewed in the same way as the manifest content of a dream. The latent dream content (the underlying wish) undergoes elaborate distortions involving primary process mechanisms. Thus, the underlying wish is probably the wish to be pregnant which, in turn, represents a denial of death's approach. The pregnancy is to come about through contact with a phallic object: the hard railing with the red knob (glans). (This is an example of the use of displacement and symbolic representation.) Touching the phallic symbol causes part of her body to swell. The swelling represents the idea of pregnancy, but it is displaced to her thumb, another phallic symbol. Thus, through symbolic representation, displacements, etc., an underlying fantasy is highly distorted and condensed into a brief somatic delusion. (This is the same patient as on p. 149 of Chapter 9).

Paleological Thought. Essential features of a thought disorder include the presence of paleological thought and concretization of the concept, and the loss of abstract capacity. In *paleological* thought, a common predicate leads to the establishment of an identity of two nouns. *Concretization of the concept* involves loss of the abstract capacity and transforming the abstract into the concrete.[5] The *abstract capacity* comprises the ability to assume a specific mental set, to imagine the "merely possible," to shift reflectively from one aspect of a situation to another, and to keep in mind several aspects of a task simultaneously, to find common denominators; and, to use concepts and symbols properly.[6] The following case illustrates a thought disorder in a patient with senile dementia.

An 80-year-old woman (without a past history of schizophrenia) complained "I have stones inside of me and it is hard for them to come out." This patient had occasional fecal impaction, and her stools were hard, *like* stones. Because her abstract capacity was impaired, she could not conceptualize the "as if," and make proper use of a metaphor. While normal thought accepts identity only on the basis of identical subjects, paleological thinking accepts identity based on identical predicates.[7] Thus, an associative link becomes an identifying link. The attribute "hard," common to both feces and stones, leads to the identity: feces = stones.

A 91-year-old woman admitted to the mental hospital, because she constantly talked about death, was suspicious that her family was "too interested in her will," and was calling various relatives "Peter"or "Judas." Following hospitalization, she expressed fear that death would come about by way of electroconvulsive therapy.

> During an interview, she declared suddenly that "Jesus comes as a thief in the night" (reference to biblical metaphor—Jesus comes unexpectedly). The explanation of her concerns and accusations was considered to be as follows. The thought of her own death is concretely personified and externalized: a thief in the night. The externalized threat is not only disarmed, but changed into its opposite: Jesus, the Savior. The notion of thief now finds its way toward some of her relatives: Judas was a thief—for some money he betrayed Jesus. But even Peter disowned, betrayed Jesus—and that, just before His death. Likewise, her own offspring might abandon, disown, or betray her for money. This patient was found to have diabetes and a duodenal ulcer. Significantly, she actively resisted diagnostic tests as well as recommended treatment. Thus, she appeared ready to die, and yet was very much frightened by that thought—Judas, Peter as well as Jesus Himself, had died a painful, cruel death.

The logical association between one thought and the next may be disturbed in thought disorders resulting in *loose associations* (derailment). A simple way of testing abstract capacity is to ask the patient "What is the same about an orange, apple, and a grapefruit?" One correct answer is that all three are fruits (the common denominator is that they belong to the general category of fruits). A person with an impaired abstract capacity might respond that his mother used to buy all these fruits; he can only think of a concrete event and cannot generalize from the particular toward the general. At times, the manifestations of a thought disorder may be quite subtle. Under routine circumstances, schizophrenia or brain-damaged patients may not reveal their impairment, in contrast to situations which require an initiative, making a choice, or shifting from one mental set to another.

> A woman in her late 50's had a 15-year history of vague psychiatric symptoms: a phobia about eating in public places; often changing jobs because she would not feel appreciated; and occasional crying spells "out of a clear blue sky." Her diagnosis had been involutional depression, but in spite of antidepressant therapy, her complaints persisted. The diagnostic riddle was eventually solved through a careful analysis of verbatim transcripts of some clinical interviews: repeated, subtle nonsequiturs suggested a thought disorder. For example she reported that her neighbor had said to her "I haven't seen you for some time—Where have you been?—I thought maybe you were shopping for Christmas." The patient had answered, "No, I have done my Christmas shopping already." Thus, she could not conceive of shopping as the "merely possible"—some general type of situation that could account for her absence from home, at any time. Instead "shopping" referred to one particular, concrete event.

Content of Thought

In addition to the formal aspects, the *content of thought* must be explored. The latter may be highly abnormal and indicative of a psychosis, but yet, this phenomenon is not restricted to the domain of thought disorders. In affective psychoses, for example, all sorts of psychotic thought contents may occur, but these delusions are considered to be secondary to, and in keeping with, the primary disorder in affect.

Ideas of Reference. Characteristic of ideas of reference is that the meaning of events or people's actions is interpreted as being especially related to oneself. The terms reference and relationship have a common etymological derivation: the past participle of the Latin *referre* is *relatus*. Thus, a reference implies a type of relatedness. Ideas of reference signify thoughts that establish a special relationship between the thinking subject and one or more external objects. The second feature of ideas of reference pertains to the nature of this special relationship. The subject (patient) may see himself as being active (influencing the other) or passive (being at the receiving end); the type of interaction may be good and pleasant, or evil and painful. In their extreme form, such ideas of reference become delusions of reference, and include phenomena such as thought broadcasting, thought insertion, and delusions of being controlled.

Paranoid Ideation. Mild, fleeting ideas of reference occur, at some time, in almost all individuals. In contrast, when their duration becomes extended and the sense of conviction more intense, they indicate a pathological relationship between oneself and the world around. This type of disordered relationship is referred to as *paranoid* (etymology: para = besides; noia = knowledge; hence paranoia denotes knowledge that is beside the point).

> A 65-year-old woman with a diagnosis of schizophrenia, since age 51, had the idea that "whenever somebody passes my window, the food in the refrigerator sours." (Illustrating a paranoid idea of reference of psychotic proportions, i.e., a delusion of being controlled, the patient being the passive victim of evil forces.) This patient also had covered every mirror in the house with towels, presumably part of a delusional schema to protect herself against the evil eye.

Delusions. Delusions represent a serious thought disorder indicating illness of psychotic proportions. A delusion is a false idea out of keeping with the beliefs generally held by society and which cannot be corrected. Delusions may be grandiose (as in manic and schizophrenic states), persecutory (paranoid schizophrenia and organic brain syndrome), hypochondriacal (depression, schizophrenia, and organic brain syndrome), etc. Delusions may be systemized, logically built up on a basic premise; but, since the premise is incorrect, the deductions constituting the delusional system are equally incorrect. In senile dementia, paranoid delusions tend to be poorly systematized due to impairment of intellect. In organic delusional syndrome, the delusions may range from poorly systematic paranoid delusions to those that are highly organized. The delusions of affective disorders are consistent with the prevailing mood, but in thought disorders, there often is a discrepancy between the delusional thought content and the patient's feelings.

DIFFERENTIAL DIAGNOSIS OF THOUGHT DISORDERS

The true thought disorders need to be differentiated from pseudo-thought disturbances, which may occur in depression, manic conditions, and obsessive-compulsive states.

Depression

In *depression*, thoughts emerge at a slow tempo, but the nature of the associative links is not affected. What may happen in profound depression, however, is that the patient replaces the verbalization of certain thoughts by a period of silence. In such a case, the first thought in a sequence of thoughts may be verbalized while the next several thought components are not verbally expressed, e.g., due to self-absorption or depressive apathy. Following the silence, the patient may verbalize the last thought in the series, one that probably shows little logical connection with the first thought. The absence of a logical connection, in this case, does not signify true incoherence, but pseudoincoherence, because the intermediate associative links between the first and the last statement were not verbalized.

Manic States

Hypertalkative patients at times seem to show incoherence or irrelevant thoughts. The manic patient, however, may think so fast that there is not enough time to verbalize all his thoughts. Thus, he may leave some of them out, resulting in an apparent loosening of the associations. Although his speech may seem rambling or incomprehensible, this does not reflect a true disturbance in logical thinking, but rather the inability of the speech apparatus to keep up with the increased tempo of thought production.

Circumstantiality

The obsessional, perfectionistic individual may depart tangentially at each station of the train of thought, going sideways into details, producing rococo verbal structures, but returning to the main trend ("as I was saying a while ago"). In spite of the baroque style, the circumstantial patient eventually gets to the point, and makes his point.

Rambling

In the case of *rambling*, the point is never made. The patient with organic brain syndrome may set out with thought 1, and proceed toward thoughts 2, 3, etc. While doing this, he loses sight of the point to be made, goes astray, and gets lost. The mental impairment may not permit him to carry out the dual task of remembering the point to be made, and the elaboration of successive steps needed to get to the point. Inasmuch as the brain-damaged patient forgets where his train of thought is heading, the essential deficit is in the area of memory, rather than in formal thought processes.

Organic mental disorders often present with symptoms that suggest schizophrenia, such as delusions, hallucinations, incoherence, and blunted or inappropriate affect. Organic delusional syndromes, in particular, may cross-sectionally resemble schizophrenia, but the presence of disorientation or memory impairment suggests an organic mental disorder.

Factitious Illness

In *factitious illness with psychological symptoms,* any seemingly psychotic symptoms are under voluntary control and are likely to be present only when the individual thinks he is being observed.

AGING AND SCHIZOPHRENIA

With regard to the relationship between aging and schizophrenia, we are interested in exploring four aspects: the usual age of onset of the clinical subtypes, the pathogenetic effects of aging, the pathoplastic effects of aging in modifying the symptomatology, and the possible effects of schizophrenia on the aging process itself.

AGE OF ONSET

Compared with other forms of schizophrenia, the paranoid type becomes clinically manifest at a later age, usually after age 30. As a subtype, it is more stable over time than the other subtypes. One plausible factor is that compared with other forms of schizophrenia, the paranoid type is relatively less severe; a disorder that, intrinsically or for whatever reasons, is less severe, would proportionately need more time to become overtly manifest. And, if the premorbid personality in paranoid schizophrenia does have relatively more strength, not only would it take longer for overt symptoms to develop, but also, once the disorder has become manifest, it would leave the overall personality more intact.

PATHOGENETIC EFFECTS OF AGING

The role which the aging process may play in terms of contributing to the etiology of thought disorders and paranoid phenomena, includes the following possibilities:

Pathological Trait Intensification

In the course of time, due to progressive accumulation of stresses, schizoid or paranoid personalities may develop an *intensification of their pathological character traits.* This process may take only a few years, or almost a lifetime. The psychodynamics and the duration of this process depend on biological, psychological, social and environmental factors, and their mutual interactions. In some cases the character disorder may decompensate in early childhood, transiently or permanently; in other cases the regression toward autism and thought disorder may not come about until the prospective patient has arrived in old age.

> An 82-year-old widow had recently developed extensive paranoid delusions. At first, the diagnosis of late life schizophrenia was considered because the schizophrenic disorder appeared to have started in old age. A careful anamnesis revealed, however, that during her early 20's, the patient had had a brief episode of hearing voices (telling her "to jump in the well"), excessive religious preoccupation, and marked ambivalence of affect. She apparently had a remission of this, and it was some 60 years later that the schizophrenic disorder became again overtly manifest.

Progressive Decompensation: Disengagement and Withdrawal

Some cases of progressive decompensation appear to take as their point of departure the midlife crisis. Normally, the awareness of entering the second half of life and the realization of its significance involve an involutional grief reaction. Failure to resolve the latter may lead to an involutional depression (second step). Such a depression may be mild or severe, short or long lasting, a "one time thing" or recurrent, and so on. Individuals differ greatly in their ability to overcome the depression and to develop mechanisms of psychological immunity against subsequent involutional losses. Some involutional depressions do not fully recover, and in fact, do not even hold their own, in terms of remaining on a level of chronic depression. Rather (and this would be the third phase), they settle down at a lower level of adjustment, i.e., hypochondriasis. This involves a *disengagement* from external objects and a *withdrawal* of interest onto the self. The distancing from others and the somatic self-absorption produce further object losses and impoverishment of the self, because the patient alienates others with his complaints. Due to the prolonged disengagement from the basic human dimensions of love and work, the patient's social and vocational skills suffer from disuse atrophy. Some patients may succeed in finding a new support base on the hypochondriacal level, depending on multiple factors. However, when the unstable, brittle adjustment does not hold up, the final phase sets in: a further withdrawal (from the realm of the body to the sphere of the inner self); regression to autism, with concomitant loss of contact with reality; and the onset of a thought disorder and paranoid ideation.

A 65-year-old divorced woman had become an overwhelming problem to all agencies in the community, because she was perenially dissatisfied with any place, person, or program arranged to meet her demands. At the age of 40, she had been admitted to a mental hospital because she had been accusing her husband of being "immoral and unfaithful," and she expressed suicidal threats (i.e., an involutional depression, with paranoid features). During her stay in the hospital, the depressive symptoms cleared up, but were replaced by hypochondriasis. She was discharged after a few months with the diagnosis neurasthenia. At the age of 43, she divorced her husband, who later remarried. She has not had any contact with him, nor with her two sons, since that time. Reportedly, the sons will have nothing to do with her, and the patient blames this on her ex-husband ("He taught them to hate and despise me"). Over the last 15 years, the patient (still an attractive, well-dressed lady) has sent out 41 formal change-of-address notes. (In one 2-year time span, she moved 15 times.) Over the past 10 years, she has lived in 30 different boarding homes. No one will allow her to return, once she leaves. The depressive symptoms never returned and were permanently replaced by hypochondriasis. At all times, her conversation revolved around herself, her ailments, doctors, medicine, and diet. After a few years of moving ceaselessly and alienating people, she also became more hostile and suspicious. She began to write letters to heads of agencies and directors of departments, explaining her plight, asking for help, and making assorted accusations. Some of her gossip was so vicious that she acquired a reputation of being like a snake in the grass, ready to strike any time. By the time she was in her late 50's, the accusations began to acquire decidedly paranoid aspects (e.g., "I heard the cleaning woman beating up some old people in the room next to mine"). She was constantly planning to litigate against various boarding homes, or to bring suit against some social service department. In her early 60's, grandiose thoughts and behavior were superimposed on the symptomatology (e.g., calling the police department to deliver her medicine to her from the drug store). By age 65, her litigious correspondence had reached for higher and higher echelons, eventually including letters to the U. S. President.

THE PATHOPLASTIC EFFECTS OF AGING

The passage of time may influence existing psychopathology in numerous ways. There does appear to be evidence suggesting certain general types of age-related effects on schizophrenic and paranoid conditions.

Hallucinations become less frequent and less exciting in chronic paranoid schizophrenia,[2] although in schizophrenia with late life onset, threatening or exciting hallucinations occur often.

Psychotic motor activity tends to decrease with aging. Patients who initially were hyperactive have a better chance for trial visits or discharge, after 20 years of hospitalization.[8]

Delusions may remain unaffected by aging, or show various changes. In one study, about half of the aged schizophrenics showed no change in their delusions; in the other half, the delusions had disappeared, expanded, or consolidated. Five possible mechanisms by which the delusions in old schizophrenics could be modified were observed: liquidation through suppression and retrenchment; shift of delusional content by restructuring of the milieu; conversion of a productive delusion into a nihilistic, depressive configuration; disappearance of the delusion, coincident with a psycho-organically induced regression; and expansion and fantastic generalization of the delusional themes.[9]

The extent of adherence to the same delusional thought content is roughly parallel to the degree of withdrawal.[8] Delusions may become less prominent or even disappear, in the course of aging, due to the development of physical illness which facilitates recathexis of the body. The switch from a persecutory delusion to a grandiose one is, psychodynamically, probably comparable to the shift from depression to mania (involving a mechanism of psychotic restitution fantasies).

There are chronic schizophrenics, who have been on phenothiazines for 10–15 years, and finally are able to leave the hospital. In these cases, it is not logical to assume that the phenothiazines became fully effective after all these years; nor, that improved community facilities can better handle such patients now-a-days. When these aged schizophrenics leave the hospital after some decades, they usually are placed in simple boarding home settings, the same kind that has existed throughout the years. This is further evidence that the aging process has a pathoplastic effect in certain schizophrenics.

EFFECT ON AGING PROCESS

With regard to the question, whether or not schizophrenia can have an effect on the aging process, there is no way of answering this in a generalizing way. Bleuler was of the opinion that organic-cerebral changes occurred less often in schizophrenics than in the average population.[2] Riemer[10] and Bychowsky[11] found no clinical evidence of organic brain syndrome in the aged schizophrenics studied by them. The notion whether or not schizophrenia would provide some type of immunity or protection against the effects of senile brain changes certainly requires a lot more systematic investigation. Apart from this, a few points can be made on a common sense basis.

First, schizophrenics, as a group, if not protected and treated by society, would show a drastically reduced life span: they would succumb to illness, accident, and deprivation. The illness is so pervasive that it is difficult to separate complications from manifestations of the impairment. Complications include failure of educational achievement, work performance below that appropriate to education, social isolation, and inability to develop or maintain close interpersonal relationships. The life expectancy is shorter than that of the general population due to an increased suicide rate and death from other causes, for example, economically deprived environments. Secondly, persons with a schizoid character structure may have a built-in protection against the stresses of old age. The withdrawn schizoid does not engage himself with others, may not acquire objects of value, in short, he travels lightly. Hence, he has little to lose, later in life. Third, the fact that many schizophrenic patients find permanent shelter in the refuge of a hospital, or protection in the custody of a family, implies that they are not being exposed to the stress and strain of the daily rat race. Finally, the idea that schizophrenics may have a special resistance to dementia is probably a deceptive mirage. Rather, it is more logical to consider the fact that a schizophrenic suffers from a functional disorder of thought. When, in old age, structural cerebral impairment sets in, the dementia is no longer functional, but organic. But, the clinical difference between not using intact brain equipment and not using not-intact equipment may be hardly noticeable.

CLINICAL TYPES

PARANOID SCHIZOPHRENIA

Symptomatology

Paranoid schizophrenia may appear as late as the middle adult years and leave the personality relatively intact, in contrast to other types of schizophrenia. The *symptomatology* includes delusions of persecution or grandeur, ideas of reference, auditory hallucinations, and frequent preoccupation with religion or supernatural topics. A distinction has been made between a hostile and a grandiose subtype. The *hostile* subtype is characterized by delusions of persecution and injustice, extensive use of projection, a tendency to develop a systematized network of inter-related delusions, and auditory hallucinations of a threatening or violent nature. The *grandiose* subtype has delusions of grandeur and occasional persecutory delusions, autistic restitution fantasies (regression to infantile omnipotence), inclusion of protective supernatural powers in the delusional system, and auditory hallucinations involving communication with the supernatural powers.

The difference between these clinical subtypes probably has little significance. Whenever an individual feels singled out for persecution, it is easy for him to rationalize that he must be "special"; and from here it is only a small step to get on the road toward grandiosity. Conversely, any one who feels grandiose, "extra special," or chosen by God, may well conclude that lesser mortals will envy him; and start imagining that evil elements are ganging up on him to get even with him, or rob him of his treasure. Because of the ideas of reference and paranoid delusions, such patients are often constantly on the move.

A 66-year-old man had started to have progressively severe ideas of reference in his mid-40's. Most of his life had been taken up by a see-saw battle with tuberculosis. When the latter was finally brought under control, at age 55, the patient had a full-fledged mental breakdown which necessitated commitment to a psychiatric hospital. Two years later, he was discharged with a diagnosis of paranoid schizophrenia. He continued to have persecutory delusions, including the idea that other people gave him their colds, and that he would catch these any time he was in a draft. Thus, he would try to maintain a no-man's land around him. However, these efforts always failed, the draft would still come across, and so he felt compelled to move else where. Over a period of 8 years, he moved in and out of 14 boarding homes.

Late Life Schizophrenia

Some authors have described schizophrenia which develops for the first time in the senium as "*late life paraphrenia.*" The term paraphrenia dates back to the early nineteenth century, and has been used by authorities (Kraepelin, Freud, etc.) in different ways. In 1911, Freud formulated his views on the relationship between paranoia and homosexuality in his analysis of the Schreber case. He suggested the term paraphrenia because he felt that Schreber was suffering from paranoia as well as schizophrenia. Kay and Roth conclude that late paraphrenia must be regarded as the mode of manifestation of old age schizophrenia.[12] Its clinical symptomatology is characterized by many schizophrenic-like disorders of thought, mood, and volition; by relatively good preservation of formal intellect, personality, and memory; systematized delusions, with or without hallucinations, in a setting of clear consciousness; onset of illness in late middle age. These patients may survive for a long period of time; recovery is the exception and prolonged hospitalization is the rule. The patient is most often female, single or widowed, and has few close relatives. Most have been living alone for many years prior to hospitalization. Few have children, and those with children have only limited contact with them. Good physical health is common, except for frequent problems with hearing and vision. The presence of these sensory losses and long-standing social isolation, along with the premorbid personality traits (usually schizoid or paranoid) appear to be the major contributory etiological factors.[12–14]

Patients with late onset schizophrenia may have had premorbid personality disorders, but the latter apparently had not prevented them from coping with their environment before the onset of their active illness.

A 71-year-old widow, with no children and no close relatives, had been living alone for several years. Reportedly, she had an episode of acting peculiarly, 7 years ago, but since then she had succeeded in maintaining an independent adjustment. Recently, however, her neighbors reported that she acted strangely. A psychiatric referral revealed that she had the delusion that men from a nearby amusement park were "making marks on her window, and sleeping on her front porch"—and that "some people were burying dead children in her back yard." On one occasion, the patient apparently under the influence of her delusions, had torn out the flowers from her neighbors' planters. It must be emphasized that, even during the acute psychosis, she maintained a social facade, visiting all over town, well known and liked by many people. Of particular interest in the delusional thoughts are the themes of sex, birth, and death (the men are sleeping on her front porch—but she is a marked woman—the child is dead — and her revenge is to destroy what grows in her neighbor's planter).

Persecutory delusions include ideas of being drugged, thoughts being read, being influenced by rays, machines, or electricity, and so on. Auditory hallucinations occur in most cases, particularly at night (threatening, jeering commentaries, obscenities, loud bangs, etc.). The delusions and hallucinations frequently have a sexual slant or erotic coloring. The responsible parties are often jealous, hostile neighbors. These experiences are intermittent; behavior and thought content during intervening episodes can be relatively undisturbed. Once hospitalized, these patients do well, but as the years go by, their adjustment becomes more brittle.[13]

A 74-year-old widow, living alone and still taking care of herself and her home, had the delusion that a night watchman, hiding in her attic, was spying on her. To protect herself, she undressed and bathed in the dark (projecting her reluctance to see her own deteriorating body, onto an evil eye). The night watchman "kept her awake for almost 3 months trying to make her think he was a bird by tapping on the ceiling. One night he even threw a bucket of water on her." She changed locks on her house, but discovered he would enter by lifting a part of the roof. A few months later, however, she reported that the watchman was acting real nicely, and she talked to him all the time. At first, he had been an old man with only one thing on his mind, her money, but now he is a young boy interested in helping her, "and he knows I have a gun that will shoot 25 times." The delusion of the watchman is overdetermined; it represents the evil eye, that sees ugly things; it is the projection of the concretized concept of loss (he is after her money); and it is the externalization of her wish to have somebody watch over her.

The figurative watch "over" becomes a literal, spatial "above, in the attic." The delusion of the man upstairs fails to reassure her; neither the old spy-thief nor the young boy would be much of a protection, and so she has her magic gun ready.

A few comments regarding the external enemy, intruder, or foreign body in this type of delusions. In the early stages of the illness, the enemy is perceived as being well outside the patient's house, beyond the perimeter of personal space. Typically, they are hoodlum types on the street, in front of the house, acting obnoxiously or speaking vulgar language. During the next phase, the undesirable elements make their way across the property line, into the garden, or onto the front porch. The third stage is that of penetration into the house. This intrusion usually involves damage, e.g., to the plumbing or wiring in the basement. During the last stage, the protective symbolic equation (body = house) breaks down and now the enemy is felt to intrude into the patient's body space itself (tactile hallucinations). This last phase may also be described by the patient as "something coming through the wall toward me."

A 72-year-old woman, with a long history of schizoid behavior and recent evidence of organic brain syndrome, was placed in a home for the aged and developed hallucinations, agitation, and depression. She had the delusion that a machine in the room next door was pushing pictures through the wall, which would then appear on her television screen. Clinical management in this case included haloperidol 0.5 mg, three times daily; encouraging her to stay in the home and to get to know the residents; and to arrange for regular visits by relatives. When the patient returned for the first follow-up, she reported that the pictures were no longer on the television screen, but just on the wall itself, and she was undecided how they got there. Two weeks later, she reported the pictures were gone altogether and she disowned any memories about the recent delusional-hallucinatory experiences. Meanwhile, she was gaining weight, looked calmer, and spoke favorably about the home. In this case, the mental decompensation producing paranoid manifestations was precipitated by a "transplantation shock." What is further illustrated is that the degree of closeness of the intruding elements, and its proximity to the self, tend to correspond with the degree of psychopathological regression.

PARANOID DISORDERS

In paranoid disorders, a delusion, usually persecutory or grandiose, is the essential abnormality. Disturbances in mood and behavior are dependent on, and determined by, this delusion. This distinguishes paranoid states from the affective psychoses and schizophrenia, in which mood and thought disorders, respectively, are the central abnormalities.[1] The paranoid disorders include paranoia, shared paranoid disorder (folie à deux), and paranoid state. A precipitating factor is often apparent which may be any of the common age-related losses. The question comes up why some individuals respond to such ubiquitous losses by developing a paranoid state. The following factors may play a role.

Premorbid Personality

The *premorbid personality* may have counterphobic features, and an inclination to use defenses of the "high energy" variety (mastery through attack; projection) with subsequent attempts to move aggressively against the externalized threat. Another type of premorbid personality, also inclined to use projection, may be less aggressive, and thus prefer to move away from the external danger (a phobic pattern).

Relative Assets and Strength

Whether the patient will aggressively move against the external enemy, or flee in apprehension, depends on whether he unconsciously views himself as being potentially stronger, or inferior vis-à-vis the persecutor; and whether or not he feels backed into a corner and becomes a desperado who has nothing to lose by attacking.

Nature of the Loss

The *nature of the loss* is important, in the sense that the tendency to respond with projection and intense hostility or fear is greater, the more the loss pertains to an exquisitely sensitive area (in the case of men, masculine attributes, such as power, "manhood," or sexual potency; and in women, notions of feeling loveless or lifeless). Also, the *acuteness* and *rate of speed* with which the loss takes place play a role. The more sudden and acute, the more likely it is that ego strength will fail, and maladaptive defenses are employed.

> A 78-year-old widow had long been a chronic complainer, accusing the operators of the boarding homes where she had been, of being mean and mistreating her. Although she was married twice, she had no children. In both marriages she was dominant and decidedly in charge. Her first husband died when the patient was in her mid-40's. She met her second husband through a lonely hearts club and married him at age 51. Over the next 15 years, the couple moved 25 times. During this period of uprootedness, the patient became a determined hypochondriac. She would see various physicians for "indigestion and arthritis," but never used their prescriptions, and instead would buy patent medications according to her own judgment. In the course of time, her tendency to be dominating and demanding became more aggressive. After her second husband's death, 12 years previously, she moved into a boarding home, but

the earlier pattern of frequent moves persisted. Finally, having run out of places to stay, and having seemingly lost everyone's goodwill, she developed an acute delusion that the water in the home was poisoned and that her roommate was trying to kill her.

Delusions pertaining to water and food are common in paranoid states.

Another patient, an 81-year-old widow, developed a fairly extensive delusional system, to the effect that somebody was putting lime in her water. Her original concern had been about the (realistic) issue of fluoridation of the water. From here on, she developed the lime delusion. As a result, she sold her house, moved into a new one, only to discover that "this time they were sprinkling lime on the snow." To protect herself, she started to buy water, and stored it in jars. But even this provided no escape from the enemy: somebody began to put deliberately too much sugar in her food—and that, while she is a diabetic.

Delusions of jealousy, often conjugal paranoia, also are common. On the basis of no or irrelevant evidence, a patient will become convinced that his or her spouse is unfaithful.

Often there is social isolation, seclusiveness, or eccentric behavior. Suspiciousness, anger, vindictiveness, letter writing, complaining about various injustices, as well as the instigation of legal action, are often seen.

PARANOID REACTIONS IN ORGANIC BRAIN SYNDROME

Organic Delusional Syndrome

Paranoid phenomena frequently occur in the setting of *organic brain syndrome,* e.g., organic delusional syndrome. In most cases, they represent nonspecific manifestations of a severe mental disorder, in the context of which the emergence of prominent primitive defense mechanisms (e.g., massive projection) is no surprise. Typical for the paranoid phenomena secondary to cerebral decompensation is the lack of sophistication and systematization, as well as their variability: it is as if the patient improvises on the spot, changing his tune without regard for consistency. The paranoid delusions or hallucinations tend to clear up, as the patient's overall condition improves (compare Organic Delusional Syndrome).

A male patient in his 70's had the delusion that he was being poisoned because of uranium in his blood which was sinking down into the veins of his legs. In actuality, his legs were swollen because of thrombophlebitis and cardiac decompensation. He had been in renal failure and attempts had been made to treat his uremia. The patient had been aware that the element of urea was poisoning him. The idea of something toxic became the focal point of a delusional elaboration. Urea was transformed into uranium, an element that is both "heavy" and toxic; this served to explain his state of being poisoned and the heaviness in the legs. A few days later, the patient casually changed this delusion onto another one: that his heart was to be cut out.

Senile Dementia

These patients may show paranoid delusions (usually persecutory); quarrelsome, demanding behavior; and chronic complaints about being mistreated.

A 74-year-old widow would phone various community agencies, complaining that neighborhood boys kept her awake at night, and damaged her property. She feared the boys would burn her house if she made any complaints (concretization and projection of her own sense of feeling "burned up" about being victimized). A few weeks later, the delusions changed: she accused the pharmacy of giving her pills with the wrong color. Again a few weeks later, she became acutely apprehensive during the night and called the police for help. After this, she complained it had taken the police many hours to come, and they had searched her house for illegal liquor. The progressive deterioration is suggested by increasingly prominent oral concerns (being poisoned, illegal liquor) and feelings of utter helplessness: even the parental symbols (pharmacy and police) are corrupt. It is significant that once this patient was placed in a boarding home, the paranoid symptoms subsided.

Alcoholic Paranoid Disorders

These disorders develop in chronic alcoholics, usually male, and are manifested by extreme jealousy and frequent delusions of unfaithfulness on the part of the spouse.

A 60-year-old man, a chronic alcoholic, was committed to the mental hospital, because of violent threats to his wife. He accused her of having had many lovers throughout their married life, and stated that of the five children born of this marriage, only the oldest had been fathered by him. In reality, the patient himself has had numerous extramarital affairs. His wife had stayed with him, in spite of his abusive behavior, "to keep the family together." In fact, when the children had grown up and left, she began to help her husband in running their small business. Thus, the patient's paranoid accusations flew directly in the face of the evidence; the delusions of jealousy came about by projecting his own impulses and fantasies onto his wife.

In alcoholic paranoid reactions (as in many paranoid states), there is a serious risk of violent, destructive behavior, even to the point of homicide. Because of this, immediate intervention, usually involving hospitalization, is indicated.

References

1. Task Force on Nomenclature and Statistics of the American Psychiatric Association:

Diagnostic and Statistical Manual of Mental Disorders, ed. 2, (DSM-III), American Psychiatric Association, Washington, D. C., 1978.
2. Bleuler, E.: *Dementia Praecox, or the Group of Schizophrenias.* International Universities Press, New York, 1952.
3. Schneider, K.: Primaere und sekundaere Symptome bei Schizophrenie. *Fortschr. Neurol. Psychiatr. 25*:487, 1957.
4. Oppenheimer, H.: *Clinical Psychiatry: Issues and Challenges,* Harper & Row, New York, 1971. pp. 227–246.
5. Arieti, S.: Schizophrenia: symptomatology and mechanisms. In: *American Handbook of Psychiatry,* edited by S. Arieti, vol. 1, chap. 23, Basic Books, Inc., New York, 1959. pp. 475–484.
6. Goldstein, K.: Functional disturbances in brain damage. In: *American Handbook of Psychiatry,* edited by S. Arieti, vol. 1, chap. 39, Basic Books, Inc., New York, 1959. pp. 770–793.
7. Von Domarus, E.: The specific laws of logic in schizophrenia. In: *Language, and Thought in Schizophrenia,* edited by J. S. Kasanin, University of California Press, Berkley, 1944. pp. 104–113.
8. Ehrentheil, O. F.: Behavioral changes of aging chronic psychotics. In: *New Thoughts on Old Age,* edited by R. Kastenbaum, chap. 7, Springer Publishing Company, Inc., New York, 1964. pp. 99–115.
9. Muller, C.: The influence of age on schizophrenia. In: *Processes of Aging,* edited by R. H. Williams, C. Tibbits, and W. Donahue, chap. 23, Atherton Press, New York, 1962.
10. Riemer, M. D.: A study of the mental status of schizophrenics hospitalized for over 25 years into their senium. *Psychiatr. Q. 24*:309–313, 1950.
11. Bychowsky, G.: Schizophrenia in the period of involution. *Dis. Nerv. Syst. 13*:150–153, 1952.
12. Kay, D. W. K., and Roth, M.: Schizophrenias of old age. In: *Processes of Aging,* edited by R. H. Williams, C. Tibbits, and W. Donahue, chap. 20, Atherton Press, New York, 1963. pp. 402–448.
13. Roth, M.: The natural history of mental disorders in old age. *J. Ment. Sci. 101*:281–301, 1955.
14. Herbert, M. E., and Jacobson, S.: Late paraphrenia. *Am. J. Psychiatry 113*:461–469, 1967.

6

affective disorders

INTRODUCTION

A discussion of affective disorders in the elderly is a difficult challenge and complex task for several reasons. First of all, there remain many obstacles to the development of a coherent and valid psychobiological theory of depression. What has been generally agreed on is that the major affective disorders are heterogeneous with regard to their nature and etiology, that there is a subclass which is probably hereditary in nature, that disordered brain chemistry is involved in certain severe affective disorders, and that no one system of classification (e.g., primary-secondary, bipolar-unipolar) meets all of the requirements for research and clinical practice.[1] Second, if the above applies to affective disorders in general, it is even more true of those in late life. Salzman and Shader[2] state that depression in the elderly may resemble the familiar clinical syndrome seen in younger adults, but that the elderly, more than their younger counterparts, may mask their depression through a variety of mechanisms. Third, depressive disorder is the most common psychiatric illness in late life. Currently, there are more than 20 million individuals over the age of 65 in the United States; in this older age group 5% (about 1 million persons) is estimated to have a clinically recognizable depression.[3]

DIMENSIONS OF AFFECT

With regard to "emotion," there are three specific dimensions: *subjective* feelings which can be communicated through speech, *physiological* concomitants in the autonomous nervous system, and *motor* behavior involving the musculoskeletal apparatus. In affect states or disorders, all of these dimensions may be manifest, or one of them may be relatively more dominant. The physiological concomitants, for example are more prominent in patients with a depressive equivalent[4, 5] (a depression masked by physical symptoms). Emotional expression primarily by way of motor behavior can be seen in the action language (acting out) of certain behavior disorders.

SUBJECTIVE EXPERIENCE

The subjective experience of an affect can be assessed by the examiner only if the feelings are formulated and verbalized by the patient. Not infrequently, active inquiry into these feelings is indicated, because some individuals are not used to putting their feelings into words. One can then help the patient by presenting him with various mood statements (e.g., sad, blue, edgy, annoyed, let down, aggravated, etc.). When the patient recognizes and acknowledges the appropriate affect, this may be accompanied by noticeable physiological concomitants or motor expressive behavior.

> A 62-year-old minister's wife, hospitalized because of depression had always been concerned about making a good impression. In her many contacts with church members she had to set a good example, turning the other cheek when she was hurt or frustrated. This pattern of suppressing anger had become second nature, until she got caught in a tug of war between two factions in the congregation, and was being slapped on both cheeks. During the interview, she could describe her feelings only as "being upset"; but at the same time she made a fist with both hands, pressing them against each other. After her attention had been drawn to this, she could verbalize the sensation of pressure and counterpressure in her fists, and recognized in this gesture her feelings of deadlock and the state of impasse in her life.

BIOLOGICAL CONCOMITANTS

Some physiological concomitants of specific affects can be directly observed during the interview (e.g., tearfulness. sighing, holding one's breath); others are obtained from the anamnesis (e.g., loss of appetite, fatigue, insomnia). Certain patients communicate primarily by way of organ language. By carefully tuning in to such an organ recital, one can be alerted to clues about the patient's affect; e.g., a heavy sensation in the chest (depression), butterflies in the stomach (anxiety), a pain in the neck (suppressed anger), feeling choked up (acute grief). Somatization is a term that has been used to describe the relative prominence of the physiological concomitants vis-à-vis the subjective-experiential aspects of specific affects.

When the biological concomitants of depression are particularly prominent, and overshadow the subjective-experiential aspects, a *masked depression* or so called depressive equivalent may be the result. In fact, physical symptoms in general, as well as hypochondriasis, are able to mask an underlying depression.[4, 5] (See also Chapter 9.)

Depression involves a *slowing down,* and any or all organ systems and personality functions may be affected by it. There are frequent exceptions to this rule, however, because an individual may try to defend against a depression by way of increased activity of particular physiological functions. Thus, changes in metabolism and energy production can vary considerably. Although appetite is usually decreased, in some cases there may be an increase, even to the point of bulimia. Most depressed patients complain of insomnia, but some tend to become more sleepy, somnolent, or even lethargic. And, while psychomotor activity is usually slowed down, the reverse is true in agitated depressions. These apparent exceptions are not paradoxical phenomena, but probably serve the purpose of warding off the depression, or facilitating its remission. Repetitious movements, for example, as in agitated depression, may not only reflect and express anxiety (co-existing with the depression), but also may involve self-stimulation and tension accumulation which is preferable to the lifeless, empty quality of the inner world of the depressed patient.

Depressive slowing of central nervous system functions may produce a clinical picture resembling an organic mental disorder.[6] Such cases have been referred to as *pseudodementia.*[7]

Total *sleep* time is decreased in depression; the patient awakens more frequently, and there is a reduction of Stage 4 sleep.[8] By and large, the extent of the sleep disturbance is in keeping with the severity of the depression.[9]

BEHAVIORAL ASPECTS

In some instances, the affect is manifested primarily through its *motor* aspects and *behavioral* dimensions. Specific action language (e.g., gestures, psychomotor patterns) will suggest the presence of depression or anxiety. Thus, acting out, and even accident-proneness have been described as manifestations of a depressive equivalent.[10, 11]

The general posture may convey lack of vitality, as if the patient is burdened down by a heavy weight. In contrast, the manic patient seems to pit himself actively against the force of gravity. For the depressed patient, personal time drags, so that the world around is perceived as going too fast.

> A 64-year-old woman with a psychotic depression was "bothered by the fact that all the clocks on the hospital ward were running fast."

In manic states, personal time flies (everything around going proportionately slower), and spatially there is an exhilarating sense of soaring. While the depressed patient is oriented backwards toward the past, the manic patient is going forward in a "flight into health." The former is a captive of the past, the latter escapes into the future.

The various dimensions of depressive affect states have been investigated by Zung and incorporated in a rating scale (Self-rating Depression Scale).[12] The specific items in the depression scale refer to subjective experience, physiological concomitants, and psychomotor behavior (see Table 6.1). Another frequently used rating scale in depression is the Hamilton Rating Scale for Depression. This scale was designed to quantify systematically the results of a clinical interview with patients who already have been diagnosed as having a depressive disorder. Thus, the Hamilton Scale should not be used for the purpose of diagnosis, but only as a tool to determine the severity of depressive symptoms.[13, 14]

AGING AND AFFECTIVE DISORDERS

Some authors state that depressions are mitigated by the aging process.[15–17] This would be particularly true for *neurotic depressions* that developed in early life. Some questions that concern us here pertain to

Table 6.1
Criteria for the Diagnosis of Depressive Disorders and the Self-rating Scale Items Using Them*

Diagnosis of depressive disorders	Self-rating depression scale items
Pervasive affect	
A. Depressed, sad and blue	1. I feel down-hearted and blue.
B. Crying spells	2. I have crying spells, or feel like it.
Physiological disturbances	
A. Rhythmic disturbances	
1. Diurnal variation	3. Morning is when I feel the best.
2. Decreased sleep with early or frequent waking	4. I have trouble sleeping at night.
3. Decreased appetite	5. I eat as much as I used to.
4. Weight loss	6. I notice that I am losing weight.
5. Decreased libido	7. I still enjoy sex.
B. Other disturbances	
1. G. I.: constipation	8. I have trouble with constipation.
2. C. V.: tachycardia	9. My heart beats faster than usual.
3. M. S.: fatigue	10. I get tired for no reason.
Psychological disturbances	
A. Psychomotor activities	
1. Agitation	11. I find myself restless and can't keep still.
2. Retardation	12. I find it easy to do the things I used to.
B. Ideational	
1. Confusion	13. My mind is as clear as it used to be.
2. Emptiness	14. My life is pretty full.
3. Hopelessness	15. I feel hopeful about the future.
4. Indecisiveness	16. I find it easy to make decisions.
5. Irritability	17. I am more irritable than usual.
6. Dissatisfaction	18. I still enjoy the things I used to.
7. Personal devaluation	19. I feel that I am useful and needed.
8. Suicidal rumination	20. I feel that others would be better off if I were dead.

* Item numbers 3, 5, 7, 12, 13, 14, 15, 16, 18, and 19 are worded symptomatically negative.
W. W. K. Zung: Depression in the normal aged. *Psychosomatics 8*:287, 1967.

the lack of unambiguous, clear operational definition of depression in these studies, and secondly, whether the data were obtained through longitudinal follow-up of certain neurotics over a period of decades, or through cross-sectional studies of various age groups. Psychoneuroses may seem to improve in late life because the severe neuroses have disappeared due to death, or decompensation into more severe psychopathology. The dropping out of severe neuroses, in the course of time, would leave available the milder types, thus creating the false impression that the neurotic process per se is favorably affected by the passage of time. This is not to say that such favorable changes cannot occur. But the only satisfactory way to study the effect of aging on neuroses is by way of longitudinal follow-up of individuals with specific neuroses.

Other authors emphasize the high incidence of late life depressions.[18, 19] There appears to be a consensus that *reactive depressions* become more frequent in old age. Loss of physical health is probably a major factor in the development of such depressive feeling states.[12, 20, 21] A reactive depression, however, is more like a grief reaction than a neurotic depression. Since aged persons often have multiple illnesses and other types of losses, it is reasonable to expect an increasing incidence of reactive depressions, with advancing age.

The onset of *manic-depressive illness* usually is in middle age, although occasionally a first episode occurs after age 65.[22] As will be discussed later, the question is whether such late life manic disorders are an expression of manic-depressive illness, or a separate entity. Apparently, manic disorders in general become less frequent with advancing age.[19] Hereditary factors apparently play a role in depression and mania, and may well be the same for both disorders.[23] Although the genotype is fixed, the phenotype may change in the course of aging. Since mania is an illness involving the use of high-energy defenses (hyperactivity, extroversion), it may become increasingly difficult to "choose" mania as a mode of expressing affective disorder in late life.[24, 25] It has been reported that the chance of a patient with recurrent depressions becoming bipolar is only about 5 percent.[26]

Relevant in this context is the finding that monoamine oxidase (MAO) levels steadily increase, and that norepinephrine-levels decrease with aging. This *relation of age to enzyme activity* might reflect a predisposing factor to depression.[27, 28] According to some epidemiological studies, the incidence of affective disorders increases with age,[29] and this has been related to the fact that MAO levels also increase with age.[30] It appears that with advancing age, bipolar depressive illness occurs with increasing frequency, severity, and duration of episodes, and with increasing resistance to treatment. Reportedly, the prognosis for recovery of recurrent depressions becomes less good in old age.[31, 32]

The difference between *unipolar and bipolar* affective disorders is reflected by differences on the neurophysiological level.[33] Thus, the administration of L-dopa can differentiate between patients with unipolar versus bipolar depressions.[34] The administration of L-dopa causes the formation of more dopamine in the brain, and this is associated with an increase in anger in patients with unipolar depression, without improving the depressive affect. In patients with a history of manic-depressive illness, however, L-dopa can precipitate manic or hypomanic behavior.[34] According to Coppen, the administration of lithium to bipolar patients causes improvement in the affective disorder, in contrast to unipolar patients.[35] On the other hand, unipolar patients respond well to tricyclic antidepressants, while bipolar patients do not. Some bipolar patients tend to become hypomanic when taking tricyclics. Finally, bipolar patients show a significantly decreased level of MAO in blood platelets, in contrast to unipolar patients.[36] Such a deficiency could produce an increased amount of biogenic amines, which in turn serves as a predisposition for mania.[34]

At the present state of our knowledge, it would be premature to make final generalizations concerning the effects of age on affective disorders. It does appear that, in the course of time, affective disorders can change by following a plurality of pathways, and that the symptomatology may be expressed through a diversity of clinical manifestations.

PSYCHODYNAMIC ASPECTS AND CLINICAL MANIFESTATIONS

INVOLUTIONAL GRIEF

An involutional grief reaction may occur in early middle age as part of the midlife crisis. Among the factors responsible for it are failure to attain ideals, realization of one's transience, relinquishing illusions of perennial progress, and other disillusionments as well as biological or social stresses emerging around this time. More than likely, this grief reaction is the first in a series, which is not to say, of course, that the second half of life consists only of successive losses and grief.

Clayton studied the bereavement of widows and widowers who were followed for 1 year after the deaths of their spouses.[37] It was found that 35 percent of the sample (76 women and 33 men, with an average age of 61) had a depressive syndrome 1 month after their bereavement, and 17 percent had the same syndrome 1 year later. The question came up whether these prolonged depressive symptoms were due to the primary loss (i.e. bereavement), or to effects of a secondary loss (i.e., living alone). In this study, the data indicated that the bereavement itself rather than the effects of living alone influences the occurrence of depressive symptoms.

Frequently, of course, one loss leads almost inevitably to another one, and to a third one, etc. For example, loss of health may bring about forced retirement (loss of job), which in turn leads to loss of income. The depressive feelings do not amount to a depression unless the grief reaction derails, e.g., into a neurotic or psychotic depression. If losses occur in rapid succession, multiple grief reactions can be superimposed. When, during a period of grief, a second loss occurs, then a third, and so on, a situation develops in which the person has persistent depressive feelings. Yet, this persistence is not to be interpreted as "chronicity," but it reflects a succession of superimposed losses and episodes of grief. A grief reaction, however, can derail in several ways and, as a result, various types of affective disorder may develop.

NEUROTIC DEPRESSION

Definition

This entity is designated in the *Diagnostic and Statistical Manual of Mental Disorders* (DSM III) as depressive neurosis or dysthymic disorder. Neurotic depression is the most common psychiatric diagnosis, but nevertheless it has multiple meanings that are often used interchangeably in clinical practice. Klerman and co-workers[38] identified at least six different meanings of "neurotic depression." These include the ideas that neurotic depressions are less socially incapacitating, are nonpsychotic, do not present endogenous symptoms, usually follow a psychosocial stress, are due to long-standing maladaptive personality patterns, and are the result of unconscious conflicts. They state that the overlap between these different meanings is higher than chance alone, but not sufficiently high to allow complete interchangeability.

Theoretical Frameworks

This lack of precision was already mentioned in the introduction of this chapter. Undoubtedly, it is related to the multifaceted nature of depression which, in turn, is reflected by the existence of several *theoretical frameworks.* Some of these will be mentioned below; it appears that these psychological theories of depression are by no means mutually exclusive.

Chodoff[39] states that depression-prone individuals are unduly *dependent* on narcissistic supplies from other people to maintain their self-esteem. Their frustration tolerance is low, and they may employ various techniques, submissive, manipulative, coercive, piteous, demanding, or placating, to maintain their desperately needed relationships with external or internalized objects that provide these supplies.

In Beck's *cognitive* approach,[40] depressive patients are seen as possessing an enduring cognitive set consisting of negative attitudes regarding the self, the world, and the future. This causes the person to expect defeat, frustration, and deprivation and to regard himself as inadequate and unworthy. Such people are highly sensitive to situations that reinforce the negative attitudes.

Another cognitive theory is that of *learned helplessness*, proposed by Seligman.[41] He noted that if dogs are unable to prevent an aversive stimulus (e.g., an electric shock), they soon elicit behavior similar to that of human depressive individuals, including withdrawal, apathy, and reduction in goal-directed behavior. Once conditioned, this behavior is very resistant to change, even when opportunities to avoid the aversive stimulus become available. This observation led to the learned helplessness theory of depression. Several major symptoms of learned helplessness are parallel to those in depression: lowered initiation of voluntary responses, negative cognitive set, lowered aggression, loss of appetite, and physiological changes.

The *behavioral* approach emphasizes the deficient instrumental behaviors of the depressive individual. Lewinsohn[42] has shown that instrumental behaviors such as social skill are significantly less developed in depressive patients than in others. He postulates that a reduction in the rate of positive behavioral reinforcements is the cause of depression. Low self-esteem is a consequence of the lack of such reinforcements. The interaction of impaired instrumental behavior and a low rate of positive reinforcements tends to perpetuate low self-esteem and dysphoria. Thus, the depressive individual is less able to influence others to receive positive attention from them.

Hirschfeld and Klerman[43] state that the excessive dependency on others described in psychoanalytic theory, the negative attitudes and learned helplessness of cognitive theory, and the deficient instrumental behaviors described in behavior theory are consistent with the profile emerging from their study. That is, the depressive is introverted, lacking in self-confidence, unassertive, dependent, pessimistic, and perceives himself as inadequate.

Integrity versus Despair

In following an approach from the viewpoint of the developmental phases of the human life cycle, we are especially interested in the clinical manifestations of what Erikson has called *despair.*[44] When a person falls short of the ultimate developmental goal of integrity, a specific type of hopelessness, i.e., despair, comes about. Little is known about the psychodynamics of integrity and despair, as well as about the clinical manifestations of despair. It does appear that there is an existential side to all this which has to do with personal values. Integrity involves the acquisition and possession of clear values, while in despair there is a loss or absence of these. The predisposition to the loss of values may well be an antecedent state of *ambiguous values.* This existential notion might be related to the sociological concept of anomie[45] and the psychodynamic concept of ambivalence. Leighton[46] and Strole et al.[47] have linked the existence of anomie and a high prevalence of mental disorders, including suicide.

The Role of Ambivalence

The significance of ambivalence in terms of interfering with successful resolution of grief is well recognized. If the individual used to have ambivalent feelings about the lost object, the grief reaction gets in an impasse. If a person had mixed feelings about having something, he will also have mixed feelings about not having it. Thus, the working through of the loss tends to get into a deadlock.

If a person had mixed feelings about, say, his father, there will be a sense of unfinished business after the latter has died. Because of the positive feelings (love, admiration), the negative emotions (hostility, envy, fear) are repressed. But in their repressed state, they maintain an influence, leading to unconscious wishes that are vindictive in nature. Now, if the father should die after a long and painful illness, the following developments may occur. Inasmuch as the patient loved his father, he experiences a major loss resulting in a grief reaction. But to the extent that he hated or resented him, he may have a sense of satisfaction that the negative wishes were fulfilled. The affection and respect for his deceased father cause him to feel guilty that the hostile fantasies came true. By way of primitive magical thought processes, he now holds himself responsible for his father's death. (What is magic here is the notion that one's wishes or thoughts can cause something to happen. Since the hostile feelings are unconscious, they are out of reach for the corrective influences of rational thought).

The next sequel in the chain is the need for a punishment that fits the crime. At this point, two currents of feelings converge. Because of his affectionate feelings, the patient tries to hold onto the lost object by introjection or identification. By becoming like his father, he is better able to retain an image of him, and maintain a sense of closeness to him. But because of the other feelings (hostility and guilt), the identification is highly selective: the patient identifies with those features that are painful, i.e., his father's illness. By including these painful elements in his identification, he suffers the way his father did and atones for his hostility.

Such a *hostile identification,* however, is not a stable, satisfactory state of affairs: the grief reaction is not being resolved and the patient develops a neurotic depression, or is suffering from physical symptoms.

> A middle-aged woman was hospitalized for disabling attacks of "asthma" which were in fact due to hyperventilation episodes. She had been married to an alcoholic man who "had been running around with other women," while she had been a "good wife." One reason she suppressed her feelings of outrage and resentment was the fact that he had heart disease, with a lot of shortness of breath.

> One day, he asked her to go fishing with him, but she refused; a few hours later, she was informed that he had drowned. Presumably, he had an acute heart attack, fell in the water, and drowned. Soon after this, she began to have "asthma." The symptom choice was determined by the husband's cardiac dyspnea and his death by drowning. Through the mental mechanism of hostile identification with her dead husband, she developed an illness of her own, which represented a punishment for her resentment toward him and alleged negligence of him ("If I had gone fishing with him, I could have saved him.").

Through a process of abstraction and generalization, the ambivalence and unresolved feelings about a specific object (e.g., a father) may proceed to ambiguity and loss of values about general ideals (e.g., fatherhood).

PSYCHOTIC DEPRESSION

The Role of Over-reaction and Generalization

A person who has experienced a loss may over-react. Having experienced one loss, the individual feels more easily threatened and may develop a mental set involving the anticipation of multiple losses. The nature of the latter type of losses is that they are not factually real, but have psychic reality. And it is the latter that counts with regard to the development of emotional responses. In addition, there may be a process of generalization, from one particular loss, to losses in the realm of general categories and ideals. For example, the loss of a spouse may be the first step on a pathway leading to the conclusion that marriage in general is no good; loss of a child, to the conclusion that parenthood in general is not worth it; loss of a job, to the feeling that it does not pay to be a good worker. In this manner, disappointments and disillusionments may wreak havoc with personal ideals and cherished sets of value.

Predisposition

The predisposition for over-reacting is related to certain premorbid character features. First, there may be a tendency to function according to the all-or-none principle, and to think in terms of black-white, instead of shades of gray. Such a rigid framework leaves no place for flexibility, relativity, and nuances. The second feature refers to overvaluation of meaningful objects and personal ideals. Because the object is overvalued, its loss becomes a disaster. The patient is not responding to the actual value, but to something inflated by fantasy. These two tendencies combined (i.e., the idea of a disaster, plus the all-or-none principle) lead the patient to believe that everything must be bad all over. This is the intrapsychic counterpart of the domino theory: once the first domino stone falls, the rest will automatically follow.

There is also evidence that the premorbid character has compulsive features. Compulsive individuals tend to be rigid and reserved. They may be emotionally inhibited and sexually incapable of attaining true intimacy. The ambivalent feelings about one's feminine or masculine role come into sharper focus during the involutional years.

In this type of premorbid character, a loss produces a depression, which feeds on itself, and may progressively decompensate into a depressive psychosis. The more pervasive the sense of disillusionment, the more the future becomes constricted, with doubts about life being worth living. The more the lost ideals and objects were once a source of pride, the more the self-esteem will be lowered.

Role of Hostility

With regard to the *role of hostility* in the psychodynamics of a psychotic depression, there are two considerations. The first one pertains to the well-known mechanism of introjection, and turning the hostility against the self. Secondly, the more the lost object had been inflated in fantasy, the more there will be an angry protest. Knowing that his anger is not reasonable is of little comfort to the patient, and makes matters even more frustrating, the thought that he only has himself to blame. The destructive elements of his anger, having little in the way of a realistic outlet, now may flow through the channels opened up by the process of generalization. As a result, the hostility is not aimed at real objects but at their abstractions: ideals and values. This may have a lethal effect on the symbols of life and love. The scene of Armageddon overwhelms the patient with remorse and guilt; he feels doomed having committed the unpardonable sin. In this context, the delusion of unpardonable sin does not only reflect the patient's guilt about his destructiveness, but also the irrevocability of the damage.

Symptomatology

In the *symptomatology,* the disturbance of affect is the outstanding manifestation with disturbances of thought and behavior being secondary. The sensorium is clear, but depressive stupor may occur due to extreme introspective preoccupation. The affect is one of profound depression, guilt, worthlessness, or hopelessness, often with agitation and anxiety. When illusions or auditory hallucinations occur, their content is in keeping with the depressive affect. The voices may tell the patient, for example, that he will be punished for an unpardonable sin. Delusions are frequent and also consistent with the depressive affect. Psychomotor activity may show retardation or agitation in varying degrees. The physiological concomitants may be quite prominent. Some cases are characterized chiefly by depression, others by paranoid ideas. The difference between the depressed and paranoid subtypes can be quite subtle, indeed.

One middle-aged man with a psychotic depression had the delusion of having given syphilis to the entire world. Certainly, a delusion that might qualify for "unpardonable sin"—but the element of paranoid grandiosity is just beneath the surface: only a sexual superman could give syphilis to the whole world.

MANIC DISORDERS

Psychodynamic Aspects

A person may respond to a loss by denying its significance (i.e., rationalization); by denying the emotions associated with the loss (suppression); or by denying the actual fact of the loss (e.g., psychotic restitution fantasies). Psychotic restitution fantasies may occur not only in manic disorders, but also in schizophrenia and dementia.

Denial and suppression are often facilitated by hyperactive behavior, the pursuit of external diversions, and a general stimulus hunger. These patterns of behavior facilitate the pushing of painful thoughts to the back of one's mind. With advancing age, it will become progressively more difficult for the individual to "select" the manic cluster of defenses and it becomes increasingly likely that the affective disorder will be manifested in terms of an agitated depression or a depressive psychosis.

The actual onset of manic-depressive illness is precipitated by a combination of endogenous (hereditary, constitutional) factors and external, situational stresses. The following case example (dating back to the prelithium era) illustrates the interaction of multiple factors: family history, premorbid personality, ambivalence toward the lost object; cyclic mood swings with clock-work regularity for 13 years following acute onset in middle age.

> A 62-year-old woman had recurrent mood swings, since the age of 49, when her husband died. Her first depression began a few days after his death and she was already receiving electroconvulsive therapy (ECT) within a week after the funeral. During the following 13 years, she had her annual fall depression and spring elation. During the first 9 years the manic episodes were treated with ECT, while ECT was given during depressive episodes only if they were severe. The family history revealed that both parents and one brother had suffered from recurrent mood swings, while a sister was chronically depressed. The patient described her father as being "superman-ic." The patient's premorbid personality was characterized by passive-aggressive traits, an inability to assert herself and to express anger ("I never ask for anything"). Her marriage had been unhappy because her husband allegedly ran around. The patient stayed with him "only to raise my children—I kept everything to myself." During her husband's prolonged terminal illness, she had taken care of him because she used to be a nurse. When interviewed during a follow-up visit in early fall, she stated:"I am getting ready for my depression."

Clinical Manifestations

Manic-Depressive Illness. In *manic-depressive illness* (bipolar affective disorder), the essential features are alternating, marked mood swings, remission, and recurrence of episodes. The manic type demonstrates increased verbal and psychomotor behavior, and rapid flow of ideas. The patient may engage in unwise business activities or inappropriate extramarital romances. The depressed type manifests depression of mood; psychomotor retardation usually is prominent, but agitation may occur. The depressed phase of manic-depressive illness is differentiated from other depressions on the basis of the cyclic pattern of the depressive episodes. In some cases, the periodicity has a seasonal character, and the patient may report, for example, that "spring is my time to feel up and autumn is my time to feel down." When the recurrent episodes of affective disturbance tend to be similar, the patient (and family members) often learn how to recognize the onset of the disorder, at an early stage.

> In the case of a 58-year-old woman, with a clear history of manic-depressive illness, the earliest sign of a manic phase was an increased preoccupation with household chores. The patient would get up at 5 a. m. and start cleaning, washing, and cooking, which would go on until midnight. During the first manic episodes, the patient thought "this was just great" and she would glow with joy about her excessive work. Only later did she learn to recognize such keyed-up behavior as being part of an illness. She also had to learn to recognize the onset of depressive episodes. During the initial stages of her manic-depressive illness, she would ignore a depression until she was suicidal.

According to Stotsky,[48] manic-depressive disorders continue into old age; most are of the depressed type with psychomotor retardation, and have a tendency toward paranoid ideation, seclusiveness, and apathy. In some cases, "pseudosenility" tends to be prominent.

The *differential diagnosis* between a manic disorder and an *agitated depression* can be rather difficult. Patients with agitated depression may report that they feel unable to resist the surge of energy that compels them to be active, and also, that "going so fast" lifts their spirits and makes them feel good. Typically, there is a pattern of decreased sleep; the appetite may be up or down, but since the patient usually "does not have time to sit down and eat," weight loss is common.

Manic episodes may be due to *drug reactions* (steroids) or idiosyncratic drug responses (e.g., tranquilizers and sedatives). Also, it may be the first sign of an organic mental disorder.

Psychotic Manic Reaction (Manic Disorder, Single Episode). When a manic disorder appears for the first time in late life (and a careful scrutiny of the past history does not reveal previous episodes of affective disorder), the diagnosis manic-depressive illness would not be appropriate. In many of these patients, there is a constellation of social, environmental, and psychodynamic factors, which we would expect to cause a psychotic depressive reaction. Instead, we are confronted with mania. In such patients, the protective aspect of the manic defense cluster (denial, flight into health, shallow euphoria) is usually rather transparent. The manic element is represented by grandiosity on the ideational level rather than elation on the emotional level. In these cases of isolated mania, there is not a joyous grandiosity, but a solemn, austere grandeur. Furthermore, since these manic conditions appear to be reactive in nature, it would be proper to designate them as a psychotic manic reaction, as a counterpart of the psychotic depressive reaction.

> A 75-year-old man was hospitalized because "he expected the end of the world." He also had the delusion that his house was surrounded by enemies. During the alleged siege, however, the patient had suddenly felt that the "Lord was on my side—so I went outside—and stood in front of my house facing my enemies—I raised my cane—and the crowd opened up, so I could walk through." This man turned out to have a carcinoma of the lung, which had not been expected by anyone prior to, or right after, hospitalization. The manic delusion replaced a depressive-paranoid one (expecting the end of the world). The latter delusion may have been precipitated by the enemy within (cancer) which would end *his* world. The projection allowed the intrapsychic gain of externalizing and concretizing the internal (physical) threat. The next defensive procedure involved the creating of enough help to defeat the external enemy: the Lord Himself came to the patient's rescue. The resulting sense of invincibility and grandiosity was expressed by his identification with Moses, who also had been beleaguered, raised his cane, and opened a path through the sea, toward the promised land.

DEPRESSIVE WITHDRAWAL

A person who has experienced a painful loss may decide that he is not willing to expose himself again to such a risk. The full resolution of the grief reaction does not take place because the bereaved person is unwilling to invest his interests into a new object. The world around does contain potential substitute objects, but the feeling is: "I won't get hurt twice—once is enough." Such a person may resolve his grief up to a point, but what remains is an emotionally sensitive scar. The absence of a new object or activity brings about an impoverishment. As with most maladaptive patterns, the process does not stop here; it may further decompensate in the direction of hypochondriasis or a narcissistic self-absorption. The patient's remaining object relationships are endangered, because he may alienate people by being self-centered and neglecting his interpersonal contacts. Withdrawal, self-absorption, and hypochondriasis, having a positive feedback on each other, become a vicious circle, and lead to progressive impoverishment of the self.

PARANOID DECOMPENSATION

Paranoid versus Depressive Position

At almost any point during the decompensation of a grief reaction, paranoid elements may enter. This is usually due to a further weakening of the patient's position, or increasing regression. Paranoid features must be distinguished from the expression of anger which can be a sign of clinical improvement in depressive states. Such outward-directed anger is not the same as the hostility frequently associated with paranoid phenomena; the latter are chiefly characterized by the use of projection and the presence of ideas of references. Thus, the development of "anger-out" phenomena is a favorable sign, while paranoid changes indicate further decompensation. The depressive position essentially conveys: "I am bad, you are good." The *paranoid position* reverses this: "I am good, you are bad"; (while the schizoid view is: "I am bad, you are bad"). Developmentally, the paranoid position precedes the depressive position, which emerges at a developmental level of 4–6 months. There is a tendency to regress, in varying degrees, to the paranoid position when the working through of depressive anxieties is interfered with.

Hypochondriasis

Not only affective disorders may undergo a paranoid decompensation, but so can *hypochondriasis*. Initially, the hypochondriac still has "faith in the system." The withdrawal from others was not primarily on the basis of depreciating them. Rather, they are perceived as valuable, otherwise the patient would not keep on making contacts, in his search for aid. After some time, however, the hypochondriac usually becomes more and more disillusioned. He begins to feel mistreated, angry, and bitter.[49] Ideas of reference exist when the patient feels especially singled out for abuse or neglect. Further decompensation produces vindictiveness, active depreciation of others, with a proportionate elevation of himself.

Depressive Bitterness

In *depressive bitterness*, the individual feels embittered by the failure of providence to allot him "the good life." There is a sense that life in general can be good but that fortune has smiled on others, not on him. While others found their place in the sun, he feels like an outsider, left out in the cold. Considering his misfortune, it is almost impossible to remain resigned and not to feel envy toward the lucky ones who are counting their blessings. A paranoid shift may occur when the "have not" accuses "those who have."

Cynical Depressions

In *cynical depressions*, the concept of a providence disappears, and is replaced by that of fate, a power, which rules blindly according to the laws of necessity. In such a fatalistic ideology, there is no place for the good life or gifts of fortune, but only submission to the inevitable, with out understanding. The cynic may sustain a misanthropic consolation, that all those happy people are merely deceiving themselves, they don't know that life is a cruel joke. He may live his life in quiet desperation, comforted only by his secret that, in his nihilism, he knows more than his fellow humans. The secret is kept intact, through arrogance and distancing. The arrogance discourages trespassers who might question him on his ideology. The patient may also resort to other behaviors to keep others away: becoming dirty, living in filth, or developing his private system of thinking (delusions).

The misanthropic depressions and their paranoid features can be regarded as manifestations of a perspective of hopelessness, or specific dimensions of despair.

References

1. Katz, M. M., and Klerman, G. L.: Introduction: overview of the clinical studies program. *Am. J. Psychiatry 136*:49–51, 1979.
2. Salzman, C., and Shader, R. I.: Depression in the elderly. I. Relationship between depression, psychologic defense mechanisms and physical illness. *J. Am. Geriatr. Soc. 26*:253–260, 1978.
3. Williamson, J.: Depression. In: *Geriatric Medicine,* edited by W. F. Anderson and T. G. Judge, Academic Press, London, 1974. pp. 67–75.
4. Lesse, S.: Depressive equivalents and the multivariant masks of depression. In: *Masked Depression,* edited by S. Lesse, chap. 1, Jason Aronson, Inc., New York, 1974.
5. Goldfarb, A. I.: Masked depression in the elderly. In: *Masked Depression,* edited by S. Lesse, chap. 14, Jason Aronson, Inc., New York, 1974, pp. 236–249.
6. Cavenar, J. O., Maltbie, A. A., and Austin, L.: Depression simulating organic brain disease. *Am. J. Psychiatry 136*:521–523, 1979.
7. Wells, C. E.: Pseudodementia. *Am. J. Psychiatry 136*:895–900, 1979.
8. Zung, W. K., Wilson, W. P., and Dodson, W. E.: Effect of depressive disorders on sleep EEG responses. *Arch. Gen. Psychiatry 10*:439, 1964.
9. Snyder, F.: Sleep disturbance in relation to acute psychosis. In: *Sleep Physiology and Pathology,* edited by A. Kales, J. B. Lippincott Company, Philadelphia, 1969.
10. Spiegel, R.: Anger and acting out as depressive equivalents. In: *Masked Depression,* edited by S. Lesse, chap. 5, Jason Aronson, New York, 1974.
11. Tabachnick, N., and Farberow, N. L.: Accidents as depressive equivalents. In: *Masked Depression,* edited by S. Lesse, chap. 16, Jason Aronson, New York, 1974.
12. Zung, W. W. K.: Depression in the normal aged. *Psychosomatics 8*:287–292, 1967.
13. Hamilton, M.: A rating scale for depression. *J. Neurol. Neurosurg. Psychiatry 23*:56–62, 1960.
14. Hamilton, M.: Development of a rating scale for primary depressive illness. *Br. J. Soc. Clin. Psychol. 6*:278–296, 1967.
15. Silverman, C.: *The Epidemiology of Depression.* Johns Hopkins University Press, Baltimore, 1968.
16. Ernst, K.: *Die Prognose der Neurosen.* Springer, Berlin, 1959.
17. Meyer, J. E.: Psychoneuroses and neurotic reactions in old age. *J. Am. Geriatr. Soc. 22*: 254–257, 1974.
18. Batchelor, I. R. C.: Suicide in old age. In: *Clues to Suicide,* edited by E. S. Shneidman and N. L. Farberow, McGraw-Hill, New York, 1957. pp. 143–151.

19. Roth, M.: The natural history of mental disorders in old age. *J. Ment. Sci. 101*:281–301, 1955.
20. Nowlin, J. B.: Depression and health. In: *Normal Aging, II*, edited by E. Palmore, Duke University Press, Durham, N. C., 1974. pp. 168–172.
21. Verwoerdt, A., and Dovenmuehle, R. H.: Heart disease and depression. *Geriatrics 19*: 856–864, 1964.
22. Davis, J. M., Fann, W. E., El-Yousef, M. K., and Janowsky, D. S.: Clinical problems in treating the aged with psychotropic drugs. In: *Advances in Behavioral Biology*, edited by C. Eisdorfer and W. E. Fann, vol. 6, Plenum Press, New York, 1973. pp. 111–125.
23. Winokur, G., Cadoret, R., Dorzab, J., and Baker, M.: Depressive disease: a genetic study. *Arch. Gen. Psychiatry 24*:135–144, 1971.
24. Prange, A. J.: The use of antidepressant drugs in the elderly patient. In: *Advances in Behavioral Biology*, edited by C. Eisdorfer and W. E. Fann, vol. 6, Plenum Press, New York, 1973. pp. 225–237.
25. Court, J. H.: Manic-depressive psychosis: an alternate conceptual model. *Br. J. Psychiatry 114*:1523–1530, 1968.
26. Dunner, D. L., Fleiss, J. L., and Fieve, R. R.: The course of development of mania in patients with recurrent depression. *Am. J. Psychiatry 133*:905–908, 1976.
27. Coppen, A.: The biochemistry of affective disorders. *Br. J. Psychiatry 113*:1237–1264, 1967.
28. Robison, D. S., et al: Aging, monoamines, and monamine-oxidase levels. *Lancet 1*:290–291, 1972.
29. Rawnsley, K.: Epidemiology of affective disorders. Recent developments in affective disorders. *Br. J. Psychiatry*, Special Publication No. 2, pp. 27–36, 1968.
30. Nies, A., Robinson, D. S., Davis, J. M., and Ravaris, C. L.: Changes in monoamine oxidase with aging. In: *Advances in Behavioral Biology*, edited by C. Eisdorfer and W. E. Fann, vol. 6, Plenum Press, New York, 1973. pp. 41–54.
31. Perris, C.: A study of bipolar (manic depressive) and unipolar recurrent depressive psychoses. *Acta Psychiatr. Scand. 41* (suppl. 1974):7–189, 1966.
32. van der Velde, C. D.: Effectiveness of lithium carbonate in the treatment of manic-depressive illness. *Am. J. Psychiatry 127*:345–351, 1970.
33. Leonhard, K.: *Aufteilung der Endogenen Psychosen*, ed. 2, Akademie Verlag, Berlin, 1959.
34. Brodie, H. K.: Affective changes associated with L-DOPA therapy. In: *Advances in Behavioral Biology*, edited by C. Eisdorfer and W. E. Fann, vol. 6, Plenum Press, New York, 1973. pp. 97–104.
35. Coppen, A., Noguera, R., Bailey, J., Burns, B. H., Swani, M. S., Hare, E. H., Gardner, R., and Maggs, R.: Prophylactic lithium in affective disorders. *Lancet 2*:275, 1971.
36. Murphy, D. L., and Weiss, R.: Reduced monamine oxidase activity in blood platelets from bipolar depressed patients. *Am. J. Psychiatry 128*:1351, 1972.
37. Clayton, P. J.: The effect of living alone on bereavement symptoms. *Am. J. Psychiatry 132*:133–137, 1975.
38. Klerman, G. L., Endicott, J., Spitzer, R., and Hirschfeld, R. M. A.: Neurotic depressions: a systematic analysis of multiple criteria and meanings. *Am. J. Psychiatry 136*:57–61, 1979.
39. Chodoff, P.: The depressive personality: a critical review. *Int. J. Psychiatry Med. 27*: 196–217, 1972.
40. Beck, A. T.: *Depression: Causes and Treatment*. University of Pennsylvania Press, Philadelphia, 1972.
41. Seligman, M.: Depression and learned helplessness. In: *The Psychology of Depression: Contemporary Theory and Research*, edited by R. Friedman and M. Katz, John Wiley & Sons, New York, 1974.
42. Lewinsohn, P.: A behavioral approach to depression. In: *The Psychology of Depression: Contemporary Theory and Research*, edited by R. Friedman and M. Katz, John Wiley & Sons, New York, 1974.
43. Hirschfeld, R. M. A., and Klerman, G. L.: Personality attributes and affective disorders. *Am. J. Psychiatry 136*:67–70, 1979.
44. Erikson, E. H.: Identity and the life cycle. In: *Psychological Issues*, edited by G. S. Klein, vol. 1, International Universities Press, New York, 1959.

45. Durkheim, E.: *Suicide: A Study of Sociology.* The Free Press, New York, 1951.
46. Leighton, D. C.: The distribution of psychiatric symptoms in a small town. *Am. J. Psychiatry 112*:716, 1956.
47. Srole, L., Langner, T. S., Michael, S. J., Opler, M. K., and Rennie, J. A. C.: Mental health in the metropolis. In: *The Midtown Manhattan Study,* vol. 1, McGraw-Hill, New York, 1962.
48. Stotsky, B. A.: Psychoses in the elderly. In: *Advances in Behavioral Biology,* edited by C. Eisdorfer and W. E. Fann, vol. 6, Plenum Press, New York, 1973. pp. 193–202.
49. Lesse, S.: Hypochondriasis and psychosomatic disorders masking depression. In: *Masked Depression,* edited by S. Lesse, chap. 4, Jason Aronson, Inc., New York, 1974.

7

personality disorders

This group of disorders is characterized by deeply ingrained patterns of behavior that are different in quality from neurotic and psychotic manifestations. By and large, they are life-long patterns recognizable by the time of adolescence, or even earlier.[1] In contrast to the neuroses, internal discomfort and a sense of anxiety from within are lacking, and maladaptive interaction with the environment is prominent. While a neurotic conflict remains contained within the boundaries of the self, in personality disorders conflicts are often acted out or externalized. As a result, the individual himself is relieved of the tension while the environment now has to put up with it. The pathology is no longer in the person, but in the society, hence the term sociopath.

The problems that society has to put up with, in terms of its relationship with personality disorders, are of the following kind: 1) the consequences of acting out of specific impulses or fantasies, intrapsychically invested with much drive energy; 2) the consequences of poor impulse control, in general; 3) the consequences of social and vocational inadequacies, resulting in the need for all types of assistance, especially money.

The broad category of personality disorders comprises numerous types, including paranoid, introverted, schizotypal, compulsive, hysterical (histrionic), narcissistic, antisocial, borderline, avoidant, dependent, and passive-aggressive personality. From a psychodynamic point of view, the common denominator in these types is considered to be a deficiency in the ego. This ego deficiency may pertain to the ego's basic tasks of adequate impulse control (delay of immediate gratification) and defense against anxiety, or to one or more of the autonomous ego functions.

In addition to reviewing the clinical manifestations of various personality disorders in late life, the issue of the relationship between aging and personality disorders (and their mutual interaction) is of particular interest and relevance.

AGING AND PERSONALITY DISORDERS

With regard to the relationship between aging and personality disorders, the following questions can be raised.

1. How does the aging process influence the various life-long patterns of personality disorder (pathoplastic effects)? 2. What are the adaptational assets and liabilities of specific character disorders vis-à-vis the stress of the aging process? 3. Which types of behavioral disorder can arise, for the first time, in the context of senescence (pathogenetic effects)?

EFFECTS OF AGING ON PERSONALITY DISORDERS

No systematic, longitudinal studies exist which would provide information about the effects of the aging process on various personality disorders. Such a study might not be feasible anyway, in view of the lack of adequate operational definitions of what constitutes a personality disorder, and because of the innumerable variables impinging on the individual, in addition to the factor of aging.

Statistical data pertaining to first admissions to U. S. public mental hospitals show that the diagnosis of personality disorder occurs most frequently in the 25–44 age range (about one out of every three admissions), while the incidence of personality disorders in the two adjacent age groups (18–24 and 45–64) is only slightly less.[2] In contrast, the frequency in the 65+ age group drops below 5 percent, while the incidence of organic brain syndromes soars to 84 percent. A similar type of distribution is obtained for neurotic disorders. Statistical data on the incidence of neuroses and personality disorders obtained from community mental health clinics are along the same lines.[3] Thus, cross-sectional studies appear to indicate that the incidence of neuroses, as well as personality disorders, gradually increases in early life, reaching a peak during the 25–44 age range, and then tapering off during senescence and old age. But such cross-sectional studies do not tell us what happens to particular individuals, over a period of many years. The statistical finding that the incidence of personality disorders decreases after middle age does not justify the conclusion that such disorders therefore ameliorate with advancing age. Although such a favorable development is certainly possible, it is just as possible that the behavior patterns undergo unfavorable changes. For example, what had been diagnosed as a personality disorder, early in life, may decompensate in various ways: an alcoholic developing organic brain syndrome; a compulsive personality developing a depressive disorder; inadequate personalities, who often also have a poor educational background, may be more vulnerable to early onset of dementia; or, a schizoid type may become paranoid or schizophrenic.

> An 85-year-old man, never married, had lived alone in a remote area, ever since age 20. During his early teens, his father was killed by a sheriff who himself was also killed in the fight. The patient's mother then became mentally ill and was unable to care for the seven children. The patient, being the oldest child, reportedly took

care of his mentally ill mother and his six siblings for a few years. Then he moved away to live by himself. During all these years (from age 20 until 85), he lived in a one-room shack, keeping other people away, and refusing all offers of medical or financial assistance. Eventually, his physical condition necessitated placement in an extended care facility. Following this, he became acutely belligerent and paranoid. Once he discovered, however, that in the rest home he could have his own private room, his behavior calmed down. His life-long schizoid patterns were restored and remained intact, by locking himself in his room and refusing contacts with others.

Finally, it is possible that a certain number of personality disorders simply do not survive until old age: they become the victim of their deficiency in adaptation, and succumb due to accidents, or lack of proper self-protection. Thus, inasmuch as personality disorders are thought to originate in early life, a pattern of repeated failure and maladjustment increasingly takes its toll as the individual is confronted with the tasks of adulthood.

Personality types which the clinician may diagnose as a "disorder" are not necessarily considered abnormal from the "patient's" viewpoint. First, since the personality defect is built-in into the character structure, it is ego-syntonic, and not perceived by the individual himself as a handicap. Secondly, the existence of certain personality assets may be used to minimize, or compensate for, the character deficiency, or even to turn the handicap into an advantage. A "manipulator," who is lacking in the area of intimacy, trust, and affiliation, may succeed in building an empire for himself, and his character deficiency may never catch up with him. A dependent personality disorder may be lucky enough to find the protective niche essential to his happiness. The inadequate personality may find out that society will take care of him, by being on welfare, by taking refuge in the sick role, or even as a career prisoner.

A 73-year-old man, whose father used to be sheriff, succeeded going through life always being taken care of by one person or another. He lived off and on with various relatives; spent time in a few sanatoriums for alleged tuberculosis; married and lived off his wife's earnings; and after her death, made a suicidal gesture which assured him the protection of a mental hospital; and finally, moved into a boarding home living off a small "disability check."

Certain types of impulse disorders (including alcoholics or habitual "trouble-makers") tend to settle down after the midpoint in life: at some time between 35 and 45 years of age. The explanation for such phenomena is probably in terms of an interaction between intrapsychic shifts and social changes. These would include changes in the drives (their aim, source, object, and intensity), changes in the ego (belated mastery of skills, increased ability to deal with drives of lesser intensity), and superego changes (mellowing, or the discovery that society's standards are not so confining that personal satisfaction can be obtained only by way of rebellion). Social-interpersonal developments can contribute to the amelioration of behavior disorders. An alcoholic may come to the point where the satisfactions of the group experiences of Alcoholics Anonymous, or of religious conversion, are felt to be more rewarding than the euphoric oblivion from alcohol. And, an individual with a long history of breaking the law may find himself at a point where he can use his inside familiarity with delinquency as the very basis for efforts aimed at rehabilitating law-breakers. In such instances, intrapsychic shifts and social opportunities interact, and complement each other, to bring about the behavioral improvements and turn a loser into a winner.

> The past life of a 75-year-old man consisted primarily of a series of defeats and rejections. He never had a steady job and spent his money as fast as he would earn it. His only son was killed in the military service. His wife left him for another man, and he does not know the whereabouts of his two daughters. By the age of 70, he had no home, no family, no belongings. Arrangements were made by the social service department for placement in a boarding home. In the first home, he courted a woman employee, but after a while, lost out to another resident who was also in the competition. After this defeat, the boarding home operator gave him added responsibilities in the home to boost his morale, but the patient felt he was being used as a janitor. Next, he focused his attention on another woman, this time a resident in the home; and again he lost out to a competitor. Thus, he went from one boarding home to another, for a period of years. The pattern of defeats and rejections stopped when he was placed in a small rest home managed by a widow. She gave him special responsibilities, and made him feel worthwhile. Since there was no "other man in the house," and no competition, he felt progressively more secure. For the first time in as long as he could remember, he felt at home and a sense of belonging.

In studying the life histories of personality disorders, we frequently see a life-long pattern of deficient personality functioning, of which the individual himself was not aware. As a result, such a person has been "losing out" all along, but without clearly realizing this. The losses are not the kind we usually have in mind (loss of something of value), but they represent missed opportunities. The individual is missing out on any number and type of basic elements in the spectrum of human experience. Since what is being missed are opportunities, he tends not to know about such a loss, and may not feel like a loser. But when such a person arrives in old age, he has little to show for: at his station in life there is a paucity of external objects, a poverty of external support systems. At this point, awareness begins to grow that something is amiss. In keeping with the life-long pattern of not seeing the deficiency as related to the self, the patient now is aware only of the deficiencies around him: somebody else must be responsible, somebody else is not giving him enough. Thus, a variety of personality disorders may end up in late life as losers, have-nots, putting the blame for this on the environment.

The clinical symptomatology of such patients is characterized by hapless complaining and a persistent bitterness. The accusations are directed at whatever people happen to be around or various community agencies. These individuals are usually in their 60's or 70's, and show no evidence of organicity, schizophrenia, or recurrent depressions. Their past history reveals lack of significant achievement in areas such as education, marriage, parenthood, work, and social relationships; failure to learn from experience; increasing impoverishment of self and milieu; and the absence of recognizable depression.

ADAPTATIONAL ASSETS AND LIABILITIES

Regarding the adaptational assets and liabilities of personality disorders vis-à-vis the stress of aging, the following points may be considered.

Low Energy Coping Patterns

Personality disorders relying largely on *coping patterns requiring little energy* may be relatively better equipped to deal with the stresses of aging. These low energy patterns (described in Chapter 3 under the heading of Retreat and Conservation of Energy) would apply to passive dependent, schizoid, asthenic, and inadequate personalities. Such individuals may feel quite comfortable with the regressive modes of adaptation, frequently encountered in old age.

High Energy Defense Patterns

Persons using primarily *high-energy defense patterns* are likely to be more vulnerable. The paranoid personality tends to react with anger and aggression. The compulsive personality requires much time and energy for pursuing perfectionism or repeating rituals. In the case of many passive-aggressive personalities, an aggressive or overly independent facade covers underlying passivity and dependency.

Inadequate Impulse Control

Personalities in which the central deficiency is *inadequate impulse control* include the explosive personality and the hysterical personality, as well as alcoholism and sexual deviations. In these personality disorders, life may act as a therapist, inasmuch as the strength of the drives declines with age. However, this is still a far from simple proposition: active and aggressive impulses may well decrease in intensity, while passive needs are becoming more prominent. Thus, whether personality disorders involving poor impulse control will improve or deteriorate with age depends on the nature of the impulses. In personalities who are action-prone or tend to act out, age-related illness interferes with their habitual activity patterns; anxiety, depression, and regressive behavior may be the result, especially if action had been used to ward off intrapsychic tension.[4]

AGE-SPECIFIC BEHAVIOR DISORDERS

Age-specific behavior disorders are those that arise for the first time in old age, and may reflect the pathogenetic effect of aging. This category includes three types of psychopathological constellations: changes in the personal time perspective; regressive ego changes leading to (re-) activation of latent conflict and acting out; and behavior disturbances secondary to other age-related mental illness.

Time Perspective Alterations

As was mentioned in Chapter 2, there are specific alterations in the *time perspective*, with advancing age. Some individuals feel that time is running out and want to make the most of whatever time remains. Those who discover that they have missed out on this or that subjectively important experience may want to catch up. Depending on many factors (ego strength, appropriateness of belatedly attaining overdue goals, situational opportunities and constraints, etc.), such endeavors will succeed or fail. For example, an old person may always have had the wish to see the world. Sir Chichester, in his 60's, succeeded going around the world, alone in a sailboat, but the goal was reached after a lifetime of preparation. Likewise, a person well-to-do and well-off in his retirement, may appropriately decide to go around the world. On the other hand, there are proverbial situations of old men and women who, having missed out on true romance, now become libidinal desperadoes, willing to exchange their fortune for a mirage of romantic love.

Persons who have been "on good behavior" all of their lives may feel that now the time has come for a reward. This may reflect a process of genuine mellowing, but it can also be a caricature of it. The latter happens when the individual used to resent being on good behavior. His resentment may have betrayed itself through getting irritated at people who did indulge without qualms in those pleasures which our patient had renounced. In such cases, the old person will reach for his reward with a vengeance as though in finally doing what he wants, he is getting back at the authority that had kept him so long in line.

> A 71-year-old woman, married to a man 24 years her senior, had acquired notoriety of being "a conniver, demanding, and bitter." The patient, the oldest of seven siblings, had wanted to become a nurse but her father had not permitted it, "since this was not considered proper for young ladies during those days." The patient was bitterly disappointed and really never forgave her father for

this. When she married a man, who was old enough to be her father, there was no doubt as to who was in charge this time. Having taken revenge in this manner, life dealt her a cruel blow when her only two children died at a young age. "They are buried in the cemetery across from my home, and I can see them from my window." During the last 10 years or so, her behavior has become more dominating. She calls her doctor, caseworker, or family members for the slightest reasons, no matter what time of the night. She also periodically puts the money allocated for attendant care for her husband in her own pocket.

Ego Changes

Ego changes in old age may affect psychological conflicts which, throughout life, had remained relatively dormant or latent. Due to age-related stresses, the ego may function ineffectively and ego strengths may decompensate. The altered time perspective may be associated with a decline in the ability to delay gratification. Due to weakening of repression or reaction formation, impulses that used to be kept in check are now coming to the fore, and find expression in specific behavior patterns. The latter tend to be the opposite of what used to be the life-long dominant ego style. In the case of acting out, we deal with a specific wish, or a cluster of wishful fantasies, which used to be repressed. When the ego's capacity to maintain repression is diminished, these wishes can gain access to the motor apparatus, and be acted upon. Related to this, and often an essential part, is the reactivation of a childhood neurosis.

A 67-year-old man was hospitalized because of combative behavior, especially toward his oldest son whom he accused of plotting to take away his 500-acre farm. The patient had taken his son into several business endeavors, the last one (ironically) a funeral parlor. In addition, the patient had grandiose delusions and a euphoric affect. He stated that he "did not feel like 67, but like 17 years old—and when I was young, I had sex four times per night." (The patient's wife had expressed her irritation at his aggressively romantic demands.) He also was preoccupied with fantasies about meeting a queen, and reported that, in fact, he had met a queen on several occasions. In the absence of a past history of affective or schizophrenic disorder, the diagnosis psychotic manic disorder was made. Of special relevance, in this context, is the role played by the reactivation and acting out of a neurotic conflict dating back to childhood. At the age of 5, he wanted to be a millionaire and had been preoccupied with fairy tales in which a poor boy marries a princess; as a millionaire he would be able to marry the queen herself. This oedipal fantasy (marrying the mother if he could be as powerful as the father) remained with the patient throughout his life. It became a near-reality in as much as he became a near-millionaire. Then, during senescence, came the painful realization that he no longer was powerful. Now, it was his son who possessed power. The patient then developed envy and jealousy toward his son, much like the mixture of envy, awe, and hostility he once had felt toward his father. This psychodynamic constellation we may call a reversed oedipal complex. The patient's manic and paranoid behavior represented a defense against depression and a sense of helplessness; regressive forces resulted in a reactivation of an early childhood oedipal conflict. As soon as the patient began to improve, the regressive forces lost their power and the childhood conflict was once more repressed. Concomitantly, he disowned any accusations toward his son. The idea of a son rising up against his father disappeared along with other derivatives of the childhood neurosis: he disclaimed any acquaintance with queens. Significantly, as clinical improvement set in, the more severe psychopathology (paranoid) disappeared first, while it took longer for the less serious psychopathological elements (mania) to clear up.

Behavioral Disturbances Secondary to Senescent Psychopathology

In these cases, the behavior disorder emerges, not as a carry over from the past, but as the result of specific psychopathology that develops in late life (organic brain syndrome, affective disorders, paranoid states).[5] Of course, in many cases, late life psychopathology will have the effect of only bringing into sharper profile behavioral traits that had existed throughout life without being unduly troublesome.

An 87-year-old woman who was known to have always had a "mean and ugly" disposition, gradually developed increasingly severe temper tantrums. During these outbursts, she would hit and flail at people, and spit on them.

Organic Brain Syndrome. In *organic brain syndrome*, behavioral disturbances are the consequence of profound regression, unlearning of previously acquired skills, loss of impulse control, impaired judgment, etc. Examples include regressive sexual behavior (e.g., pedophilia), combativeness, loss of social decorum, incontinence, tendency to hoarding, deterioration of personal hygiene and personal milieu, and excessive wandering.

The main problem in the case of a 78-year-old woman with early signs of dementia was her constant moving around. Over the last several years, she had moved more than 30 times, in four southern states. The patient was born on a deep South plantation. "I lived in a big house with many servants, and had everything I wanted." In contrast to this fairy tale childhood, her adult years were marred by tragedy. Her two marriages ended in failure. Her only child, a boy, died at age 11. When asked about this, the patient responded: "I don't know—I can't think about that, it is too sad—I tried to forget—I have forgotten" (illustrating the role of "forgetting" and "loss of memory" in depressive reminiscing). In old age, she ended up lonely and penniless. Her constant moving around represented a search for the utopia she once had known in childhood.

Manic Disorders. In contrast to mania in younger age groups, hyperactivity is less prominent. What may be striking, however, are behavior patterns reflecting an underlying sense of grandiosity or invulnerability (for example, expansive business transactions, inappropriate romantic pursuits).

Depressive Disorders. These disorders may cause behavioral disturbances, such as self-destructive activities. In cases of extreme depression where the element of hopelessness enters, the ultimate act of despair is to take one's loved ones along in death (homicide-suicide).

Paranoid Disorders. These are frequently associated with outward aggression; tendencies toward malice, ill-will, vicious gossip, and litigation. There is a risk of combative, and occasionally even homicidal, behavior.

CLINICAL TYPES

Schizoid

The *schizoid* personality (schizotypal, introverted) avoids close involvement with others and has difficulty in being normally assertive; he is seclusive and sometimes eccentric.

Paranoid

The *paranoid* individual has certain schizoid traits and a tendency to use projection which results in suspiciousness. Emotional stress, including age-related losses, may increase the tendencies toward withdrawal and projection, resulting in overt symptomatology.

A 63-year-old unmarried woman was hospitalized because of hallucinations, delusions, and "arguments with her family about a piece of land." The patient had always been a shy, reticent person, who preferred staying close to home. Her father had died when she was 2 years old. The mother remarried and, when the patient was 16 years, she and her stepfather began to have sexual relations. This continued until, at age 30, she became pregnant by her stepfather and gave birth to a daughter. The family knew all about it and "forgave" her. In fact, the patient lived without interruption with her mother continuously, until the latter died. This happened a few years prior to admission, and forced the patient to live on her own and support herself for the first time in her life. Meanwhile, disagreement was building up about a sizeable piece of land which the stepfather had left to the patient, who in turn had given it to her illegitimate daughter. The combined stresses of life-long social isolation, constant bickering about her status and estate, and being forced into independence, exceeded her coping ability. The dynamics and symptomatology of her mental illness included. 1) *Regression and withdrawal*: she stayed in her home, refusing to go out; increasing preoccupation with her self, and a regressive drift into the past, led to reactivation of feelings about her stepfather, especially guilt. 2) *Projection*: the guilt about her stepfather, and the suspicion that her family would take her land, were projected in the form of a single delusion ("People are following me") which lacked any elaboration or systematization. 3) *Perceptualization of the concept*: There had been visual and auditory hallucinations in keeping with the delusion of being followed: she "saw" and "heard" the people following her around. 4) The psychological test data showed a surprisingly low intelligence (70). It was obvious that her intellectual potential was not that low: the lowered I.Q. and the feature of *concreteness* in the test findings were interpreted as a consequence of the regressive drift and autistic withdrawal. When proper environmental support was given to this patient, her symptoms quickly disappeared.

In the loneliness of old age, an individual with mild schizoid tendencies may well feel relatively comfortable. Such persons have traveled lightly through life, with a minimum of belongings. They had not much to begin with, and have not much to lose in the end.

On the other hand, a severely schizoid person may become a recluse living in marginal circumstances. Some old persons, often female, are hospitalized because of paranoid delusions. Typically, such a woman is unmarried, childless, has long been living alone, and has few social contacts. Age-related physical problems add the element of helplessness to the isolation. The resulting anxiety is dealt with by way of projection: the internal threat is externalized and becomes an "enemy out there." This enemy is given attributes which the patient always considered particularly threatening or alien. In unmarried, isolated women, these often pertain to sexual-erotic notions; thus, the troublemakers have sexual schemes. But this autistic fantasy is usually not expressed in a direct fashion. By way of (primary process) symbolization, another distortion is added: the patient's body is symbolically represented as a house, and the evil designs of the trouble-makers as a foreign body coming inside. The sexual aspect is illustrated by the frequent delusion that the foreign man intrudes in the basement and messes up the plumbing or electric wires. When such paranoid delusions are chronically persistent, in the absence of organic brain damage, the diagnosis of late life schizophrenia would be appropriate.

In some cases, the patient's isolation is seemingly not as absolute or severe: there is another person around who shares the patient's house, or life, and sometimes the delusions as well. This is the condition of *folie à deux*, a paranoid illness involving two individuals. However, since their relationship is typically a primitive symbiosis, the two persons function as one unit; and, as a unit, they are just as isolated (perhaps more so even) as the above described cases.

Schizoid and avoidant personalities may view illness as a secure bridge leading toward another human being. They may wish to hang onto their illness, or their sick role, because the contacts with nurses and physicians provide them with closeness which, however, does not necessarily involve true intimacy. In the course of an illness, they may develop an attachment to the hospital or clinic in general, rather than to specific members of the staff.

Hysterical

The *histrionic (hysterical) personality* is excitable, dramatic, and attention-seeking. These individuals are immature, vain, egocentric, and tend to erotize relationships, but their emotions are shallow. Underlying this changeable surface behavior, there are often strong dependency needs. In the language of psychoanalysis: oral dependency needs are being gratified by genital-sexual means; the sexuality of the hysterical personality is in the service of pregenital oral needs. What suffers, due to age-related decline in energy and attractiveness, is the individual's ability to effectively use dramatization, seductiveness, and over-reactivity. The aging process may predispose them to depressive disorders, hypochondriasis, and hysterical exaggeration of physical illness. Prior to the onset of a depression, there may be periods of heightened sexual inclinations and romantic activities, or attempts to deny the existence or significance of involutional processes. On the other hand, it is possible that age-related improvement occurs in terms of decreased excitability and dramatization provided such behavioral changes are felt to be ego-syntonic, and are reinforced by the environment.

The aging process, especially the involution of the genital apparatus, may have a profound effect on the adjustment of such persons. It becomes more difficult or inappropriate to employ the instrument of genital sex for pregenital aims (e.g., dependency wishes). Hence, such persons are predisposed to involutional depressions and hypochondriasis, as well as factitious disorders. Ideally, such individuals would learn (through life's experiences, or through psychotherapy) that closeness, intimacy, or dependency can be achieved in many different ways, not just through the experience of genital sexuality.

Narcissistic

Narcissistic personalities operate on the premise that they are exceptional. Life's inevitable losses deflate their undue self-esteem and make it progressively more difficult to maintain belief in one's special status. When their sense of invulnerability is punctured by the discovery of the "Achilles heel," such persons react with depression (due to unresolved involutional grief), hypochondriasis, or more severe psychopathology (manic-like conditions, paranoid decompensation).

Dependent

The *dependent* personality may not fare too badly, in the course of life. If the dependency features are out in the open, the issue is at least unambiguous. Some people, for whatever reasons of their own, may feel attracted to a passive, dependent person; a strong marital partner may provide the needed gratifications. And if the latter should die, various substitutes may be available (children, the security of a home or hospital, etc.). A dependent individual may welcome illness as a means of permitting him to gratify his dependency needs. When bolstered by a supportive environment, dependent, inadequate, and immature personalities may maintain themselves for a long time. They may feel quite contented about retirement (often an early or forced retirement), because they do not have to cope with the demands of work any more. Likewise, illness may provide a welcome escape from adult role responsibilities. Many such persons depend for their happiness on the support from social service and other agencies.

Inadequate

The behavior pattern of *inadequate personalities* is characterized by the lack of efficiency and efficacy. Even though the individual is not physically inadequate, nor mentally retarded, his overall adaptation is deficient, as manifested by lack of physical and emotional stamina; by socioeconomic instability, and a paucity of object relations.

Passive-Aggressive

The mental mechanisms of reaction formation and/or overcompensation may produce, in a basically dependent person, a facade which is precisely the opposite: undue self-reliance and aggressiveness. The *passive-aggressive personality* is characterized by passive as well as aggressive behavior. The aggressive feelings, thoughts, or tendencies are expressed by passive means: oppositional behavior (obstructionism, stubbornness); being out of step with the environment (procrastination, intentional "faux pas," deliberate misunderstandings); and a tendency toward brooding and cherishing of old hurts. The element of passivity does not only apply to the method of expressing aggressive impulses, but also pertains to underlying passive-dependent wishes. Thus, the surface behavior may be the opposite of deeper, hidden tendencies.

The repertoire of dependency wishes does not only center on the functions of the upper gastrointestinal tract (lips, mouth, stomach), but also includes submissive wishes (to be held and to follow), passive wishes (e.g., stimulation by touch and warmth), and narcissistic wishes (to be in the center of attention).

Conflicts may develop because the aggressiveness and independence are not genuine, and therefore difficult to maintain. In addition, the underlying dependency needs are not being met. An individual who covers his dependency needs with a facade of self-reliance is pseudoindependent. But the facade of strength has the effect of attracting others who are passive or dependent. The day of reckoning comes when there is no longer enough energy to maintain the independent facade. The patient will fight the loss of face, first by way of an increase in the very aggressiveness or appearance of self-reliance, then often suddenly giving way to helpless dependency and depression.

> An intelligent and attractive woman, in her mid-50's, had tried to commit suicide several times, over a period of 5 years. She was married to a professional man of some prominence and had two grown daughters. Throughout the years she had worked in public relations jobs. During the interview she appeared outgoing and quickly took control. She claimed she was "the dominant type," while her husband was "passive." Her first depression (age 20) occurred right after her father's death. He had been a strict, strong man who had kept her on the straight, narrow path. After his death, she searched for similar men who were strong and dominant. When she met her husband-to-be, she was "impressed by his silence." After having been married to him for some years, she discovered that the silent type is not always the strong type. The depressions recurred, each episode being more severe. This patient's aggressive, dominating exterior covered a core of intense wishes for dependency, passivity, and submissiveness. The choice of marital partner was made on the basis of a mutual misunderstanding: she mistook his silence for strength; he felt attracted to her aggressive, extrovert facade. In this neurotic mismatch, the patient's real needs were not being met; and, feeling hopelessly trapped in the marriage, she became suicidal.

Emotionally Distant

Individuals whose premorbid personalities showed prominent reaction formations may react to physical illness in a surprising way. The *emotionally distant* personality, whose coldness is the result of reaction-formation against tender feelings, may use the illness situation for the expression of emotional warmth and experience of intimacy. Thus, physical illness may come to be the currency that permits the exchange of emotional warmth between persons who otherwise have a distant relationship. The same constellation may develop in the case of *avoidant* personalities who have deep-seated fears of rejection. Physical illness may be used in a similar way by patients who are *overly self-reliant.* They may publicly protest but secretly enjoy being sick, because the illness "forces" them temporarily into a position of dependency and receptivity.

Compulsive

The *compulsive* personality is characterized by undue concern with conformity and adherence to standards of conscience. They are rigid, inhibited, and unable to relax. Those who were able to make a virtue out of necessity and use their compulsiveness adaptively may, in old age, draw the benefits from this orderliness and regularity. But, if the emphasis was on rigidity and inhibition, the losses in old age may precipitate a depressive disorder. This personality disorder is considered to have more than average susceptibility to involutional depressions and a greater tendency to react maladaptively to the stress of intellectual decline in later years.[6]

In the area of work, the *perfectionist* pays more attention to the detail than the overall pattern. He works in order to do things right, at the right time, in the right place; it is more important how he does it, than what he does. When, however, the details can no longer be attended to, he feels at a loss and his productivity comes to a halt. In senescence, the decline in the energy required to live up to high standards, may result in feelings of helplessness, and shame. Thus, physical illness may bring about anxiety and depression in these personalities. On the other hand, sometimes physical illness is the lesser of two evils. For example, an ambitious, hard-striving, middle-aged man, who discovers that he has fallen short of the goals set by his ego-ideal, may find in illness an alibi that covers his shortcomings, be they real or imagined.

References

1. Task Force on Nonmenclature and Statistics of the American Psychiatric Association: Diagnostic and Statistical Manual of Mental Disorders, ed. 3 (DSM-III), American Psychiatric Association, Washington, D. C., 1979.
2. U. S. Department of Health, Biometry Branch, Washington, D. C., No. 7, 1971.
3. U. S. Department of Health, Biometry Branch, Washington, D. C., No. 59, 1970.
4. Spiegel, R.: Anger and acting out as depressive equivalents, In *Masked Depression*, edited by Stanley Lesse, chap. 5, Jason Aronson, Inc., New York, 1974.
5. Gianturco, D. T., Breslin, M. S., Heyman, A., Gentry, W. D., Jenkins, C. D., and Kaplan, B.: Personality patterns and life stress in ischemic cerebrovascular disease: I. Psychiatric Findings, *Stroke* 5:453–460, 1974.
6. Wolk, R. L., Rustin, S. L., and Scotti, J.: The geriatric delinquent, *J. Am. Geriatr. Soc.* *11*:653–659, 1963.

8

psychological responses to physical illness*

The psychological responses to physical illness include coping and defense mechanisms, as well as emotional reactions subjectively experienced as "feelings." The type and intensity of these somatopsychic reactions, adaptive or maladaptive, depend on the interaction of a great many factors, which can be grouped into three categories: (*a*) stresses pertinent to the physical illness per se, (*b*) characteristics of the "host," and (*c*) situational factors. Processes of interaction among the foregoing factors may be considered as yet another category.

CHARACTERISTICS OF THE SPECIFIC PHYSICAL ILLNESS

SEVERITY OF THE ILLNESS

This factor includes considerations regarding the magnitude of the actual physiological disorder, the severity of subjective symptoms, the degree of anticipated disability, and the extent to which the illness is life-threatening.[1, 2]

TIME FACTORS

Severity of the illness at a given moment is not a reliable basis for accurate prediction of the psychological response. One must also take into account the *duration* of the illness and its *rate of progression* in the course of time. A study of cardiac patients,[3] for example, showed that the severity of the depressive response varied inversely with the length of the illness. Both in mild and in severe cardiac disease severe depressive symptoms were apt to occur early in the course of the illness. These symptoms tended to disappear in patients with mild cardiac disease after 3 years. Severe cardiac illness, on the other hand, was associated with severe depressive symptoms throughout its course. Thus, it appears that in its early phases any cardiac illness is interpreted by the patient as something very serious, and the initial psychological response tends to be in the nature of a "shock reaction," based on the patient's feeling that an

* Portions of this chapter, which originally appeared as "Psychological Responses to the Stress of Physical Illness" in *Adv. Psychosom. Med. 8:* 119–141, are reprinted by permission of S. Karger Ag Basel.

organ of vital importance has been damaged. Only after some time (in this particular study, 3 years) does the patient begin to recognize that the illness has different degrees of severity.[4]

Another time factor is the *rate of progression* of the pathological process. Slowly developing conditions allow more time for adaptation, both on the organic and psychological level. A rapidly progressing illness, on the other hand, may have an overwhelming psychic as well as somatic effect. For example, patients with fast-growing malignancies show more evidence of anxiety than patients with slow-growing malignancies.[5] One specific measure in which the time factor is used retrospectively is *distance to death.* This is the interval between the point in time at which the investigator observes certain phenomena about the patient and the time at which death occurs. This longitudinal approach was used in an investigation of 30 patients thought to have a fatal illness.[6] They were studied with regard to feelings of hopelessness, changes in time sense, and other variables. A follow-up study 1 year later revealed that 22 patients had expired, the median distance to death being 2 months. Patients who had died within 2 months had manifested more evidence of hopelessness and had been less future-oriented than those who had died from 2–9 months after the time of testing.

ORGAN SYSTEM INVOLVED

Some organ systems (e.g., cardiopulmonary) are essential to biological functions; others (e.g., musculoskeletal) are vitally less important. Systemic diseases have widespread repercussions throughout the entire organism; in other conditions, the effects remain more or less localized. Some illnesses (e.g., skin disease) affect body parts accessible to the patient's sight; others, such as intestinal malignancies, are hidden. Nevertheless, it is reasonable to assume that disease in any organ system produces specific "signals" which originate at the site of the disturbance and are transmitted along somatic or visceral afferent pathways to the central nervous system, where they are registered as messages about the state of the "interior."

> A woman who suffered from periodic diarrhea due to diverticulitis of the colon would dream about "falling in a mudhole," 1 or 2 days before the onset of each episode.

In some patients with a disease that has widespread, systemic repercussions such as carcinoma of the pancreas, a careful history reveals that the very first symptoms consisted of a vague, ill-defined depression. Thus, it would be wise to suspect early systemic disease when one encounters a patient complaining of nonspecific depression, especially if there have been no depressive episodes in the past.[7]

The apperceptive capacity of the central nervous system can be defined as its capacity to evaluate the significance of afferent stimuli by comparing them with past experience. Because apperception is often impaired in organic brain damage, it is important to distinguish between illnesses involving *cerebral* impairment and those involving *extracerebral* pathology. In the former, the "organ of adaptation" itself is affected, so that the final psychological response reflects the specific distortion caused by the mental impairment.

> A man in his 50's who had chronic brain disease was constantly preoccupied with that time in his life when he was an airplane pilot. He actually would appear to relive the experiences of that era. This preoccupation and reliving represented a primitive attempt to deny the impact of the present illness. The mental mechanisms of denial and negation require a certain amount of abstract capacity, and having lost this capacity, the patient substituted a reliving of the past.

CHARACTERISTICS OF THE "HOST"

Among the personality-related variables contributing to the final psychological response are constitutional endowment, including intelligence and other "ego apparatuses," as well as preferred response patterns,[8] experiential factors and interpersonal relationships, educational level, and vocational achievements. All of these interact in the process of personality development and maturation, as well as in the response to illness.

A person free from major intrapsychic conflict will possess flexibility, resilience, and an adequate repertoire of effective coping strategies. Individuals with intrapsychic conflict, on the other hand, must expend valuable energy in dealing with the internal, neurotic pressures; the range and efficacy of their coping mechanisms tend to be reduced.[9] As long as they do not encounter stresses too great for the narrow range of their homeostatic capacity, they may present an appearance of well-being and psychological equilibrium. Even minor stresses, however, can throw this tenuous balance out of kilter. The psychic economy of such individuals does not have the reserve capacity to absorb and buffer the impact of stressful events.

The capacity to adapt is also greatly influenced by congenital defects or acquired disabilities. Patients with mental retardation, for example, may respond to illness-related stresses in a primitive fashion (by projection or primitive motor patterns) or, they may decompensate, becoming agitated and confused.

AGE AND SEX

The role of age is illustrated by the observation that, at age 7, the loss of a tooth signifies growth and is a source of pride, while at 70 it signifies decline and is a cause of grief. Various mental and physical capacities develop at different rates of speed, reaching peak performance levels at different points in the life cycle. In considering the influence of age upon a particular illness, therefore, it is necessary to go beyond merely chronological age, and to define age in terms of the *maturational level* of specific biological, psychological, and social capacities.

Because general homeostatic capacity, recuperative ability, resilience, and energy gradually decline with advancing years, stresses in late life may have a greater impact than those occurring earlier. The stress involved in sexual involution serves to illustrate the roles played by both age and sex. Women usually cope with the stress of menopause during their 40's. Sexual involution in men tends to occur later, when the overall capacity for coping may not be as great as during the middle years. The advantage to the male of a longer period of reproductive ability may well be offset by the advantage that women have of coping with the stress of involution while they still have many other resources. [10, 11]

THE BODY IMAGE

Sociocultural conditions being what they are, disabling illness may present a more specific threat to men; disfiguring illness, to women. In both instances, the psychological reaction depends not only on the actual impairment but also on its symbolic significance. The latter is determined by many personal and interpersonal factors, one of these being the body image. This is the conceptualization of the body's structure and functions, and includes the ego's perceptions, ideas, and feelings in reference to its own body.[12]

As illness interferes with different physiological functions, different psychological concerns are activated. Patients with emphysema, for example, often present somatopsychic phenomena based on fears of suffocation.

> One patient with long-standing emphysema had repetitive anxious dreams of being underneath a house, in the narrow space between floor and ground, with just enough space to crawl along on his stomach.

Less intense in the immediate anxiety it produces, but profound in its disruption of body image, are illnesses which affect psychically significant sites. Involvement of the reproductive organs may bring loss of sexual capacities and disturbance in sexual identity; disease in the lower intestines may result in bowel incontinence and concomitant fears of helplessness and losing control in general. Many fears and fantasies associated with diseases which impair organ function are *somatopsychic elaborations* of the physiological disturbances. Such psychological manifestations cannot be separated from their basic physiological causes. Hence, they must be distinguished from body image disturbances which occur on a purely psychodynamic basis, such as cancerophobia, conversion reaction, hypochondriasis, and the somatic delusions encountered in schizophrenia and psychotic depression.

The psychological reaction to the loss of a body part or the loss of a function includes grief and depression, shame and embarrassment, as well as apprehension about the future impact of the body alteration on interpersonal relations, occupational performance, etc. Patients with a colostomy, for example, experience a serious narcissistic injury; embarrassment can be intense, and the patient is anxious about the effects of the colostomy on sexual intimacy. It may be difficult for him to *reorganize the body image* and to integrate the colostomy as part of it. When the colostomy is not accepted, it continues to be viewed as something alien, a foreign body. Such lack of integration into the body image sets the stage for psychological "rejection" of the foreign element, often in the form of denial. This response is maladaptive because the patient's negative attitude poorly equips him for the task of adjusting and attuning the physiological processes of elimination to the structural limitations of the colostomy. The result may be chronic discomfort and dysfunction.

Another example of discomfort associated with altered body image is the painful phantom limb. Apparently this phenomenon is frequently related to unresolved emotional conflicts concerning the loss of the limb, the circumstances in which the injury occurred, as well as the type of premorbid personality.[13]

> A 71-year-old man had undergone an amputation of his left arm because of a malignancy, at the age of 44. Soon after the surgery, he developed a painful phantom limb, which persisted through the years, and about which he still is complaining. Psychiatric consultation revealed that the patient had always been considered as "the queer one in the family." He never had a regular job, but became a self-styled preacher. He did not go beyond the third grade in school, but he taught himself to read "after he had heard the call to preach." Reportedly, his preaching was not bad, but he never was called to a church, and this caused him much bitterness. The patient's mother had walked out on his father, leaving him and the 12 children behind. Shortly after that, the father became embroiled in a lawsuit against a neighbor. At the day of the trial, the father was shot and killed from ambush. The patient was married and divorced twice. The last few years he has been living alone. He is constantly afraid that someone will burglarize his home, and for protection he has two vicious dogs, one gun, and seven locks on the door. None of his relatives visit him anymore.

Psychodynamically, this patient illustrates a paranoid personality disorder who in the course of his life, gradually decompensated into a chronic schizophrenic. His past history shows exposure to violence, and presently he is excessively preoccupied with violence and the threat of being attacked. The occurrence and persistence of the painful phantom limb in this context of violence is plausible.

When a relatively minor physical injury triggers a major psychological response, the explanation may lie in the symbolic significance of the physical trauma. When the premorbid personality includes conflicts regarding fear of physical injury, castration, or aggressive competition, even minor injuries may acquire tremendous significance. The types of injuries (traumatic or surgical) which, in men, are likely to precipitate such neurotic reactions are those involving the hand, the inguinal area (hernia repair, appendectomy), and the nose. In such cases, the accidental or surgical alteration of the body image may have become symbolic of genital injury.

CHARACTERISTICS OF PREMORBID PERSONALITY

Knowledge concerning the premorbid personality may enable the clinician to anticipate the psychological responses to stress. In some cases, a premorbid behavior pattern will be intensified under the impact of the illness. A *passive-dependent* individual may welcome illness as a means of permitting him to gratify his dependency needs. Physical illness may also be welcome to *guilt-ridden* or *masochistic* personalities; since the disease satisfies their need for punishment, their emotional state may actually improve during the illness. For *immature* and *inadequate* persons, illness can provide escape from adult responsibilities.

Sometimes physical illness is the lesser of two evils. For example, an *ambitious*, hard-striving, middle-aged man, who discovers that he has fallen short of the goals set by his ego-ideal, may find in illness an alibi that covers his shortcomings, be they real or imagined.

Individuals whose premorbid personalities showed prominent reaction-formation against tender feelings, may "use" the illness situation for the expression of emotional warmth and experience of intimacy. Thus, physical illness may come to be the currency that permits the exchange of emotional warmth between persons who otherwise have a distant relationship. Physical illness may be used in a similar way by patients who are *overly self-reliant.* They may publicly protest but secretly enjoy being sick, because the illness "forces" them temporarily into a position of dependency and receptivity. If, however, the illness becomes prolonged or disabling, so that the reaction-formation of excessive self-reliance is jeopardized, the patient may first fight back with an exaggeration of the very traits of self-reliance. Later, when he no longer has enough energy to sustain this behavior, this rigid line of defense may suddenly give way to regressive behavior such as excessive helplessness and dependency.

> An elderly male patient had been a most prominent and respected citizen of his community before an accident resulted in quadriplegia. Every time he was cleaned following defecation, he unleashed a torrent of invectives and profanities at the male attendant, but as soon as the procedure had been completed he quieted down. His rage at the attendants was overdetermined and involved: (1) projec-

> tion of the cause of his discomfort onto the attendants; (2) a regressive, primitive attempt to be the "big shot" he used to be; (3) a desperate, paroxysmal exaggeration of the reaction-formation against passive-dependency wishes; (4) an attempt to ward off homosexual feelings and thoughts stimulated by the enforced passivity and fostered by the regular attention from male attendants.

Schizoid personalities, or lonely and isolated persons, may view illness as a secure bridge leading toward another human being. They may wish to hang onto their illness, or their sick role, because the contacts with nurses and physicians provide them with closeness which, however, does not necessarily involve true intimacy. Such patients may, in the course of their illness, develop an attachment to the hospital or clinic in general, rather than to specific members of the medical or nursing staff.

Schizophrenic patients occasionally display a most interesting reaction to the development of a physical problem.

> A skin lesion appeared on the foot of a male patient suffering from chronic undifferentiated schizophrenia. This was treated effectively by his physician. As soon as the skin had closed over the wound, however, the patient became acutely psychotic. When the foot lesion broke down again a short time later, the patient's mental condition improved. Each time the lesion healed, the schizophrenic symptoms flared up; when the lesion broke down again, the schizophrenia improved. It finally became clear that the patient himself reopened the wound as soon as the bandages were removed.

This example illustrates the fact that the body represents an "intermediate station" between external reality and the inner realm of the mind. In autistic regression, the ego withdraws from external reality and the body may become the recipient of the withdrawn cathexes, a situation that tends to manifest itself as hypochondriasis. When this last anchorage point in reality, the physical body, is given up, the patient withdraws into his inner realm, where memory and fantasy images are cathected. A physical condition, especially one which is painful or visible to the patient, draws his attention back toward the sphere of the body, a part of actual reality.

In personalities who are *action-prone* or tend to *act out*, illness interferes with the habitual pattern of activity. Anxiety, depression, and regressive behavior may be the result, especially if action had been used to ward off intrapsychic tension. Physical illness may also bring about anxiety and depression in personalities who are *obsessive-compulsive, or perfectionistic*. It simply becomes impossible for the perfectionist to live up to his high standards; likewise, the compulsive individual may no longer have sufficient energy to maintain repetitive behavior rituals.

For *narcissistic* personalities, physical illness is a special threat, because it represents an attack on the integrity of the body and the body image. Such individuals may have prided themselves on possessing unusual attractiveness, physical strength, or sexual prowess. The loss (either real or imagined) of these attributes leads to lowered self-esteem.

SITUATIONAL FACTORS

THE ILLNESS SITUATION

Sick Role

The individual with a physical illness is confronted with the necessity of assuming the *sick role*. The patient must adapt to his restricted pattern of living by withdrawing from many of the usual pursuits engaged in by healthy people. He transfers the right to make decisions concerning his welfare to his physician and family and society frees him from the discharge of ordinary duties. For many people, this new pattern of dependent behavior is not easy to adopt, because dependency may connote inferiority and create feelings of guilt and hostility. Nevertheless, the physically ill patient generally responds by gradually surrendering to dependency needs. When strong denial and counterphobic mechanisms are active, however, this adaptive device is obscured and the patient tends to resist appropriate regression, ignore limitations imposed by the disease and the treatment program, and reject support and supervision by the physician.

Physician-Patient Relationship

The physician-patient relationship is an important factor in shaping some of the patient's reactions to illness. Difficulties in the doctor-patient relationship may arise from a great variety of sources.[14] For example, the greater the class differences between physician and patient, the more difficult it becomes to communicate. On the patient's side, dissatisfaction is the result, which in the lower classes often takes the form of evasiveness in deference to the doctor's status, while in the middle and upper classes, it may be expressed with more self-assertiveness. Other obstacles to communication result from cultural differences. For example, a patient from a cultural group given to overt expression of feelings may make much of his pain and create the impression that he is a complainer. Some ethnic groups attach little importance to time as a regulator of behavior. When a person from such a background is told to take his medicine "twice-a-day," he may translate this as "any time it occurs to me."

Hospitalization

Hospitalization may be refused by the patient who interprets it as confirmation of the seriousness of his illness. The patient who accepts hospitalization is usually faced with difficult adjustments, separation from home being the most consistent traumatic factor.[15] The hospital tends to foster an impersonal atmosphere; for many, it represents a strange environment where one loses personal identity for the sake of institutional efficiency. Hospitalization can also produce stress through informational overload or excessive sensory stimulation. Preconceived anxieties are often reinforced by fearful sights, smells, and sounds, by undue proximity to other patients, lack of privacy, routines that clash with the patient's personal habits, and by the expectations of the medical staff concerning his behavior.[16]

FAMILY RELATIONSHIPS

The family may not easily accept the patient in the sick role. They may resist decisions made by medical personnel which tend to remove the patient from his usual activities, and attempt to view his symptoms within the framework of normality. When it becomes necessary to hospitalize the patient, the family may feel that they have in some way rejected him. This feeling of guilt causes some families to make undue financial sacrifices or give the patient an excessive amount of attention.

If the patient is hospitalized for a long time, it is often necessary for the family to reorganize itself, establishing new patterns of relationships to fill the gap left by the patient. These may work out so well that problems arise when the patient returns home.

Problems of an *intergenerational* nature are not uncommon between elderly patients and their adult children. The latter have to recognize that they can no longer look to their parents for the support they used to receive in earlier years. The ability to relate to one's parent as a mature adult involves seeing him as a person separate from his role as head of the family. Thus, the adult child ceases to be dependent and becomes dependable. It is a critical point, when a person realizes that his aging parents are no longer pillars of support but that they themselves now need the support of their children. If the relationship between adult children and their parents has been mature, the transition of roles can be made without difficulty. But when the adult child has remained immature or dependent, a crisis occurs, and he may not permit the aging parent to become dependent. Because he continues unrealistically to regard his parent as capable and competent, the latter is subjected to the stress of having to play a role he does not want, nor would be capable of. In other cases, the problem originates with the parent, who may cling to an obsolete set of roles or outdated self-concept. In most instances, however, difficulties in the role reversal are due to psychological factors in both the aging parent and his adult child.

PROCESSES OF INTERACTION

Physical illness is associated with disturbed function on three different levels.

Intrasystemic level refers to processes taking place within the molecule, the cell, or the organ. *Systemic level* refers to that of the organism as a whole, and the personality (ego, character). *Intersystemic level* includes interpersonal phenomena such as dyadic relationships (marriage), small groups (nuclear family), and larger groups (extended family, community).

Functional integrity on a particular level depends on the *structural* intactness of the preceding "lower" levels. Damage at one level affects the functions of other levels, the effect depending on the properties of these adjacent levels. For example, prostatic hypertrophy requiring a prostatectomy represents physical illness on the organ level. The extent to which the patient can continue to function sexually after the operation depends not only on the structural and functional properties of other components of the genital apparatus, but also on systemic characteristics of the patient (e.g., psychosexual maturity) and intersystemic factors (e.g., marital adjustment).

The interactional processes among these various levels must be viewed in a *sociopsychosomatic* framework. Even the manifestations of organic brain syndrome can be more adequately understood when the illness is studied in this framework. The clinical picture of organic brain syndrome depends not only on the nature and extent of the brain damage, but also on the patient's educational level and emotional maturity, on the quality of interpersonal relations, and on environmental support.[17]

To varying degrees, chronic illness in general (for example, cardiovascular disease, stroke, diabetes) interferes with sexual interest and activity. The majority of men, however, who have had a coronary occlusion or a prostatectomy continue sexual activity.[18, 19] When illness interferes with the capacity for sexual initiative or sustained performance (secondary consequence), the patient and his (or her) spouse face the task of seeking new ways of sexual intimacy. This requires a spirit of open-mindedness and cooperativeness which permits experimentation with new sexual techniques. For aggressive men, the change from an active role to a less active one may mean a difficult adjustment. If a mutually satisfactory readjustment cannot be achieved, marital conflicts may develop. These problems are not an immediate (secondary) result of the illness, but represent more remote (tertiary) consequences. Now, when these third-order problems (the lack of marital harmony) are not effectively resolved, another set of repercussions is set in motion. These fourth-order reverberations in the interactional network may consist of maladaptive coping behavior (regression, withdrawal) and further problems within or outside the marriage (sexual acting out). This last set of events is likely to have an unfavorable (positive feedback) effect on the primary condition (such as coronary heart disease).

Similar *cause-and-effect sequences* involving other functional capacities are also set in motion by physical illness. Decreased work capacity, for example, often causes lowered self-esteem and depression, which in turn can affect sexual interest and capacity. Conversely, sexual problems may adversely affect work capacity.

A 60-year-old man with heart disease had become progressively short of breath. Eventually, he had to stop work and was hospitalized because of violent coughing spells caused by pulmonary congestion. During a psychiatric interview, he was tearful and depressed. The immediate cause for this was his feeling of loneliness in the hospital; but he had already been feeling dejected for some time prior to hospitalization. He admitted, with visible embarrassment, that since he had quit work, his wife had gone to work to make a living. The patient stayed at home doing household chores. Somewhere along the line he lost his potency. He related that his family physician had explained the heart condition by comparing the heart valves with the worn out valves of a car. Since then, the patient had come to think of his heart as an engine, and the coughing spells as the ominous sounds of a machine ready to explode. Finally, he mentioned that he "probably only had himself to blame for getting in this shape, because he never took care of himself when he had a cold."

This case illustrates the wide range of somatopsychic reactions: a reactive depression (due to loss of physical health, loss of job and social role, and separation from home due to hospitalization); changes in body image (fearful fantasies about the illness); complex phenomena (such as the loss of potency) caused by the interaction effect of physical illness, depression, changed social role and self-concept, and fear of exertion; and finally, feelings of guilt (holding himself responsible for his predicament). Psychiatric treatment in such a case would aim at preventing the patient from settling down permanently in the sick role. This would involve giving the patient adequate information about his symptoms without frightening him, reassurance about the prognosis and his ability to continue to do some type of work, correction of his fearful fantasies about his symptoms, removal of guilt feelings, exploration of ways in which sexual intimacy can be continued, etc.

Complexity is a fact of life and, in the living system, countless forces interact dynamically.[20-22] One "cause" may have "effects" in several directions, or may even have repercussions throughout the entire system. Further, an "effect" can become a "cause" for new "effects." Eventually, some kind of end-state develops, when a balance of forces is reached in the interactional network. Although it is impossible, in view of the infinite complexities of a living system, to trace the nature, intensity, direction, and interaction of all factors operating at a given moment, the big lines and major themes can usually be discerned without too much difficulty. Clinical judgment involves this capacity to see the essential phenomena and grasp their interaction. The experienced clinician utilizes the comprehensive approach, or sociopsychosomatic framework, to his advantage and that of the patient.

References

1. Verwoerdt, A.: *Communication with the Fatally Ill*, Charles C Thomas, Springfield, Illinois, 1966. p. 183.
2. Gottheil, E., McGurn, W. C., and Pollak, O.: Awareness and disengagement in cancer patients. *Am. J. Psychiatry 136*:633–635, 1979.
3. Dovenmuehle, R. H., and Verwoerdt, A.: Physical illness and depressive symptomatology. I. Incidence of depressive symptoms in hospitalized cardiac patients. *J. Am. Geriatr. Soc. 10*:932–947, 1962.
4. Dovenmuehle, R. H., and Verwoerdt, A.: Physical illness and depressive symptomatology. II. Factors of length and severity of illness and frequency of hospitalization. *J. Gerontol. 18*:260–266, 1963.
5. Beigler, J. S.: Anxiety as an aid in the prognostication of impending death. *Arch. Neurol. Psychiatry 77*:171, 1957.
6. Verwoerdt, A., and Elmore, J. L.: Psychological reactions in fatal illness. I. The prospect of impending death. *J. Am. Geriatr. Soc. 15*:9–19, 1967.
7. Koranyi, E. K.: Morbidity and rate of undiagnosed physical illnesses in a psychiatric clinic population. *Arch. Gen. Psychiatry 36*:414–419, 1979.
8. Fries, M. E., and Woolf, P. J.: Some hypotheses on the role of the congenital activity type in personality development. *Psychoanal. Study Child 8*:48–62, 1953.
9. Tennant, C., and Andrews, G.: The pathogenic quality of life event stress in neurotic impairment. *Arch. Gen. Psychiatry 35*:859–863, 1978.
10. Szalita, A. B.: Psychodynamics of disorders of the involutional age. In: *American Handbook of Psychiatry III*, edited by S. Arieti, chap. 5, Basic Books, New York, 1966.
11. Verwoerdt, A., Pfeiffer, E., and Wang, H. S.: Sexual behavior in senescence. II. Patterns of sexual activity and interest. *Geriatrics 24*:137–154, 1969.
12. Hinsie, L. E., and Campbell, R. J.: *Psychiatric Dictionary*, ed. 4, Oxford University Press, New York, 1970.
13. Kolb, L. C.: Disturbances of the body image. In: *American Handbook of Psychiatry*, vol. 1, chap. 38, edited by S. Arieti, Basic Books, New York, 1959.
14. Bogdonoff, M. D., Nichols, C. R., Klein, R. F., and Eisdorfer, C.: The doctor-patient relationship. *J. Am. Med. Assoc. 192*:45, 1965.
15. Verwoerdt, A., and Dovenmuehle, R. H.: Heart disease and depression. *Geriatrics 19*: 856–864, 1964.
16. Schottstaedt, W. W., Pinsky, R. H., Mackler, D., and Wolf, S.: Prestige and social interaction on a metabolic ward. *Psychosom. Med. 21*:131, 1959.
17. Wang, H. S.: Organic brain syndromes. In: *Behavior and Adaptation in Late Life*, edited by E. W. Busse and E. Pfeiffer, chap. 13, Little, Brown, Boston, 1969.
18. Hellerstein, H. K., and Friedman, E. H.: Sexual activity and the post-coronary patient. *Med. Aspects Human Sexuality 3*:70–96, 1969.
19. Finkle, A. L.: Sex after prostatectomy. *Med. Aspects Human Sexuality 2*:40–41, 1968.
20. Surawicz, F. G., Brightwell, D. R., Weitzel, W. D., and Othmer, E.: Cancer, emotions, and mental illness: the present state of understanding. *Am. J. Psychiatry 133*:1306–1309, 1976.
21. Solomon, G. F., Amkraut, A. A., and Kasper, P.: Immunity, emotions, and stress. *Ann. Clin. Res. 6*:313–322, 1974.
22. Schiair, R. C., Camerino, M.: Influence of brain and behavior on the immune system. *Science 191*:435–440, 1976.

9

somatic expression of psychiatric illness

SOMATIC ASPECTS OF PSYCHIATRIC DISORDERS

The somatic aspects of psychiatric disorders can be considered under various headings depending on the type of etiology (physical versus psychogenic), the site of pathology (cerebral versus extracerebral), and the temporal factor in the cause-and-effect sequences (primary versus secondary). Following this approach, four major categories can be delineated.

Organic mental disorders, due to organic-cerebral etiological factors or secondary to extracerebral-somatic pathology (see Chapter 4).

Functional psychiatric disorders, in the absence of organic mental disorder, e.g., schizophrenia, depressive psychosis, neurotic disorders (see Chapter 5, 6, and 7).

Somatopsychic reactions: psychological responses secondary to physical illness, the central nervous system being structurally intact, for example, a reactive depression in cardiac illness[1,2] (see Chapter 8).

Psychophysiological disorders, in which neither the physical nor the psychological factor alone is sufficient to lead to illness, but both are necessary. Again, there is no structural impairment of brain tissue. In the *Diagnostic and Statistical Manual of Mental Disorders* (DSM III), these are listed as Psychological Factors Affecting Physical Condition.

Several psychosomatic aspects of psychiatric illness were already menmentioned in previous chapters. At this point, it will be useful to review those types of physical symptoms which represent the outward manifestations of an underlying mental disorder. These somatic expressions of psychiatric illness represent the somatoform disorders, and include conversion disorder, somatization disorder, psychogenic pain, hypochondriasis, and atypical somatoform disorders, as well as some factitious disorders with physical symptoms.[3]

SOMATOFORM DISORDERS

CONVERSION DISORDER

The classical conversions appear to occur less frequently nowadays than a few decades ago; specifically, they are considered to be rare in old age.

Psychodynamics and Manifestations

In a conversion reaction, a psychological conflict is converted into a physical symptom. This mechanism decreases anxiety (primary gain) and often also produces a secondary gain (a gain derived from the sick role). Characteristic of conversion are the following *psychodynamics* and *manifestations.*

The psychological conflict is converted into a somatic symptom, which at the same time expresses the conflict.

The somatic symptoms involve components of the motor system whose innervations are under voluntary control, or the sensory organs of the perceptual system. There is no primary physical impairment, but secondary disuse atrophy may develop in rare cases.

The nature of the symptom is in terms of a loss of function (e.g., hysterical paralysis, hysterical blindness) or an alteration of function (e.g., hysterical paresthesia).

The hysterical symptom expresses the psychological conflict in a symbolic way. Related to this is the fact that the nature, location, and extent of the conversion symptoms do not correspond with objective, anatomical facts. Instead, the somatic manifestations correspond with the body image.

The physical discomfort from the hysterical symptom can serve as atonement for the guilt from the unacceptable impulses.

Since the unacceptable impulse is indeed expressed (symbolically, through conversion) while the patient at the same time does penance through his suffering, the net sum total amounts to a balance of forces. The patient may have a peculiar equanimity vis-à-vis the physical symptom (la belle indifference).

Differential Diagnosis

Psychophysiological Disorders. Conversion reactions must be differentiated from *psychophysiological disorders* (psychological factors affecting physical condition). In the latter, there is no symbolic expression of psychic conflict. These disorders are located in organs under control of the autonomous nervous system and have a physiological origin (mediated through the limbic system, hypothalamus, etc.). Anatomic-structural changes may develop that can be even life-threatening; and the physical symptoms do not relieve anxiety or guilt as in conversion. The diagnosis of conversion can be established only by meeting two basic requirements: (1) *positive* evidence of a psychological conflict, and its symbolic, somatic expression; and (2) *negative* evidence, in terms of ruling out possible physical pathology, which of course is particularly relevant in the case of aged patients.

Neurological Disease. It is especially important to rule out *neurological* disease since so many conversion symptoms can mimic these.

Drug Side-Effects. By the same token, it is necessary to keep in mind the possibility of *side-effects of psychotropic drugs,* e.g., dyskinesia, akathisia. Included in the general class of side-effects is the "negative placebo effect" which can manifest itself in innumerable types of physical distress.

> A 62-year-old woman, who had always lived in an isolated rural area, had recently started to have persistent chewing movements. She herself was not bothered by these, and her hospitalization had been prompted by a cardiac problem. The psychiatric interview revealed that she had been feeling neglected by her husband. When asked how she felt about this, she shrugged her shoulders indicating that she was resigned to it. She was then asked if she ever felt like "wanting to chew him out." The patient looked up surprised and acknowledged remembering having felt just that—but she had dismissed the idea of chewing her husband out, because of a mixture of fear and love for him. Significantly, her chewing movements stopped the moment she remembered the wish to chew her husband out. To establish the diagnosis of conversion in this particular case, it was also necessary to rule out lingual-facial-buccal dyskinesia, either the spontaneous type or as part of tardive dyskinesia.[4]

SOMATIZATION DISORDER

Somatization disorder (Briquet's syndrome) is thought to start early in life, often before age 25. Thus, age-specific somatization disorder, by definition, is rare in late life. No research data are available concerning the effect of time and aging on the symptomatology of this entity. It would be expected, however, that in a substantial number of cases the symptoms become more depressive or hypochondriacal in the course of the aging process.

HYSTERICAL EXAGGERATION OF PHYSICAL ILLNESS

Much more frequent among elderly patients is the phenomenon of hysterical exaggeration of physical illness. In some cases, this entity may correspond to the Factitious Disorder with Physical Symptoms of DSM III. As mentioned above, the primary gain in a psychodynamic constellation is an intrapersonal gain: the re-establishment of an intrapsychic equilibrium. Secondary gain is interpersonal and refers to advantages that secondarily accrue from the sick role, to unexpected fringe benefits from a neurotic illness. A patient may exploit any illness (emotional or physical) for ulterior motives, and usually this involves an hysterical exaggeration of the symptomatology. In the case of physical illness, the primary motive would be to obtain effective treatment. But, if an ulterior motive is operating, the patient is interested in receiving not only treatment, but also something more, such as attention, commiseration, or financial assistance.

This type of patient can be recognized fairly readily. In a typical case, the patient has been quietly sitting in the waiting room, until his name is called; it is his turn to see the doctor, and now a dramatic display of distress is suddenly enacted. A cardiac patient may clutch his chest, as if in pain; assorted types of dyspnea may appear (often the dyspnea is slightly histrionic, inasmuch as the type of dyspnea is contrary to what one would expect, e.g., a shallow, superficial blowing out of air, almost like a puffing or whistling). By the same token, a patient with a mental illness may exaggerate his psychiatric symptoms, for example, by appearing dazed, by answering ordinary questions with "I don't know," or even by cheerfully volunteering, on the way from waiting room to office, that the "voices keep me awake all night long." The purpose is to convince the physician or nurse (or other parental and authority symbols who have the power to give and to take away) that he, the patient, is sick indeed, and does deserve help. This exaggeration of symptoms is not malingering, which is conscious and deliberate. Instead, these patients are unaware of their dramatization and, furthermore, we are talking about individuals who have an illness to begin with. In view of the dramatic, naive over-reacting, of which the patient himself is not aware, it is appropriate to designate such exaggeration of illness as hysterical. This phenomenon is related to the "search for aid," described by Goldfarb.[5] This may be a rational search for skilled aid, or an irrational search, prompted by dependency striving, for parental substitutes. Part of the irrational search for aid is the element of regressive behavior, and the appeal to powerful caretakers by the display of personal suffering. Occasionally, the search for aid is less dramatic, more conniving, and borders on malingering.

> A 68-year-old woman had been confined to a wheelchair since an accident, at age 38, caused a paralysis of both legs. For some reason, she disliked her present nursing home and made no secret of her wish to be admitted to the local, general hospital. Then, because of a urinary infection, her wish came true. In the hospital, an indwelling catheter was inserted in the bladder. A few days later, a nurse discovered that the patient periodically cut the catheter with her fingernails, in the apparent belief that this would prolong her hospitalization. On subsequent occasions, this patient was observed to pick at her decubitus sores, again in the apparent hope that, if these did not improve, she would return to her favorite hospital.

The development of secondary gains and ulterior motives may complicate not only a conversion neurosis or a physical illness, but also other conditions, e.g., phobic states, traumatic neuroses, and depression. An individual may have a *phobia* about staying by himself at night. A deeper fear of death is being displaced onto an external symbolic substitute: being alone in the dark. This phobic displacement leads to the primary gain (remaining unaware of death-anxiety); but once the phobia is a *fait accompli*, other people may be moved to stay with the patient (secondary gain). Some traumatic neuroses (caused by war, accidents, etc.) develop into protracted *compensation-neuroses*, when the patient receives financial compensation because (or, as long as) he is disabled. Such a patient may conclude that he is being rewarded for being sick.

The differential diagnosis between conditions of hysterical exaggeration versus true conversion is not always easy, as is illustrated by the following case.

> A 66-year-old married woman was hospitalized because of an inability to walk for the past 2 months. Prior to this, she had been able to walk a mile every day to the local shopping center. A neurological consultation was requested and the conclusion was that the patient had no neurological disease. A consultation from the cardiologist stated that the patient had no exercise intolerance and could take the stress of walking quite well. The only positive finding was x-ray evidence of an old, partially healed fracture of the fifth metatarsal of the left foot. This fracture was incurred in a fall 3 years ago, and she had continued walking until 2 months ago. The reasons why this minor, old injury suddenly became a major disability appeared to be as follows. Shortly before her "paralysis," an elderly lady next door had fallen, broken her leg, and died. The idea of falling and becoming disabled and dependent frightened the patient who saw herself as a strong, independent person. She would resent her husband's inadequacies and accuse him of "putting on" a lot of his problems. Since she repressed her own dependency wishes, she would be all the more irritated by her husband's pattern of dependency gratifications. The combination of her anger and envy toward him, and the sudden frightening reminder (the neighbor's accident) that she would have nobody to depend on, resulted in the hysterical inability to walk. Inasmuch as the symptom was an exaggeration of the disability from the old fracture, we could make the diagnosis of hysterical exaggeration of physical illness. On the other hand, the classical features of conversion were also present: the converting of her psychological conflict (involving anger toward her husband, and repressed dependency wishes) into a physical symptom (the loss of a motor function). The latter expressed the psychological conflict in a symbolic way ("I can't walk,

so I am helpless—Sorry, I can't take care of you any more—Why don't you do your best, for a change?").

PSYCHOGENIC PAIN

Persistent physical complaints including chronic pain are common in schizophrenia, organic mental disorders, depression, and hypochondriasis. The physical complaints of the schizophrenic patient, often strange or bizarre, may represent his attempt to give expression to his chaotic inner world.

While idiosyncratic descriptions of pain suggest a "psychic signature,"[6] in organic mental disorders, this rule does not apply. The expression of pain by these patients may involve delusions, hallucinations, or bizarre behavior. The mechanism responsible for this revolves around the loss of abstract thinking.

The diagnosis and management of chronic pain should involve a consideration of the intimate connections between anxiety, depression, tension, and pain. The fact that perception of pain and reaction to pain-inducing stimuli decrease with age may be a complicating factor. Compared with younger people, the aged person may not as readily perceive the early onset of pathological changes and this presents a handicap in diagnosis and treatment. Organic pain conforms in a characteristic manner to what one would expect on the basis of anatomical lesions. Psychogenic pain, however, is related to anxious fantasies about an illness, to mental conceptions of progression of pathology, and to body image disturbances. The regressed or hypochondriacal patient may be so preoccupied with bodily overconcern that almost any sensation of distress can be perceived as painful. It should not be forgotten, however, that many older persons do suffer from one or more chronic illnesses, which may cause a variety of distressing symptoms. A long-standing pattern of psychogenic pain should not tempt the clinician to be less alert to the development of an authentic organic illness: even a hypochondriac can get physically sick.[7]

ATYPICAL SOMATOFORM DISORDERS

The term somatization apparently was introduced by Stekel who referred to it in terms of organ language.[8] The concept of somatization is based on the assumption that "emotion" has several dimensions (subjective experience, physiological concomitants, action and motor behavior, and interpersonal-communicative functions) and that individuals may vary considerably with regard to the relative prominence of these aspects.[9] The term somatization used to be reserved for those cases when the physiological concomitants of an emotion (or affective disorder) are conspicuous while the other affective dimensions are proportionately less distinct. It was thought that the mechanism of somatization could influence an emotional disorder so that the clinical picture shows a paucity of subjective, inner experiences, and a prominence of physiological manifestations. Since the emotional disorder does not express itself openly, but indirectly through physical distress, the term affective "equivalent" has come to be used. In the differential diagnosis of various illnesses, two affect-equivalents must be considered: depressive equivalent and anxiety equivalent.

Depressive Equivalents

The somatic equivalent of a depression[10] is a special instance of a masked depression. The masking effect is due to the predominance of the physiological concomitants of the depression, and the relative paucity of subjective depressive feelings.

> This characteristic discrepancy was strikingly illustrated during an interview with an elderly male patient, hospitalized because of multiple physical complaints. When asked how he felt, the patient responded by talking at length about his headaches. Having finished that, he was again asked how he felt, and now the patient recited the discomforts in his chest and around his heart. The interviewer then inquired about his stomach ("It hurts all over, it is swollen, I feel sick"); about his back ("It always hurts, down in my lower back"); about his arms and legs ("They ache and feel stiff"). Thus, in effect, the patient was hurting all over. At the finish of the organ recital, he was asked once more: "Now with all this going on, how do you really *feel*?"; to which the response was: "Feel?—Oh, I feel fine!"

Usually, however, the physiological symptoms do not represent such a formidable, impenetrable barrier. In many cases, the depressive affective experience is just behind a thin facade of physical symptoms.

> A 58-year-old woman, recently widowed, would begin each interview with a quick matter-of-fact rundown of numerous physical problems. Following this, she would talk about her two children, both of whom were a source of pride and satisfaction. Only after these prolegomena, the topic of her husband's death would come up. It was necessary for her to approach this topic gingerly, and after some preliminary circumlocution, because of her intense ambivalence toward him. By the end of the interview, she was usually able to experience the feelings of grief and sadness, and tearfully express these in words.

Anxiety Equivalents

Somatization may also pertain to anxiety, and the following case illustrates an anxiety equivalent.

> Following a coronary attack 2 years previously, a 65-year-old man had been suffering from frequent angina. This was poorly relieved

by nitroglycerin, which he took in large amounts. Sometimes he would wake up during the night feeling that he "could not catch his breath" and try to relieve the pressure on his chest by "gasping for breath." He stated that he did not feel frightened at such times; all his attention was focused on the sensations of his chest. His father had died of a heart attack at an age close to the patient's current age. Significantly, he emphasized that this did not bother him. When, during his hospitalization he had another episode of shortness of breath, it was clear that he was hyperventilating. This case illustrates that anxiety can be manifested physiologically without the patient being subjectively aware of the anxiety (caused, in this patient, by the psychological threat of having heart disease and the fact that his father had died of a similar illness). Hyperventilation is a common physiological concomitant of anxiety and, in this patient, the disordered breathing aggravated his anginal pains.

Other physiological concomitants of anxiety which can be dominant manifestations in the clinical picture (and so mask the underlying anxiety state) may be cardiovascular (e.g., palpitations), gastrointestinal (overeating, "butterflies" in stomach; episodic urgency to defecate), urogenital (urinary frequency, sexual dysfunctions), and neuromuscular (tension, tremors), as well as episodes of weakness and insomnia.

Somatic Delusions

Somatic delusions are frequent in schizophrenia, psychotic depression, organic brain syndromes, and senile dementia. Interestingly, there appear to be significantly fewer somatic delusions in manic and paranoid conditions. This is probably related to the fact that the latter two disorders tend to be "centrifugal": the patient tries to escape from his problem, in an extrovert flight away from the center of his being. In contrast, schizophrenia, depression, and dementia are "centripetal," as it were, the patient becoming more introvert and absorbed in the self.[2]

Somatic delusions involving sex, pregnancy, and childbirth are not uncommon among aged female patients, with a diagnosis of chronic paranoid schizophrenia, or senile dementia.

An 82-year-old woman with a diagnosis of chronic paranoid schizophrenia had the delusion she was 2½ months pregnant. She even identified the alleged father by name. Her delusional system included various "schemes that would make her have intercourse with this man, while under a spell, and so make her receptive to him."

Even in the presence of the somatic delusions of psychotic disorders, one has to remain alert to the possibility that actual physical disease may develop and that the idiosyncratic somatic delusions may obfuscate the signs of physical illness.

An elderly schizophrenic woman had been conplaining of "flashes of electricity shooting through her body." She had been on phenothiazines for many years. Recently, she began to add complaints of feeling "washed out." Since she had had so many bizarre somatic complaints for so long, not much attention was given to this, until she returned for a routine follow-up and appeared to be jaundiced. The prime suspect, of course, was the phenothiazine drug; but it turned out that she had metastatic liver cancer. In retrospect, the complaint of feeling "washed out" was a realistic symptom of the malignancy, not a somatic delusion.

HYPOCHONDRIASIS AND RELATED STATES

Clinical Definition

Hypochondriasis refers to excessive preoccupation with the body or a portion of it, whether physical illness exists or not. The crucial element is bodily overconcern and the manner in which the patient relates to his body; the self-absorption and undue attention focused on the body is at the expense of interests in other objects. The hypochondriacal position may be associated with negative feelings, such as anxiety, depression, loneliness, bitterness, shame, guilt, and hostility. Or, the hypochondriac may derive certain private, narcissistic pleasures from cherishing and nurturing (part of) his body. In the context of hypochondriasis, such pleasurable aspects represent secondary developments and fringe benefits.

Normally, individuals with a physical illness continue to be interested in other people; they can maintain their interpersonal relationship in spite of their suffering and may even feel a greater need to be close to others. Likewise, in cases of regression, the patient withdraws from certain adult role responsibilities, but this does not mean that he is withdrawing from people. To the contrary, since the regressed patient is more dependent, his interpersonal relationships tend to be more, rather than less, intense. In hypochondriasis, however, there is a disengagement, a shift in cathexes, away from external objects, in the direction of the self. In this light, the somatic self-absorption does not have a symbolic significance or communicative function (as in hysterical conditions); nor does it reflect the patient's preoccupation with the physiological concomitants of an affective disorder (as in a depressive equivalent).

Psychodynamic Factors

Hypochondriasis may occur at any age, but in late life it is more common. It has been estimated that 10–20% of the elderly living in the community are hypochondriacal to some degree.[11] There are several possible factors playing a role in the development of hypochondriasis in later life.

Chronic Physical Diseases. These can serve as nuclei around which hypochondriacal concerns can be precipitated and crystallized. Physical illnesses do not cause hypochondriasis, but may facilitate the redistribution of cathexes. In cases of physical illness, we can speak of hypochondriasis only when the somatic preoccupations are out of keeping with the realities of the physical illness. It is fitting, in this context, to remind ourselves of the risk of *iatrogenic hypochondriasis.* The casual mentioning by a physician of what may happen (a future complication) may become a focal point around which hypochondriacal fantasies are elaborated.

Disengagement. The fact that many old persons are socially isolated sets the stage for increased preoccupation with the one object that remains available: one's own body. Isolation per se is not sufficient to bring about the disengagement of interest inherent in hypochondriasis. Although the absence of human objects is a potentially serious psychological stress, an isolated person may protect himself in two ways against a drift toward pathological self-absorption. First, one can establish a relationship with the memories of objects, once present in one's life. Inasmuch as this stored information represents an ensemble of reasonably accurate historical records, contact with historical reality is maintained. Secondly, in the absence of human objects, one can nevertheless relate to the world (inanimate or animate) by engaging one's self with it. Through the instrumentalities of his body and mind, a person can create his own world and recreate himself. There are many examples of isolation, involuntary or self-imposed, illustrating that such modes of existence are feasible, and that the drift into self-absorption is not inevitable.

In addition to the actual loss of external objects, the self may be isolated by a loosening or a rupture of the ties between oneself and those objects. This may come about in several ways. Failure in the area of intimacy may, through distancing from people, bring about loneliness and isolation. Failure in the area of generativity, through disengagement from work, may result in stagnation of the self. Thus, disengagement either from love or from work leads to self-absorption, of which hypochondriasis is a specific example.

Flight into the Sick Role. An individual may feel that a particular relationship is too difficult or demanding. Not being able to keep up one's end of the bargain generates a sense of failure and guilt, of letting the other down. As a result, one may wish to terminate the partnership, not a happy solution, but the lesser of two evils. However, the persisting lack of closure, and the situation of unfinished business, ask urgently for repair. And now a regressive (pseudo) solution presents itself. The combination of various free-floating negative feelings and undue self-attention produces hypochondriasis: the feelings of unpleasure attach themselves to the mental contents of the self-image, specifically, the body image. The next step is the rationalization: "I am not feeling well—no wonder that I failed in this or that (marriage, parenthood, work, etc.)—it's because I was sick." Thus, hypochondriasis becomes an alibi which removes responsibility for failure, an alias that restores self-esteem. This defense may be successful until others discover the excuse of illness as being physically unjustified and see through the patient's alibi. By this time, additional maneuvers, defenses, or coping are called for, in order to reestablish closure or self-esteem.[12]

Atonement for Guilt. The self-absorption and disengagement of the hypochondriac has the effect of irritating and alienating others. The patient now experiences further losses of affection and approval; his feelings of being neglected increase in strength, so do his feelings of anger. Thus, any discomfort associated with the hypochondriacal concerns may serve for the *atonement for guilt*, not only for his failures, but also for hostile vengeful feelings. (This is related to the common neurotic pattern in depression and masochism in which the patient himself provokes a certain amount of misery to avoid punishment at the hands of somebody else. It is the lesser of two evils: by punishing oneself, one can choose the type of suffering and titrate the amount.)

Thus, hypochondriasis may play an important role in attempts to avoid responsibility for shortcomings, real or imagined. And since the question of whether one has been a success, or a failure, is often a critical issue during the later years, we are prepared to encounter hypochondriasis with greater frequency during this period of the life span.

> A 66-year-old woman reportedly "had been enjoying ill health" since a hysterectomy at the age of 54. In spite of her numerous, persisting physical complaints, the family physician could find nothing wrong, and he told the family so! Following this, the patient declared that she could hardly take care of herself anymore, let alone, her husband. The latter had been moderately disabled by a stroke and the patient had become more and more resentful about helping him (mostly in getting him dressed). She began to seclude herself in her home, allegedly because she lacked money to buy proper clothes. In reality, she had both enough money and clothes: her withdrawal into the home expressed her sense of having been short-changed in life. She vented the anger which followed in the wake of her disillusionment on her husband: by accusing him of never giving her any money, being oblivious to his presence, and covering the floors and furniture with newspapers ("So he won't be able to mess things up").

Devaluation and Depreciation of Others. When one's experiences lead to the conclusion that this or that object is "no good," the crucial issue is whether one can find a new object that really *is* all right. The repudiation of objects that have become truly obsolete is a sound move, provided one can find an adequate substitute. But, declaring another person to be "no good" may represent an act of self-deception (involving rationalization and protection). The devaluation pertains to the other, not to me myself, as in decreased self-esteem. In fact, I may conclude (e.g., because of unrealistically high expectations) that there is no use in trying to find a substitute object (or new relationship, or interest area) because "people are all alike—no good—and I am tired of getting hurt and disappointed." This form of disengagement is more serious because of the underlying narcissism and premise of arrogance. The hypochondriasis developing in this way may have a selfish, demanding streak: "Don't you see I am suffering? Why don't you do something? Obviously, you are no good either, like all the rest."

> A 75-year-old divorced man lived alone in a hotel room, eating all his meals in a nearby cafe. The daily menu is always the same: a cup of coffee for breakfast, a bowl of soup for lunch, a hamburger for supper. At the age of 56, he stopped working, explaining that he was physically ill. He was "examined by 12 different doctors, and was told there was nothing physically wrong." Following this, his wife left him and remarried a younger man. The patient still often talks about his wife's leaving him ("There is no one to take care of me, but I am against all women"). Over the years, he moved from one boarding home to another. Not long ago, he bought a gun and threatened some relatives if they refused to keep him. It was after this blow-up that he moved into the present hotel. At all times, he carries with him two objects: a large bottle containing different pills (always eager to explain what they are for) and, a brown briefcase containing a change of clothes ("I never know when I may have to spend the night away from home").

A common type of hypochondriac who combines various of the above described features is the chronic complainer: often a woman who has reached middle age. She is the martyr type, sacrificing for her children, yet demanding certain compensations. She has neglected those dimensions of her life which could remain a source of satisfaction when her children have become adults. The undue amount of satisfaction gained from her children was neurotically determined. When her main source of satisfaction is gone, the extra energy has no pathway other than toward herself.

> A 58-year-old woman had a long history of multiple physical complaints. In the course of the years, her husband had obtained a divorce and the children had left home. The patient had had physicians, and medications too numerous to mention. She would present herself at the clinic with a long-suffering look on her face. In the office, she would, without saying a word, place empty medicine bottles on the desk, then sit back. The long-suffering look on her face was now compounded by stubbornness and defiance. The therapist, aware of his own sense of irritation, nevertheless tried to convey to her that he was available to help in any possible way

offering her a new prescription, as well as regular time to review her problems. Her curt response was: "Just write the prescription." When the physician showed some hesitation, she unleashed a vicious barrage of rage, leaving no question about her resolve to persevere in the martyr role, and to go to any length to provoke rejection.

Further Decompensation: Autism

For elderly persons who have become disengaged or isolated, the world around has become empty. What remains is the world of the self: the concrete, physical body, and the intangible, invisible mental self. The bodily self is more directly in touch with the outside world. In fact, to the mind or inner self, the body is perceived as a peripheral zone that extends toward the physical world, of which it becomes a part. In this framework, the body is a bridge extending from the intimate center of "me," toward what is out there, the "not me." Using the analogy of bridge, we can think of traffic in two opposite directions: toward external objects and toward the self. In a general way, this corresponds to extroversion and introversion, respectively. The withdrawal of cathexes from external objects onto the self is narcissistic in nature. It may be due to actual loss of the object per se, loss of love of the object (real or imagined), devaluation of the object, and depletion of energy.

If, in the course of a traffic pattern, from external objects toward the self, the units of energy remain at the halfway station of the body, they will be invested at this point. This hypercathexis of the body results in hypochondriasis. If, however, this movement pattern is not halted at the halfway point, but proceeds on its inward course, the consequences will be more profound. The last contact point with the real world, the body, is abandoned; and the psychic energy is now mostly used to cathect the inner domain of the self, its thoughts, images, fantasies, and memories. This pathological immersion in the inner self is *autism* and signifies a rupture with the real world. Thus, both hypochondriasis and autism are instances of pathological self-absorption; the former, in the body, and the latter in one's innermost self. What makes autistic immersion especially pathological is the fact that the individual now is out of touch with his environment and his own body, and out of reach for the people around him. In autism, the focus of attention is no longer on the real object world, but on psychic reality. The consequences of such progressive withdrawal include: (*a*) loss of contact with reality, (*b*) disturbance in time perspective (due to hypercathexis of memories, the past becomes a new present, a new temporal reality), and (*c*) a progressive unlearning of acquired skills, including loss of abstract capacity; secondary process functions become less effective, and primitive manifestations of the primary process type of mental functions emerge. Such processes of disengagement and decathexis are typical of schizophrenic disorders, and probably also occur in many cases of senile dementia.

Corresponding to the above two phases of introversion are two phases of extroversion. The hypochondriac may emerge from the preoccupation with his body and become engaged in the world out there. Or, the autistic, severely withdrawn person may proceed on a pathway leading back to the real world. On this pathway, the body is encountered as the first object, external to the innermost self. Thus, we see sometimes that when withdrawn, autistic, or schizophrenic patients improve, they first become hypochondriacal.

> The psychodynamics of a 55-year-old man with paranoid schizophrenia involved a latent homosexual conflict. The patient made extensive use of projection: he felt followed around by "the element—men in bars who were clean and well-dressed and who'd offer him beer and bargains." Finally, a homosexual panic erupted and the patient called the hospital emergency room requesting help in contacting the FBI. Fortunately, help could be provided in a more realistic way: physical examination revealed the presence of a mild heart disease. The decision was made to have the patient come to the clinic at regular times, for treatment of his heart condition. The element of physical illness was emphasized in terms of its potential seriousness, so as to persuade the patient of the need for regular out-patient visits. Almost immediately, the paranoid panic subsided. Thus, a treatment plan based on the notion of trying to convert an autistic person into a hypochondriac appeared to be successful (see also case example of schizophrenic patient with skin lesion in Chapter 8, p. 136).

References

1. Hall, R. C. W., Gruzenski, W. P., and Popkin, M. K.: Differential diagnosis of somatopsychic disorders. *Psychosomatics 20*(6):381–389, 1979.
2. Verwoerdt, A.: Psychopathological responses to the stress of physical illness. In: *Advances in Psychosomatic Medicine*, vol. 8, Karger, Basel, 1972. pp. 92–114.
3. Hyler, S. E., and Spitzer, R. L.: Hysteria split asunder. *Am. J. Psychiatry 135*(*12*):1500–1504, 1978.
4. Weiner, W. J., and Klawans, H. L.: Lingual-facial-buccal movements in the elderly. *J. Am. Geriatr. Soc. 21*:314–320, 1973.
5. Goldfarb, A. I.: Masked depression in the elderly. In: *Masked Depression*, edited by Stanley Lesse, chap. 14, Jason Aronson, New York, 1974. pp. 236–249.
6. Engel, G. L.: Psychogenic pain and the pain-prone patient. *Am. J. Med. 26*:899, 1959.
7. Hall, R. C. W., Popkin, M. K., DeVaul, R. et al.: Physical illness presenting as psychiatric disease. *Arch. Gen. Psychiatry 35*:1315–1320, 1978.
8. Stekel, W.: *The Interpretation of Dreams*. Liveright, New York, 1943.
9. Wittenborn, J. R., and Buhler, R.: Somatic discomforts among depressed women. *Arch. Gen. Psychiatry 36*:465–471, 1979.
10. Ewalt, J.: Somatic equivalents of depression. *Tex. J. Med. 60*:654, 1964.
11. Busse, E. W., and Blazer, D.: Disorders related to biological functioning. In: *Handbook of Geriatric Psychiatry*, edited by E. W. Busse and D. G. Blazer, chap. 18, van Nostrand Reinhold, New York, 1979. pp. 403–405.
12. Busse, E. W., and Pfeiffer, E.: Functional psychiatric disorders in old age. In: *Behavior and Adaptation in Late Life*, edited by E. W. Busse and E. Pfeiffer, chap. 183, Little, Brown and Company, Boston, 1969. pp. 202–208.

10

psychopharmacology: some theoretical and practical considerations*

GENERAL CLASSES OF PSYCHOPHARMACOLOGICAL AGENTS

The psychopharmacological agents of interest to the geropsychiatrist include a great number of drugs which can influence the central nervous system (CNS) directly or indirectly. These psychoactive drugs can be grouped in the following categories: *antipsychotics*, *antidepressants*, *antimanics*, *antiparkinson agents*, *antianxiety agents*, *sedatives* and hypnotics, *stimulants*, drugs alleged to improve *cognitive* function, and a *miscellaneous* group including vitamins, hormones (e.g., anabolic agents), vasodilators, anticoagulants.

The clinical significance of some of these drugs is reflected by the fact that they are therapeutically potent, can cause major side-effects as well, and are in widespread use. A survey conducted at 12 Veterans Administration hospitals revealed that 61 percent of the elderly patients studied were receiving psychoactive drugs. Psychoactive drugs were administered to 55 percent of the patients with organic brain syndrome, 70 percent of those with schizophrenia, and 66 percent of those with other mental illness. Antipsychotic drugs were prescribed most frequently (44 percent), followed by antidepressants (11 percent), antianxiety drugs (10 percent), and cerebral vasodilators and dihydroergotoxine (10 percent). Of the patients receiving antipsychotic drugs, 20 percent received antiparkinson drugs. In this particular survey, 16 percent of the patients received multiple drug combinations.[1]

In a recent review, Prentice documents the disproportionately high use of tranquilizers, sedatives, hypnotics, and antidepressants in the elderly; especially the hypnotics and the sedatives. This high rate of use was observed both in those living in the community, as well as in those institutionalized, with women getting far the greater quantities of these drugs.[2]

* In collaboration with Alan D. Whanger, M.D.

Much basic and clinical research is conducted in psychopharmacology. Thus, it has been found that the mode of action of psychotropic drugs (antipsychotics and antidepressants) probably is in terms of altering the chemical substrates of synaptic transmission or axonal conduction within the central nervous system.[3] The synaptic transmission may be mediated by a biogenic amine, such as acetylcholine, norepinephrine, serotonin, or dopamine. Norepinephrine and dopamine are synthesized, in the neuronal cytoplasm, from the amino acid tyrosine; serotonin, from tryptophan. In the CNS, ascending and descending pathways have been identified which are noradrenergic, dopaminergic, or serotonergic in nature.[4]

The *antipsychotic* agents probably exert their tranquilizing effect by inhibiting certain noradrenergic and dopaminergic receptor sites in the CNS. It has been hypothesized that these drugs make the reticular system in the midbrain less sensitive to impulses from the sensory pathways. The blocking of dopaminergic receptors in the corpus striatum is responsible for the extrapyramidal side-effects of antipsychotic drugs. The pharmacodynamic action of *monoamine oxidase* (*MAO*) *inhibitors* occurs by inhibiting the deamination of biogenic amines, resulting in increased amounts of norepinephrine, dopamine, or serotonin at receptor sites in the CNS and other tissues.[5] The *tricyclics* are also considered to have an effect on the catecholamines in the CNS. They may exert an influence on the balance between the central cholinergic and adrenergic mechanisms.[3, 4, 6] By blocking the reuptake of catecholamines into presynaptic terminals, and by inhibiting the deamination of biogenic amines, the latter become available at central receptor sites in increased amounts.

Other important and exciting research areas include, for example, tardive dyskinesia, the increasing ability to measure tissue levels of enzymes and drugs, and a group of new drugs including the tetracycline antidepressants, cerebral metabolic stimulants such as Pyritinol and Naftidrofuryl, various memory-facilitating drugs such as Isoprinosine, Piracetam, choline chloride, and neuropeptide fragments of adrenocorticotropic hormone, physostigmine, and vasopressin.[7–10]

All of this leaves no doubt that psychopharmacology will play an increasingly important role in geropsychiatric practice.

In order to be adequately prepared to make optimal use of these psychoactive drugs in treating elderly patients with mental illness, essentially three requirements must be met. First, it is necessary to have sufficient theoretical knowledge concerning the pharmacodynamic properties of specific drugs. Second, the clinician needs to know the characteristics of the "host"; that is, in which ways the elderly patient responds differently to drugs, compared with patients in younger age groups. Third, the application of theoretical knowledge in the clinical setting is another indispensable skill. Such practical know-how is acquired through clinical experience, over a period of years. In this chapter, the main emphasis will be on the latter two points. Information on the pharmacodynamics of specific drugs will be presented, in the appropriate context, in subsequent chapters.

DRUG RESPONSES IN THE ELDERLY

Although many aged patients are treated with psychotropic drugs, comparatively little evidence is available from well-controlled studies on the effectiveness of these drugs in specific geropsychiatric conditions. The factors which influence drug responses in elderly patients can be categorized, depending on whether they are specific (age-related) or nonspecific (unrelated to age), and whether they are physical or nonphysical.

AGE-RELATED FACTORS

Physical Determinants

With increasing age, drug reactions in the individual change. This is related to specific factors such as changed absorption and distribution patterns of the drug, alterations in its metabolism, decreased capacity of the liver to detoxify, reduced renal capacity to excrete, decreased cerebral blood flow and cerebral metabolism, organic brain syndrome, etc.[11, 12] In addition to considering these functions separately, it is important to keep in mind that the overall capacity for homeostasis, or physiological stability, as a general systems characteristic, is reduced in range and resilience. Hence, the margin for error is narrowed and the probability of side-effects is increased; and once side-effects develop, they tend to be rather incapacitating. Since the homeostatic mechanisms of the component organs and of the system as a whole are diminished, the threshold for toxic side-effects is proportionately lowered.[13] Drug responses in older persons are often comparable to those in the very young. This has been related to renal function which is undeveloped in the young and declining in the aged, and to age-related changes in the capacity to metabolize drugs (microsomal enzyme activity, for example, may decrease in old age).[14] It must be kept in mind, however, that such age-related decrements are not equally applicable to all individuals in a given age group.

Absorption. The absorption of drugs may be slowed or diminished in aged persons because of various reasons such as a decrease in gastric acid output with an associated reduction of drug solubility, reduced abdominal blood flow, reduction in size of absorbing surfaces, and impairment of enzyme systems responsible for transport across gastrointestinal membranes.[13]

Drug Distribution. Once a drug reaches the circulation, its distribution depends on the extent to which the drug is protein-bound in the plasma, the distribution patterns of blood flow, the ability of the drug to pass through various membranes, and the specific properties of tissue affinity. Drugs in circulation may be bound to plasma proteins, especially albumin. Since plasma albumin decreases with advancing age, the amount of bound drug may be reduced proportionately.[15] With regard to the factor of peripheral blood flow, a lowered cardiac output in older patients results in a redistribution in favor of cerebral and coronary circulation at the expense of blood flow to the liver and kidney.[16]

Excretion and Metabolism. Once a drug is in the circulation, its concentration in the blood reflects the rate at which it is eliminated. The kidney is the primary route for elimination. Increasing age is accompanied by diminished glomerular filtration and tubular secretory capacity. Likewise, the ability of the liver to metabolize drugs decreases with advancing age. The effect of age on the blood level and half-life of the drugs indicates a decrease in the rate at which drugs are metabolized and eliminated, especially in relation to their generally less impaired absorption. The resulting higher blood levels may contribute to the higher incidence of adverse drug effects.

Other Age-related Effects. Altered drug activity in older individuals may occur in the absence of changes in the drug level in blood. This may be due to changes in the number of receptors, structural changes in the responsive tissue, and less effective homeostatic capacity.[13] Drugs with central nervous system effects, for example, show changed activity with advancing age, which is probably due to a reduction in the number of receptors.[17] Thus, the action of stimulants is reduced with age, while the action of depressants is enhanced.[18] Barbiturates, for example, tend to have erratic or paradoxical (stimulating) effects. Changes in homeostatic capacity may also influence the overall response to a drug. For example, elderly persons have an impaired capacity to respond effectively to orthostatic stress, resulting in blood pressure drop on standing. This particular homeostatic loss may be aggravated by phenothiazines and antidepressants.

Nonphysical Determinants

The aged individual probably also reacts differently to drugs as a result of age-related psychological and behavioral factors. Research efforts aimed at comparing therapeutic effectiveness of psychotropic drugs in younger and older patients may be hampered by the probability that psychopathological processes (and hence, psychiatric syndromes and target symptoms) in the two age groups are not comparable. For example, there may well be profound differences in the etiology, pathogenesis, psychodynamics, and clinical symptomatology of depression in old people as compared with younger adults. In previous chapters, the question was raised if and how the aging process can modify the overt manifestations of a psychiatric disorder, and to what extent the age-specific psychiatric disorders (developing for the first time in old age) fit the diagnostic cubbyholes designed several decades ago when the psychiatric problems of old people and late life were not as much in focus as nowadays. The new diagnostic nomenclature for psychiatry is attempting a more practical approach to the etiological and clinical aspects of the various disorders.[19]

NONSPECIFIC FACTORS

Physical Determinants

This category pertains, by and large, to the *interaction between drugs* and drug-drug toxicity. A thorough review of this important topic would go far beyond the scope of this text. Only a few points will be presented, to illustrate and emphasize the need to familiarize oneself with information already available and keep informed about future research findings.[20, 21]

Therapeutic effects can be antagonized by compounds interfering with absorption of the drug, increasing the rate of its metabolism, or blocking the transport mechanism to the drug's site of action. On the other hand, inhibition of the drug's metabolism facilitates transport of the drug to its site of action, enhancing therapeutic as well as adverse effects.

Interference with Transport of Drug to Site of Action. *Interference with Absorption.* Antacids interfere with the gastrointestinal absorption of antipsychotic agents.[22] Diphenylhydantoin and other anticonvulsants impair the absorption of folic acid.

Induction of Hepatic Microsomal Enzymes. The action of many drugs depends on the rate at which they are metabolized by enzymes in the liver endoplasmic reticulum (microsomes). The activities of these enzymes can be increased by several drugs; e.g., phenobarbital, other barbiturates, glutethimide (Doriden), many hypnotics, smoking, and caffeine. Drugs which induce microsomal enzymes decrease the action of many other drugs. Phenobarbital, for example, can facilitate the metabolizing of chlorpromazine, heparin, coumarin, corticosteroids, and diphenylhydantoin, thus lowering their plasma levels.[23] Methylphenidate (Ritalin), on the other hand, inhibits the liver microsomal enzyme system,[24] and may reduce the metabolism of diphenylhydantoin, tricyclic antidepressants, phenothiazines, and anticoagulants. As a result, the blood level of these drugs is increased.

Blocking Drug Transport. Guanethidine (Ismelin), an antihypertensive drug, is concentrated at its site of action in adrenergic neurons by a transport system in the membrane of the neuron. Antidepressant drugs inhibit the uptake of guanethidine into the neuron terminal and thus prevent its action. In hypertensive patients who are taking antidepressants of the imipramine type, this type of drug-drug interaction can be quite serious. Antipsychotic agents, especially chlorpromazine, also antagonize the hypotensive action of guanethidine, probably by the same mechanism as that of the tricyclic antidepressants. Haloperidol (Haldol) and thiothixene (Navane) have a similar effect, although less prominent.

These antipsychotic agents probably prevent the access of guanethidine to the neuron, by blockade of the amine uptake pump.[25]

Transporting Undue Amounts of Drug to Site of Action. *Displacement of Drugs Bound to Plasma Proteins.* Drugs may be reversibly bound to plasma protein (especially albumin) and not be active pharmacologically. Another drug can have the property of competing for the same binding sites. When one drug is competitively displaced by another drug, the former becomes pharmacologically active, intensifying its effect. For example, tolbutamide (Orinase) is mostly bound to plasma proteins, but can be displaced by sulfaphenazole; the resulting increase in pharmacologically active tolbutamide may cause critical hypoglycemia. In a similar way, the hypnotic agent chloralhydrate may cause an increased bleeding tendency in a patient who already is on anticoagulants.[26]

Inhibition of the Metabolism of Drugs. This will increase their action. The metabolic inactivation of diphenylhydantoin (Dilantin), for example, is decreased by bishydroxycoumarin (Coumadin) and isoniazid; thus, signs of diphenylhydantoin overdosage may occur if the patient is taking these drugs in combination.

Change in Response at Site of Drug Action. In patients taking monoamine oxidase (MAO) inhibitor antidepressants (e.g., Nardil, Parnate), hypertensive crises may result from ingesting certain foods (e.g., aged cheese or chicken livers) which contain tyramine, or from indirectly acting sympathomimetics, including even caffeine. Excessive release of norepinephrine is the cause of the hypertensive crises in patients receiving MAO inhibitors. The clinical signs of such attacks essentially consist of the manifestations typical of a pheochromocytoma, such as headache, nausea, sweating, palpitations, rapid pulse, and constricting chest pains. In view of this, the appropriate treatment consists of administering phentolamine (Regitine), which is an α-adrenergic blocking agent.

In rare cases, the combination of a MAO inhibitor with a tricyclic antidepressant, or the starting of a tricyclic within a few days after stopping a MAO inhibitor, causes hyperthermia, delirium, and coma. Although this occurs infrequently, the combination of these drugs should be prescribed with great caution.

Gender. That *gender* may play a role in the effect of a drug is suggested by the finding that methylphenidate is a more effective antianxiety agent for females than for males, while in the case of diazepam, the reverse is true.[27] Elderly male patients appear to be more responsive to the antidepressant effects of imipramine.[28]

Nonphysical Determinants

Law of Initial Value. According to the *law of initial value*, the response of an organism to a stimulus depends, among other things, on the prestimulus (baseline) condition of the organism. Thus, a stimulating drug is likely to be less effective if the organism already is in a state of excitation and a sedative is less effective in a state of inhibition. In fact, there may be a paradoxical reaction: the excited patient may become less excited following administration of a stimulant and the inhibited patient may become restless from a sedative. An example of the latter situation is seen in patients who are inactive, take frequent daytime naps, and then cannot sleep at night; a sedative at nighttime is likely to have no effect or, paradoxically, may result in restlessness or confusion. The proper approach here is to promote activities during the daytime so that the patient is fatigued in the evening.

Personality Characteristics. Characteristics such as extroversion, introversion, aggressiveness, passivity, emotionality, and obsessiveness undoubtedly also contribute to interindividual differences in drug responses.[29] In patients who are intelligent, introspective, and self-observing, certain physical side-effects of antipsychotic drugs may accentuate depersonalization, resulting in further instability of the body image. In other cases, a drug may specifically affect a major defense or interfere with a coping mechanism, such as obsessive-compulsive behavior.

> In the case of an elderly man, preoccupied with his sexual impotence, antidepressant drugs had the effect of energizing his tendency to act out and precipitating pedophiliac behavior.

Passive types of men are probably less disturbed by side-effects interfering with ejaculation or erection than aggressive, "cocky" characters. Narcissistic types of women may be quite upset about the weight gain due to certain phenothiazines. Hypomanic, extrovert, active, and compulsive individuals of all ages tend to feel guilty when, under the influence of tranquilizers, they slow down, work less, and spend more time in bed.

Social Class. Related to the factor of personality characteristics is the variable of *social class*. In a study of comparing the effects of magnesium pemoline versus methylphenidate, it was found that middle class patients responded better to both drugs than lower class patients did.[30]

Placebo-Effect. The *placebo-effect* refers to any reaction not due to specific pharmacodynamic effects but derived from the subjective meaning that the drug has to the patient. The doctor-patient relationship is one of the most important factors in determining which meaning the patient unconsciously assigns to the drug. Therapies and drugs appear to be more effective when the physician himself is convinced of their usefulness. Depending on these factors, the placebo-effect will be favorable or unfavorable. In the latter case, the placebo-effect may be described as a "side-effect." In some instances, the placebo-effect overshadows the pharmacodynamic effects.

> A chronically depressed woman, who was showing a progressive shift toward hypochondriasis, expressed enormous trepidation about taking an antidepressant medication (amitriptyline). She insisted that, some years ago, she already had been given this drug,

and it had not helped. Now she was afraid that it would make her "violently sick." She finally agreed to try taking just one tablet daily—as if it were a favor on her part. During subsequent weekly follow-ups, she would relate how "that pill makes me sick—it makes everything back up on me—it is like getting choked." The only indication that she did ingest and assimilate some of the drug was her improved appearance, and a gain in weight.

CLINICAL APPLICATION: SOME GUIDELINES

SIDE-EFFECTS

Definition

Side-effects are all those drug effects which are "undesirable, adverse, unwanted, untoward." The precise definition of a side-effect is not always possible, because the patient and his physician may disagree as to what constitutes an "untoward, unwanted" drug effect, versus a therapeutic desirable one. In certain situations, the sedative effects of psychotropic drugs could be welcomed by the busy personnel of a geropsychiatric ward; but it is clear that any sedative effect that amounts to a chemical straight jacket is antitherapeutic. On the other hand, many outpatients who are maintained on antidepressant drugs, and function well during the day at home and at work, welcome the sedative side-effects of tricyclics, such as doxepin (Sinequan) and amitriptyline (Elavil), when the hour of sleep arrives.

Incidence

Generally, aged patients have a lower tolerance for psychotropic drugs, and require smaller doses than younger patients to reach a desired therapeutic effect. Likewise, side-effects in the elderly usually develop at lower dosage levels. The incidence of side effects reported in the literature depends on the definition of side-effect, the particular patient population under study, and the accuracy of the assessment techniques. The issue of accuracy of measurement techniques involves the reliability of the various rating scales being used, the problem of achieving inter-rater reliability, and the nearly impossible task of controlling the innumerable variables encountered in a clinical setting. In spite of all these constraints which limit precise determination of the incidence of side-effects, there is general agreement that the incidence of serious adverse drug reactions is simply too high.[31, 32]

The risk of adverse drug reactions increases with age. Seidl et al.[33] observed an increase with age in the incidence of adverse drug reactions, from 11.9 percent in the 41–50 year age group, to 24.9 percent in the 80+ age group. In Hurwitz's study, 7.5 percent of patients in the 40–49 age group had side effects, and 21.3 percent in the 70–79 age group.[34] Examples of drugs which tend to produce a higher incidence of adverse reactions in older patients include digitalis, barbiturates, thiazide diuretics (more risk of potassium depletion), and phenothiazines (a higher incidence of extrapyramidal symptoms).[2, 13, 35]

Not only does the incidence of adverse drug reactions increase with age, but also the extent of their severity. In addition, some side-effects can cause new complications, e.g., postural hypotension causing a fall with resulting fracture, or causing a cerebrovascular accident.

Differential Diagnosis

At times it may be difficult to distinguish between a "true" side-effect and a placebo-effect. In addition, it is possible to mistake side-effects for a worsening of the primary psychiatric disorder. For example, motor restlessness and akathisia (inability to sit still) are side-effects of antipsychotic drugs, but may prompt one to increase the dosage on the assumption that the psychosis is worse, thereby setting up a vicious circle.

A good example of the complexity of differential diagnosis is presented by the central anticholinergic syndrome. There are many causes of confusion in the aged, but one is basically an atropine-type toxicity caused by the *anticholinergic effects* of the phenothiazines, tricyclic antidepressants, or antiparkinson agents. Hence, patients using combinations of these drugs are even more likely to develop anticholinergic side-effects.[6]

The *central anticholinergic syndrome* is characterized by marked disturbance of short-term memory, impaired attention, disorientation, visual and auditory hallucinations, and increased psychotic thinking. The syndrome can be associated with peripheral anticholinergic signs; e.g., dry membranes, tachycardia, flushing, dilated pupils, and urinary retention. It can present a difficult diagnostic problem in psychiatric patients because the anticholinergic toxic signs may resemble the symptomatology of the primary psychosis. This may prompt one to increase the dosage of the psychotropic drugs with a resulting aggravation of the symptomatology. By keeping alert to the possibility of central anticholinergic toxicity, and performing careful mental status and physical exams (especially looking for peripheral anticholinergic signs), a correct diagnosis can be established and appropriate intervention started (lowering the dosage or stopping the drug). Antiparkinson drugs are perhaps the most frequent cause of the central anticholinergic syndrome. This is especially relevant because many patients do not really need these drugs in conjunction with antipsychotic medications.

Physostigmine reverses the toxic symptomatology but does not modify the symptomatology of the primary underlying psychosis itself. The central anticholinergic syndrome can be treated by 0.5–1.0 mg of physostigmine, intramuscularly, to be repeated every 2 hours as indicated.[36] In the exceptional case where the diagnosis remains obscure, physostigmine salicylate can be used as a diagnostic tool. Physostigmine may be used only after thorough medical evaluation because of the danger of excessive parasympathetic stimulation. Since atropine sulfate is effective in reversing cholinergic toxicity, it is wise to have this drug ready when the physostigmine test is done. The importance of this test is to obtain proof that the confusional syndrome indeed represents atropine toxicity.[6]

SOME GENERAL GUIDELINES

In view of the multiple factors influencing drug effects in aged patients, it is not surprising that there is such a great variety in drug requirements, therapeutic responses, and side-effects. The correct type and amount of drug usually is determined by a cautious trial and error approach.

Drug-free Baseline

The discontinuance of current psychotropic medication to get a *drug-free baseline state* is useful to obtain an accurate assessment of the efficacy of a prospective drug. Once this behavioral baseline is known and a specific drug is administered, the behavioral changes are recorded at regular intervals. The optimal setting for this would be the hospital, but this procedure can also be carried on an out-patient basis, provided the patient returns regularly to the clinic for follow-up evaluations.

Medical Status

Evaluation of the patient's *medical status* and of the drugs used for his medical problems is essential to be alert to potential future drug-drug interactions. Multiple physical illnesses being treated with multiple drugs increases the risk of drug-drug toxicity in a near geometrical fashion.[37] Side-effects in aged patients may be difficult to differentiate from actual age-related physical disorders, including organic brain syndrome, cardiac disease, neurological disorders, glaucoma, prostate hypertrophy, impotence, etc.

Treatment Specificity

In clinical practice, the selection and dosage of psychotropic drugs are usually determined by the presenting psychological symptoms and behavioral signs, rather than the specific underlying psychiatric syndrome. Yet, in planning the treatment, it is important to be as *specific* as is possible. The physician must formulate some explicit notions concerning the etiology, pathogenesis, and psychodynamics of the disturbed behavior. By adhering to these general principles, several risks can be reduced or prevented: overmedication, undermedication, and the "shot-gun" approach.[38]

Polypharmacy

Polypharmacy clouds clinical signs. It may become impossible to distinguish among the intended effect of the drug, its side-effects, the placebo-effect, and the manifestations of the patient's initial symptoms. Since aged patients frequently have several chronic conditions simultaneously, overmedication is especially likely to occur in their management. A number of elderly patients are actually hospitalized due to multiple drug-related symptoms. In these cases, hospitalization is required to discontinue the questionable drugs, evaluate the patient's physical and psychological baseline on this drug-free (or reduced drug) status, and determine what medications are really indicated. Learoyd emphasizes the hazards of polypharmacy.[32] His study showed that 16 percent of the elderly patients, who were on psychotropic drugs before hospitalization and showed abnormal behavior, improved dramatically when the drugs were stopped. About 20 percent of the geropsychiatric admissions were precipitated by adverse effects of psychotropic drugs.

Undertreatment

Another risk is *undertreatment*. Many psychotropic drugs begin to exert their maximum therapeutic effect only after some weeks following the initial doses. To stop treatment before that time, or to fail to increase the dosage to optimal levels, may be worse than no treatment at all. Friedel has reviewed the concept of the "therapeutic window" wherein there is little therapeutic effect below a certain blood level, but also toxic effects predominate above it.[11]

Shot-gun Approach

The *"shot-gun" approach* refers to the practice of indiscriminately blanketing the target symptoms with a barrage of drugs, in the hope that at least one of them will be effective. Drug combinations should be used with caution, because the side-effects may multiply. If a second drug must be used, it is wise to give the first medication alone long enough to be able to evaluate its therapeutic and side-effects.

Consistent Drug Prescription

In view of the many different types of psychotropic drugs available, it is advisable to develop an *in-depth acquaintance* by working consistently with a few representative drugs, selected from the major drug categories, that appear to have withstood the test of time.[39] Such a systematic approach stands in contrast to "browsing around" with drugs. What happens often is that the patient is subjected to inconsistent drug patterns, because he is periodically transferred from one doctor to another. And each physician may decide to try out "his own" drug.

Inconsistent Drug Prescription

The opposite of therapeutic inconsistency is *therapeutical obstinacy*: the continuation of a particular drug while the clinical evidence does not support its efficacy, or even suggests possible harmfulness. This is a risk in some outpatient clinic settings with a high turnover of physicians and with revolving door type of consultants. Each new physician is likely to start off by continuing the drug (and its dosage) prescribed by his predecessor. Changing the drug or the dosage would be time-consuming and require a series of visits at regular intervals, and the new physician is usually more involved in getting acquainted with his overall caseload. By the time he has accomplished that, 6–12 months have passed, which is pretty close to the "half-life" of psychiatric consultants in some outpatient settings. Thus, by the time review and reappraisal of the patient's drug regimen would be possible, a new consultant arrives, who again starts off by continuing the same drug and dosage prescribed by his predecessor, and so on.

> An elderly woman with a "psychotic depression" turned out to be taking perphenazine (Trilafon) 16 mg three times daily (t.i.d.). Over a period of several weeks this was reduced to 4 mg t.i.d. By then, the "depression" had begun to lift, but it took about 3 months before the improvement in her mood and attentiveness had stabilized. Essentially, this patient was schizophrenic, with minimal residual symptoms. Unfortunately, she also began to have, at the lower dosage level, a moderate degree of orobuccolingual dyskinesia. The patient, however, preferred this type of disability to her zombie-like status at higher dosage levels.

Dosage Level

Since in a given elderly patient, neither the optimal dosage nor the maximum dose tolerated are known beforehand, it is useful to follow an individualized approach. Starting with low doses, one gradually increases the amount, while observing the patient's response and remaining alert to the development of side-effects, until therapeutic effects are achieved. Generally, it is best to start treatment at a dosage level about one-quarter to one-third of the recommended adult dosage, particularly for the more debilitated patients. The dosage can be increased according to tolerance.[40]

In the acute phase of a psychosis, it is wise to start at a low level but move rapidly to effective dosages of the drug; during the chronic phase, the dosage should be gradually reduced to the required minimum. Not infrequently, the dosage level may be too low during the acute phase of a psychosis, and too high during the chronic phase. It is particularly easy to leave a hospitalized patient on a high dose of psychotropic drugs, even after the acute phase of the psychosis has subsided. In the case of antipsychotics, this will increase the risks of dyskinesia, parkinsonism, and other complications. Therefore, periodical review and readjustment of dosage levels are required.

Dosage Patterns

Particular attention must be given to instructing the patient (and/or family, or responsible others) regarding the amount of drug to be taken, the times of day, etc. It is frequently useful to write instructions on a prescription form, so as to be clear and to emphasize the importance of the regimen. There is no general agreement about the practice of spreading the dosage of psychotropic drugs throughout the day, versus taking the entire amount at bedtime. The latter is sometimes recommended for the sake of convenience and to obtain maximum benefit from any sedative effects, e.g., in the case of tricyclics. However, aged patients may be less able to tolerate the sudden absorption of a relatively large drug dosage into their blood circulation. In addition, the physician's emphasis on precise regularity of drug schedules enhances the patient's respect for the therapeutic regimen, and results in optimal use of the placebo-effect.[41]

Side-Effects and Drug-Drug Interactions

When patients are being maintained on psychotropic drugs in the community after release from the hospital, it is good practice to inform both the patient and the relatives (or boarding home operator, etc.) of the manifestations of possible side-effects, and to caution them regarding certain drug-drug incompatibilities.

Regular Review

Patients maintained on psychotropic drugs should be *regularly reviewed* with regard to indications to adjust dosage (up or down), the risk of insidious, progressive side-effects, the possibility of a developing physical illness that would require other drug treatment with subsequent increased risk of drug-drug interactions, and making sure that the patient indeed is taking the drug as instructed. Some geropsychiatric patients who are maintained on antipsychotic drugs may undergo a change in their responsiveness to the drug, either in terms of greater or lesser sensitivity. Such variations in responsiveness usually involve time periods of several months and point out the necessity of regular checkups, at least three or four times a year.[42]

Prolonged Action of Drugs

Certain drugs (e.g., barbiturates, antihistamines, tranquilizers, lithium) can have a *prolonged action* resulting in confusion, ataxia, or other side effects. In the case of an out-patient setting, the patient himself may stop (or "forget") taking the drugs, without disclosing this to the physician at the time of follow-up. It is useful to ask the patient to describe the drugs he is supposed to be taking, how often he takes each one, and at what times of the day. When the drug regimen has been delegated to a relative (or rest home operator, etc.), the information should be obtained from them.

Individualized Drug Therapy

Finally, while the need for drug maintenance varies from patient to patient, and an empirical, individualized approach is called for, a few general points may be kept in mind:

Aged schizophrenics seem to tolerate discontinuation of antipsychotic drugs better than younger schizophrenics.

Patients maintained on antianxiety drugs report rather often that the efficacy of the drug seems to decrease in time. In such cases, one may try periodic switching to other, related drugs, and after an interval (usually several months) start the patient again on the original drug. The same approach may be useful in the case of sedatives and hypnotics.

Antiparkinson drugs should not be used routinely to prevent extrapyramidal side effects, since not all patients will develop these. While antiparkinson drugs may play a primary role in producing the central anticholinergic syndrome, they also happen to be the type of drug which can be most easily discontinued.[6]

In maintaining patients on antipsychotic drugs for long periods of time, the benefits of the drug must be weighed against the risk of tardive dyskinesia in the future.[43]

References

1. Prien, R. F., Haber, P. A., and Caffey, E. M.: The use of psychoactive drugs in elderly patients with psychiatric disorders: Survey in twelve Veterans Administration hospitals. *J. Am. Geriatr. Soc. 23:*104–112, 1975.
2. Prentice, R.: Patterns of psychoactive drug use among the elderly. In: *The Aging Process and Psychoactive Drug Use,* Services Research Monograph Series, No. 79-813, United States Department of Health, Education and Welfare, Washington, D. C., 1979. pp. 17–41.
3. Sourkes, T. L.: Biochemical effect of psychotropic drugs. In: *Principles of Psychopharmacology,* edited by W. G. Clark and J. D. Giudice, ed. 2, Academic Press, New York, 1978. pp. 97–104.
4. Friedel, R. O.: The biochemical basis of psychopharmacology. In: *Drug Issues in Geropsychiatry,* edited by W. E. Fann and G. L. Maddox, The Williams and Wilkins Company, Baltimore, 1974. pp. 9–17.
5. Quitkin, F., Rifkin, A., and Klein, D. F.: Monoamine oxidase inhibitors. *Arch. Gen. Psychiatry 36:*749–760, 1979.
6. Davis, J. M., Fann, W. E., El-Yousef, M. K., and Janowsky, D. S.: Clinical problems in treating the aged with psychotropic drugs. In: *Advances in Behavioral Biology,* edited by C. Eisdorfer and W. E. Fann, vol. 6, Plenum Press, New York, 1973. pp. 111–125.
7. Ban, T. A.: Vasodilators, stimulants, and anabolic agents in the treatment of geropsychiatric patients. In: *Psychopharmacology: A Generation of Progress,* edited by M. A. Lipton, A. DiMascio, and K. F. Killam, Raven Press, New York, 1978. pp. 1525–1533.
8. Branconnier, R. J., Cole, J. O., and Gardos, G.: ACTH 4–10 in the amelioration of neuropsychological symptomatology associated with senile organic brain syndrome. *Psychopharmacol. Bull. 14(1):*27–30, 1978.
9. Davis, K. L., Mohs, R. C., Tinklenberg, J. R., Pfeffenbaum, A., Hollister, L. E., and Kopell, B. S.: Physostigmine: improvement of long-term memory processes in normal humans. *Science 201:*272–274, 1978.
10. Legros, J. J., Gilot, P., Seron, X., Claessens, J., Adam, A., Moeglen, J. M., Audibert, A., and Berchier, P.: Influence of vasopressin on learning and memory. *Lancet 8054:*41–42, 1978.
11. Friedel, R. O.: Pharmacokinetics in the geropsychiatric patient. In: *Psychopharmacol-*

ogy: *A Generation of Progress*, edited by M. A. Lipton, A. DiMascio, and K. F. Killam, Raven Press, New York, 1978. pp. 1499–1505.

12. Beattie, B. L., and Sellers, E. M.: Psychoactive drug use in the elderly: the pharmacokinetics. *Psychosomatics 20(7)*:474–479, 1979.
13. Bender, A. D.: Pharmacodynamic principles of drug therapy in the aged. *J. Am. Geriatr. Soc. 22*:296–303, 1974.
14. Kato, R., Vassanelli, P., Frontino, G., et al: Variation in the activity of liver microsomal drug-metabolizing enzymes in rats in relation to age. *Biochem. Pharmacol. 13*:1037, 1964.
15. Rafsky, H. S., Brill, A. A., Stern, K. G., and Corey, H.: Electrophoretic studies on the serum of "normal" aged individuals. *Am. J. Med. Sci. 224*:522, 1952.
16. Goldman, R.: Speculations on vascular changes with age. *J. Am. Geriatr. Soc. 18*:765, 1970.
17. Domino, E. F., Dren, A. T., and Giardina, W. J.: Biochemical and neurotransmitter changes in the aging brain. In: *Psychopharmacology: A Generation of Progress*, edited by M. A. Lipton, A. DiMascio, and K. F. Killam, Raven Press, New York, 1978. pp. 1507–1515.
18. Verzar, F.: The age of the individual as one of the parameters of pharmacological action. *Acta Physiol. Acad. Sci. Hung. 19*:313, 1961.
19. American Psychiatric Association Task Force on Nomenclature and Statistics. *DSM-III: Diagnostic Criteria Draft*, American Psychiatric Association, Washington, D. C. 1978.
20. Fann, W. E.: Interactions of psychotropic drugs in the elderly. *Postgrad. Med. 53*:182–186, 1973.
21. Kral, V. A.: An overview of psychopharmacology of old age. *Psychopharmacol. Bull. 12*:51–52, 1976.
22. Fann, W. E., Davis, J. M., Janowsky, D. S., and Schmidt, D. M.: Chlorpromazine effects of antacids on its gastrointestinal absorption. *J. Clin. Pharmacol. 13*:388–390, 1973.
23. Conney, A. H., and Burns, J. J.: Factors influencing drug metabolism. *Adv. Pharmacol. 1*:31–58, 1962.
24. Wharton, R. N., Perel, J. M., Dayton, P. G., et al: A potential clinical use for the interaction of methylphenidate with tricyclic antidepressants. *Am. J. Psychiatry 127*: 1619–1625, 1971.
25. Janowsky, D. S., Fann, W. E., and Davis, J. M.: Chlorpromazine reversal of guanethidine hypotension. *Am. J. Psychiatry 130*:808–812, 1973.
26. Piland, B.: The aging process and psychoactive drug use in clinical treatment. In: *National Institute on Drug Abuse. The Aging Process and Psychoactive Drug Use: Services Research Monograph Series*. Publication No. 79-813. United States Department of Health, Education and Welfare, Washington, D. C., 1979. pp. 1–16.
27. Salzman, C., and Shader, R.: Responses to psychotropic drugs in the normal elderly. In: *Advances in Behavioral Biology*, edited by C. Eisdorfer and W. E. Fann, vol. 6, Plenum Press, New York, 1973. pp. 159–168.
28. Prange, A. J., Wilson, I. C., Know, A. E., McClane, T. K., Breese, G. R., Martin, B. R., Alltop, L. B., and Lipton, M. A.: Thyroid-imipramine interaction: Clinical results and basic mechanism. In: *Brain Chemistry and Mental Disease*, edited by B. T. Ho and W. M. McIsaac, Plenum Press, New York, 1971. p. 197.
29. Di Mascio, A.: Personality and variability of response to psychotropic drugs: relationship to "paradoxical effects." In: *Non-Specific Factors in Drug Therapy*, edited by K. Rickels, Charles C Thomas, Springfield, Illinois, 1968. pp. 40–49.
30. Rickels, K., Gordon, P. E., Gausman, D. H., and Weise, C. C. Pereria-Organ, J. A., and Hesbacher, P. T.: Pemoline and methylphenidate in mildly depressed outpatients. *Clin. Pharmacol. Ther. 11*:698–710, 1970.
31. Maddox, G. L.: Drugs, physicians, and patients. In: *Drug Issues in Geropsychiatry*, edited by W. E. Fann and G. L. Maddox, The Williams and Wilkins Company, Baltimore, 1974. pp. 3–6.
32. Learoyd, B. M.: Psychotropic drugs in the aging patient. *Med. J. Aust. 1*:1131, 1972.
33. Seidl, L. G., Thornton, G. F., Smith, J. W., et al: Studies on the epidemiology of adverse drug reactions, III. Reactions in patients on a general medical service. *Bull. Johns Hopkins Hosp. 119*:299, 1966.

34. Hurwitz, N.: Predisposing factors in adverse reactions to drugs. *Br. Med. J. 1*:536, 1969.
35. Petersen, D. M., and Thomas, C. W.: Acute drug reactions among the elderly. *J. Gerontol. 30*:552–556, 1975.
36. El-Yousef, M. K., Janowsky, D. S., Davis, J. M., and Sekerke, H. J.: Reversal by physostigmine of antiparkinsonian drug toxicity. *Am. J. Psychiatry 130*:141–145, 1973.
37. Fraccia, J. et al: Combination drug therapy. *J. Am. Geriatr. Soc. 13*:508–511, 1975.
38. Kenny, A. D.: Designing therapy for the elderly. *Drug Therapy 9(7)*:49–64, 1979.
39. Whanger, A. D., and Busse, E. W.: Geriatrics. In: *The Therapist's Handbook: Treatment Methods of Mental Disorders*, edited by B. B. Wolman, Van Nostrand Reinhold Company, New York, 1976. pp. 287–324.
40. Fann, W. E., Wheless, J. C., and Richman, B. W.: Treating the aged with psychotropic drugs. *Gerontologist 16*:322–328, 1976.
41. Prange, A. J.: Use of antidepressant drugs in the elderly patient. In: *Advances in Behavioral Biology*, edited by C. Eisdorfer and W. E. Fann, vol. 6, Plenum Press, New York, 1973. pp. 225–237.
42. Whanger, A. D., and Busse, E. W.: Care in hospital. In: *Modern Perspectives in the Psychiatry of Old Age*, edited by J. G. Howells, Brunner/Mazel, New York, 1975. pp. 450–485.
43. Crane, G. E., and Smeets, R. A.: Tardive dyskinesia and drug therapy in geriatric patients. *Arch. Gen. Psychiatry 30*:341–343, 1974.

11

psychotherapy and sociotherapy

CHARACTERISTICS OF THERAPY WITH THE AGED

Psychiatric therapy with the aged involves more than the average number of emergencies: complex problems of scheduling (time, place, duration), problems related to the fact that the patient, although an adult, is often dependent on other members of his family, the typically multigenerational nature of the problem, and the frequent coincidence of organic brain disease and psychogenic trauma. Home visits, in view of the physical difficulties of the patient, are a necessity to the practice of geropsychiatry as well.[1–3]

GOALS OF TREATMENT

The characteristics of the illness, the patient's environment (family, economic resources, etc.), and the aging process itself usually determine what are rational treatment goals. Sometimes, the primary goal may be to provide relief for the relatives rather than for the patient.

> One woman, in her 60's, had visited, every day for years, her demented husband in the hospital. The nursing personnel disliked her because she was bossy, and interfering with the institutional routine. But this demented husband was all this woman had: she had no children, no nearby relatives, and only a few friends. The treatment goal here would be in terms of helping her to develop new interests.
>
> In another case, a professional woman, in her early 50's, consulted the psychiatrist regarding her 80-year-old mother. The latter had been living with her for 15 years, and had become quite "senile." The mother's confusion had become so severe that the daughter realized a new arrangement was in order. In talking about the alternatives, it became apparent how much feeling she had invested in her mother. She stated she was happily married, "but all my time is spent on my work and taking care of my mother." When it was pointed out that nursing home placement for her mother was already overdue, she wondered instead how much longer she could

keep her mother at home. The question was raised to what extent she tried to avoid the inevitable loss of her mother, and to what extent the attention focused on her mother for so long had served to avoid grief about not having children. After thinking this over for a while, she agreed that this was both plausible and probable. Finally, the point was brought up that, not only would she soon face the loss of her mother but also the unsettling prospect of an essentially empty marriage.

On the other hand, some aged patients can be helped by insight therapy, when, for example, deterioration is minimal, ego strength is adequate, the patient is motivated, and adequate environmental support is present. Usually, however, treatment goals with elderly patients are more limited in scope. Once this has been realized and accepted by the physician, he is likely to find that geriatric therapy can indeed be quite rewarding in terms of obtaining tangible improvements in the patient and professional satisfaction for himself. Therapeutic failures with the aged do not have to be more frequent than in many categories of younger patients. Many failures are caused by inadequate diagnostic formulation, deficiencies in the comprehensive treatment plan, or prematurely abandoning the therapeutic program.

PATIENT FACTORS

Communication Difficulty

Due to age-related sensory decrements, intellectual impairment or slowing of central nervous system processes, the patient often has *difficulty in communicating* and cooperating with the physician during the anamnesis and physical examination. It may take him longer to comprehend and respond to questions; he is more likely to forget treatment instructions, etc. Therefore, one may need to talk more slowly (not necessarily louder), to repeat questions and instructions, and to write down advice and suggestions, or date of return visit.

Transference

Since the older patient often "lives in the past," the therapist may be seen more as a person in the patient's past. Thus, the patient may not be able to distinguish the therapist as a real person from the therapist as a *transference* figure. In contrast to therapy with younger adults, the use of transference which can be subjected to analysis is less feasible in the aged.

Transference factors play a role in most interpersonal relations, including an ongoing doctor-patient relationship. Only in insight-oriented psychotherapy is the transference analyzed; in other types of doctor-patient relationships, the transference is left, by and large, untouched. Of practical importance is that an (unanalyzed) positive transference can play a significant role in the patient's clinical improvement.

PHYSICIAN FACTORS

Empathy

Younger physicians may have some difficulty in understanding the experiences of their aged patient. The understanding of another person usually involves the mental process of *empathy*: a transient identification, imagining what it would be like to be "in the other fellow's shoes." For physicians who have not (yet) had the experience of being old, empathic understanding becomes more difficult.

Countertransference

The counterpart of the transference in the patient is the *countertransference* in the physician. Countertransference is common; it may represent a counter-role to the patient's transference roles and expectations. If the roles are fitting and appropriate, the participants in the relationship have something to offer to each other. An elderly woman patient, for example, may unconsciously regard the physician as "the son she never had." If the physician's behavior toward this elderly woman contains elements dating back to the relationship with his own mother, then there may be a fit between mutual expectations and roles. A countertransference, like a transference, becomes a problem in the relationship when it contains relatively strong neurotic components or unconscious ambivalence.

Gerophobic Attitudes

The possible existence of *gerophobic attitudes* on the part of the physician, or his own unresolved fears of aging and death, will make it difficult for him to approach disorders in the aged with enlightened detachment and rational compassion. The obvious constraints in having to set limited therapeutic goals and the lack of opportunity for modifying lifelong patterns of adaptation are added burdens; and so is the contemporary cultural emphasis on youth and attractiveness.[4–6]

Finally, early emotional conflicts which existed between the physician and his own parents may be reactivated causing specific countertransference attitudes. In such cases, effective therapeutic intervention is likely to be seriously handicapped. From a practical point of view, the physician then has two options: refer the patient to a colleague or have counsel with himself regarding the nature of his personal countertransference attitude. As a rule of thumb, it is not wise to continue treating patients for whom one has either excessive likes or dislikes.

REFERRALS TO THE GEROPSYCHIATRIST

Many aged patients have minor emotional problems; the majority of these patients are seen by the nonpsychiatric practitioner. The frequency of psychiatric referrals depends on a number of factors including availability of psychiatrists in the area, the physician's own knowledgeability in the field of geropsychiatry, the attitudes of the patient and his family, socioeconomical factors, etc. When, then, should a psychiatrist be called in? Psychiatric referral and consultations may be needed for two reasons: diagnosis or therapy.

Diagnostic

Some questions and conditions likely to lead to *diagnostic referral* are:

To what extent do psychological factors contribute to physical symptoms (psychophysiological reactions, conversion reactions, depressive equivalent, hypochondriasis, etc.)?

What are the effects of the patient's physical illness on his psychological functions? These somatopsychic reactions include reactive depression, regressive behavior, paranoid reactions, acute confusion, etc.

Evaluation of aged patients preoperatively, and of postoperative complications.

Diagnosis and differential diagnosis of organic brain syndrome, senile regression, depressive states, paranoid phenomena, etc.

Behavior disturbances, such as vindictiveness, combativeness, self-destructive tendencies, overt sexual acting-out, or "geriatric delinquency."

Determinations of mental competency.

Referrals for Treatment and Management

These include the following:

Management of psychotic conditions that require electroconvulsive therapy, lithium therapy, etc.

Advice concerning disposition, e.g., admission to mental hospitals, commitment, release from mental hospitals, placement in specific types of extended care facilities, and counseling the relatives with regard to implementation and implications of such decisions.

Periodic follow-up and re-evaluation of outpatients maintained on psychotropic medications, recommendations for changes in the spectrum of various treatment modalities.

Individual psychotherapy for selected patients such as reactive depressions, identity crisis of late life, marital counselling, and family therapy involving multigenerational conflicts.

PSYCHOTHERAPY

GENERAL CONSIDERATIONS

Basic Skills

Psychotherapy is the planned application by a professional therapist of specific psychological techniques to help the patient, by decreasing or removing psychological disability or misery, and facilitating optimal functioning and well-being. The *basic skills* involved in conducting psychotherapy include the ability to make accurate observations of behavior and to draw from these proper inferences, to synthesize the inferences in a tentative psychodynamic formulation, which serves as a theoretical model and has implications for the type of therapy indicated, to apply specific psychotherapeutic techniques in the therapist-patient relationship and observe the effects of such interventions on the patient, to use this feedback information for the purpose of testing out (confirming, refining, rejecting, etc.) the adequacy of the initial psychodynamic formulation, and to recognize one's personality limitations to avoid creating additional conflict in the patient.[7]

Therapeutic Communication

Basically, psychotherapy is *therapeutic communication.* The goal of the therapist is, first of all, understanding and comprehension, rather than sympathetic agreement or polite disagreement. He must try to discover why the patient is reacting in this way, and at this time. Thus, insight pertains, first and foremost, to a requirement for the therapist, regardless of the type of psychotherapy (insight-oriented versus supportive). Whether or not the therapist communicates his insights to the patient is a separate issue.

Changing and Modifying Behavior

All forms of psychotherapy have in common that they are essentially aimed at *changing and modifying behavior.* They do differ with regard to their specific techniques, and the theoretical premises that represent the framework for, and the basis of, these psychotherapeutic techniques. Not infrequently, there appears to be a tendency to overemphasize alleged differences between various schools of thought, and to create artificial dichotomies. In the case of psychoanalytically oriented therapy, for example, the ultimate goal is not insight per se. Insight, like an x-ray picture, makes translucent what is inside, but such elucidation is not an end in itself. The reason that insight-oriented therapy takes so long is that so much time is needed to apply the newly acquired insights to practices of everyday living. Thus, the psychoanalytical concept of "working through" involves many procedures which can also be understood in the framework of learning theory, behavior therapy, reality therapy, etc.

Formulate a Plan of Action

There are many ways in which elderly people with psychological disturbances can be helped. It is both necessary and possible to determine for each patient which factors contribute in producing a psychological disorder. Only then will it be possible to *formulate a plan of action*, which will contain one major therapeutic aim and appropriate subsidiary ones. Usually, psychotherapy with aged patients is supportive in nature. Few patients need or want an extensive personality change; some are content with solving a minor problem, others are capable of little change.

PSYCHOTHERAPEUTIC APPROACHES

Insight-oriented Psychotherapy

The distinctive feature of *insight-oriented psychotherapy* is the use of free association, and the analysis of the transference. The goal is not primarily the solution of practical problems but the alteration of the personality structure so that it may function more effectively. Through intrapsychic alterations, the ego emerges as a more mature and effective mental agency. This involves conscious recognition of maladaptive defenses and reduction of character rigidities. Regression and transference (brought about by the patient's free associations and the therapist's relative inactivity) are characteristic. Early memories are reactivated; these mobilize the feelings associated with them which makes it possible to explore their role in the present. Insight-oriented therapy is much like an in-depth learning experience. To recognize the problem, its cause and effect, is intellectual insight, whereas true insight includes a reasonable solution. It is this latter point, i.e., attaining a practical solution, which so often represents a problem and constraint in therapy with elderly patients. It may be easy to arrive at insight, but there may not be much opportunity to do anything with it.

> A 62-year-old woman was hospitalized because of a progressively severe neurotic depression. She had been the youngest of four children, and being the only girl, she was "her father's darling." At the time of her birth, the father was 62 years old, being 29 years older than the patient's mother. As a young girl, she felt very close to her father, and looked up to him with awe and admiration. Then, when she was 5 years old, he suddenly died, leaving the family behind in financial chaos. During the next few years, the patient learned that her father really was not all that admirable, but rather irresponsible. This discovery had been a painful disillusionment for her. At the age of 22, she married a prominent, respectable man who was financially well-off, and who was 29 years her senior (attempt to repair the disappointment she had as a little girl). When her husband, now 91 years old, reached his 80's, he became gradually senile. The resulting personality changes on his part (becoming less dependable, more irresponsible, etc.) reactivated the patient's original childhood conflict. She became gradually more and more depressed, and received psychotherapy for several years. She did fairly well in therapy and depended a great deal on her therapist. Then, a few months ago, he suddenly died. Since then, the patient's depression has been significantly worse. The psychodynamics of her depression are rather transparent. Intellectual insight might be

achieved in a short period of time. But the issue is: What would this woman, at age 62, with her 91-year-old senile husband, actually do with her insight? In fact, it is conceivable that this type of knowledge about herself, and the course of her life, could exacerbate her depression.

Thus, it is not surprising that insight frequently comes about when the patient intuitively feels that he can, as it were, afford it.[8]

A well-to-do business man, now in his late 60's, had his first major depressive episode at the age of 48. His premorbid personality was characterized by extreme ambitiousness, aggressiveness, and obsessive-compulsive features. His first goal in life (during his 20's and 30's) had been to make a lot of money (which he did), and to become number one in his field (which he did, too). He married a socialite, mostly as a way to facilitate his commercial endeavors. At the apex of his career, his wife left him, and the patient had a major depressive episode (age 48). After recovering from this, he found himself unable to return to his previous work patterns. The next crisis was an acute myocardial infarct, at age 55. The pattern of semiretirement now changed into full retirement. About this time, the patient married his second wife, 20 years his junior. He needed her youth; she needed the economical security. The marriage worked out surprisingly well, but the patient continued to have recurrent depressive episodes. The origin of these depressions could be understood in the context of what happened in his second marriage. First, a daughter was born, the patient then being 60 years old. This event made it possible to explore his feelings about his mother who had died when he was still a little boy. Then, at 65, he became the father of a son. Having a son was a source of intense pride for him. And, it was only now that he was prepared to come to grips with the ultimate source of his neurotic problem: his own "old man." He had never been able to resolve the ambivalence toward this powerful, capricious man: a mixture of intense admiration and hatred. Being now, himself, the father of a son, he was able to transcend the ambivalence toward his father, an act involving a retroactive conciliation and forgiveness. Thus, at the age of 65, he accomplished what optimally should have been done 60 years earlier (the resolution of the oedipal conflict). He reported that, for the first time in his life, he was experiencing a sense of serenity and gratitude. He retrieved a picture of his father's, framed it, and placed it side by side with that of his son.

Supportive Therapy

In *supportive therapy*, regression and transference are carefully kept within boundaries and not interpreted. The goal is not insight, but support of existing coping mechanisms in the face of current hardships.

Adaptive defenses are strengthened so that they can replace maladaptive ones. In supportive therapy, the goal is to bring the patient back to a satisfactory condition, which for example, could be a prepsychotic neurotic equilibrium. Insight is not achieved deliberately. In order for the patient to be involved in supportive therapy, he should be able to develop positive transference feelings, or feelings of trust and confidence in the physician. Guidance and counseling are forms of supportive therapy which aim at resolving external problems, strengthening ego functioning and enhancing the self-image.

Counseling. In *counseling*, one assists the client or patient in problem-solving by suggesting a course of action and providing support in following that direction. The interviews, usually few in number, are focused on actual interpersonal or situational problems. Likewise, explanations are reality-oriented. Solutions are considered according to the opportunities and constraints of the patient's situation. Although the counselor actively functions as a "teacher," the best solution is the one at which the learner arrives through his own efforts. Counseling is based on the assumption that the patient's ego can deal with the problem once a course of action has been outlined and that, in implementing it, there is minimal interference due to anxiety or other disturbing emotions.

Guidance. In *guidance*, the emotional factors involved are of such magnitude that the ego cannot function effectively until they are brought to light and their nature and role understood. Because of the disturbing emotions, the individual finds himself unable to carry out solutions which he himself may already have thought out. The support of the therapist, who can exert leverage as an authority or parent substitute, and his permissiveness act to free resources restricted by intrapsychic or situational impediments. Clarification of the problem often cannot be achieved without elimination of guilt, fear, or anger. Since these are not traced to their unconscious resources, improvement is accomplished by the therapist's support (empathy, acceptance, and permissiveness) which permits the patient to develop a new emotional perspective.

SOCIOTHERAPY

GENERAL CONSIDERATIONS

Group Context

Usually, supportive psychotherapy with aged patients is best carried out in a *group context.* Group experiences enhance a sense of belonging, an appreciation for the value of external sources of satisfaction, and the effectiveness of reality testing. The group provides an opportunity for ventilation of emotions and discussion of relevant issues (retirement, societal attitudes, religion, "the good old days," complaints about the institution, etc.). Patient groups may also be engaged in activities such as occupational therapy, art therapy, etc. Recreational therapy, carried out in a group setting, may employ a form of psychodrama in which elderly patients are assigned specific roles to play; these may be therapeutic inasmuch as the roles entail the expression of specific emotions and ideas. In the setting of role playing, the patient may experience catharsis, without undue feelings of inhibition or guilt.

Group Size

The *membership* of a therapeutical group preferably should number between 6 and 12, and provide enough variety and stimulation between group members, as well as protection against disruptive factors. The criteria for selecting patients for group therapy include an explicit wish to join, relative alertness, ability to communicate, adequate personal hygiene and locomotion, and some degree of emotional responsiveness.[9] In institutional or out-patient settings, however, ideal criteria are often outweighed by practical considerations. Frequently, groups are started with elderly patients that happen to be available, and this can work out surprisingly well. The group evolves into an organism that eliminates those elements that don't fit and takes in those types which do fit. Once such a group has developed into a relatively cohesive structure, it may go on for a long time.[10, 11]

> One rather loosely structured group in a retirement home has been in continuous existence for many years now. The group survived periodical changes both in its membership and leadership. In this case, the group became, in the sociological sense of the word, an institution all of its own. The secret of its longevity probably was the high calibre of its constituency and the *leitmotiv* of the discussions: counting one's blessings in the present, and a tendency to see the past in an aura of gold.

Setting for Group Therapy

Group therapy can be carried out in many different *settings*, such as out-patient facilities, day care centers, psychiatric clinics, geriatric wards, or homes for the aged. It can be conducted by a psychiatrist, nonpsychiatric physicians, clinical psychologists, social workers, nurses, and other health personnel, provided they have had some training in this area. There are several types of group therapy, characterized by differences in goals and methods.

SPECIFIC APPROACHES

Remotivation Groups

These groups are aimed at reaching out toward, and getting in touch with, chronic patients who are withdrawn or apathetic. A few such patients meet at regular, frequent times with members of the ward team. The latter are selected on the basis of specific qualities, in particular, emotional warmth and natural friendliness. Through the medium of this warm relationship, the patient is brought in contact with elements of reality, such as pictures and objects closely related to his background (things typical of his work in the past, or his home area). In this manner, he may be drawn out, and his interest in the world around him rekindled.

Resocialization Groups

In *resocialization groups*, the therapeutic goal is on a level just above the previous one. Given a patient who is still interested in his surroundings, it may be useful to maintain or relearn basic social skills and the instrumentalities required for daily living activities (grooming, eating, cleaning, cooking, etc.).

Discussion Groups

On a next higher level, *discussion groups* may be formed, focusing on problems pertaining to the here-and-now setting of the hospital, or on current relationships with family, or even abstract topics such as politics and religion.

Predischarge Groups

Patients improving to the point of being able to leave the hospital, especially after having been there for a long time, usually face many difficulties and anxieties about re-entering the community. This type of group deals with these concerns, not only by talking about them, but also by actually visiting a boarding home, going out shopping, and getting acquainted with local agencies, such as the social service department, the mental health clinic, senior citizens organizations, and so on.

Marital and Family Therapy Groups

Marital and family conflicts are common problems among elderly patients. The stresses of chronic illness and hospitalization frequently have the unfortunate result of depleting the family's economic resources as well as its reservoir of good will. When it appears that the damage can still be repaired, conjoint meetings can be set up including the patient, the immediate family, and the therapist-counselor.

Therapeutic Community

The concept of the *therapeutic community* has been applied to elderly, institutionalized patients.[12] The traditional hospital expects the patient to be "good and cooperative" in playing the sick role. However, an extended sick role fixates the patient in a regressed mold. To prevent such regression and to maintain optimal function of remaining assets, the therapeutic community provides the patient with meaningful tasks and demands; the role of worker, decision-maker, or neighbor. The patient may be active in the hospital workshop, receiving pay for his work. Patients retain individuality and dignity by wearing their own clothes, and by collaborating with the staff in decision making. The hospital ward is transformed into a home-like place, with opportunity for privacy and belonging.

Recreational Therapy

The value of *recreational therapy* is the group context in which it takes place, the enjoyments of spectator entertainment, and in particular, the exercising of physical and mental functions. The latter include "walk and talk" groups, rhythmic activities with dancing and singing, games, picnics, parties, artwork, fishing, and gardening. Of special interest are programs bringing the aged closer to nature and living things, e.g., working with flowers and vegetables in a garden or plants indoors, having a pet, and, bringing them in touch with children or young people. In this context, foster grandparent programs may be mentioned, although here of course much more than recreation is involved.

Occupational Therapy

Occupational and *industrial therapy* aim at maintaining or restoring specific skills. The rehabilitation of various functions and capacities involves programmed activities such as weaving, woodwork, arts, and crafts. In addition, occupation and industrial therapy provide opportunities for self-expression, enhancing self-esteem, and setting the stage for socialization. The fact that elderly patients are often handicapped by psychomotor slowness, short attention span, forgetfulness, and sensory impairments points up the need for occupational, recreational, and industrial therapists with special expertise in the field of aging.

Reality Orientation

Reality orientation refers to a planned program involving the reorientation of confused patients. During daily meetings, the instructor presents, in a small group context, elementary information pertaining to time, place, person, and situation. Each patient is addressed individually, in a pleasant and unhurried manner. Patients may be asked about key items in their present perspective of time and space: the weather, holidays, meals, etc. The instructor rewards accurate responses by giving praise. Reality orientation can be extended beyond the group meeting through orientational devices, such as clocks, calendars, name tags, explanations of procedures, and bulletin boards.[13, 14]

SOME COMMENTS ON TECHNIQUES IN PSYCHOTHERAPY

NONVERBAL COMMUNICATION

Metacommunication

Inherent in all techniques are two basic forms of communication: verbal language and *metacommunication.* The latter represents everything in the communication experience, other than actual words, that provides a clue for the correct interpretation of the verbal message. Metacommunication is reflected in the tonal qualities of the voice, the emotional significance of the word patterns, facial expression, etc. This metalanguage is usually more meaningful than words themselves. Since variations of metalanguage are legion, a comprehensive discussion of them is beyond our scope, but a few abuses of metacommunication are worth mentioning.

Often, a question is phrased in such a way that instructions for the answer are given at the same time. People who are busy or in a position of authority may be especially prone to do this. If one enters a patient's room and asks with an air of cheerful determination, "Feeling pretty good today?," the implied message is "I am too busy to find out how you really feel, so be a good patient and tell me you feel fine." Such questions have built-in answers and few of them provide real information.

An aged patient is often seen in the presence of an adult child or a relative. It is then not uncommon to address oneself more and more to the relative who, after all, can communicate so much better. The patient himself is by-passed; at the end of the session, the prescription may be handed to the relative; and the patient will feel like a nonentity, who has no say-so about his own affairs.

Or, one might greet an elderly patient by saying: "You really are looking good." The patient has no choice but to accept this as a compliment, even though he may think: "I may look good all right, but I sure feel bad." Thus, the above greeting has the metacommunicative aspect of instructing the patient not to talk about his feelings. A better statement would be something like: "You look good—I wonder if you feel as good as you look."

Empathy

Empathy, being a transient identification with the patient, should remain just that. An extended identification is a source of undue distress for oneself, and of no help to the patient. While overinvolvement is an occupational hazard in the treatment of children and younger adults, the other extreme, i.e., defensive withdrawal from the patient, is more likely to occur in clinical work with old patients. Such a protective detachment on the part of the clinician would foster in the patient a sense of loneliness or rejection. An attitude of optimal empathy may be facilitated by keeping in mind that "this old person once had the same age I have now."

Physical Touch

In contrast to our professional contacts with younger adult patients, *physical touch* plays an important role in the therapeutic communication with older patients. Such physical contact between therapist and patient comes about in the most natural way. Very often, the patient will initiate it by making a gesture of reaching out. At other times, the therapist himself will become aware of a spontaneous impulse to touch his patient. The physical touch reflects a basic, natural way of getting in touch with the patient.

OPTIMAL ATTITUDE

Detached Concern

For the purpose of therapeutic communication, it is necessary to view disturbed behavior as a malfunction of the total organism, just as one would regard physical symptomatology as a manifestation of malfunction of a particular organ. It is then easier to preserve an attitude of *detached concern*, and to remain both objective and helpful. This is especially useful when the patient's behavior is irritating, for example, when dealing with the communicative barriers, encountered in aged patients.

Maintaining a Realistic Approach to Treatment

Overenthusiasm on the physician's part sets the stage for a letdown for himself and the patient. While it is unethical, and therapeutically unwise, to promise a patient too much, a pessimistic or fatalistic attitude may be even worse. A realistic approach is based on the recognition that, no matter what symptoms the patient presents, there is always something the physician can do to give relief. It is important that personnel involved with the care of the aged maintain an attitude which combines realism based on scientific knowledge with the humane desire to alleviate suffering. Only then is it possible to avoid extremes of detachment and overinvolvement.

Consistent Approach

A *consistent approach* combines gentleness and firmness. Such an attitude makes it possible to set limits to undesirable behavior (e.g., hyperactivity based on denial). Effective persuasion usually does not come about by forcing or commanding a patient to respond in certain ways. On the other hand, firm insistence may be effective, for example, in certain withdrawn and underactive patients.

Attitude Therapy

Attitude therapy involves the assuming of a specific behavioral attitude on the part of the staff, toward a particular patient. These include kind firmness, active friendliness, passive friendliness, matter-of-fact approach, and no demand attitude.[15, 16]

Dual Roles

There are several clinical settings and types of therapist-patient relationships which involve a set of dual roles on the part of both participants. This duality has nothing to do with the type of duality of feelings in ambivalence. Some examples of therapeutic relationships in which dual roles are important, include the following.

Sometimes, the patient may not only be older than the therapist, but he also may have had superior social or professional status. This may pose a problem for both; the therapist may feel constrained by feelings of awe, and the patient hesitates to settle in an appropriately dependent position. In such cases, it is useful to remember that a patient's wish for support from a competent helper cuts across all ages and classes, and that one can make appropriate use of this ubiquitous tendency toward a spontaneous "positive transference." Yet, some of this should remain tacit. On the surface level of the interaction, social amenities can be carried on in keeping with the overt differences in status, class, and seniority. Thus, the therapist may comfortably assume a deferential attitude, especially at the beginning and the end of the contact; and, as a junior, not challenge any pronouncements, but accept them with a mix of respect and matter-of-factness. And yet, somewhere during the interview, he will shift his weight, easing both himself and the patient into the other dimension of their relationship, for example, by giving specific advice, or changing a medication.

In the therapeutic contacts with hypochondriacal patients, there can be an explicit, formal understanding to "do something" about the patient's physical complaints; while on a deeper level, there is a tacit, mutual understanding that things are not going to be that simple and that there is a lot more than meets the eye.

In the therapeutic management of patients with bitter, vindictive depressions, it is often necessary to be supportive, without being obvious about it. Thus, the patient is given surreptitious support, and when he improves, he can allow himself to think that it was his own accomplishment, and that he is not beholden to anybody else for this. On a deeper level, of course, both he and the therapist know that there is more to it, but this knowledge remains tacit.

MANAGEMENT OF MALADAPTIVE DEFENSES

Maladaptive defenses aggravate the patient's suffering by exacerbating the very problem toward which they are directed. The aim of therapeutic intervention is to break up such vicious circles by removing or mitigating the maladaptive coping pattern. This can be accomplished by alleviating the underlying anxiety that prompted the particular defense, or by replacing the latter with a more appropriate coping technique. A patient's defenses should not be exposed or removed without first ascertaining what he is defending against. To remove defenses can be compared with taking away crutches from a paralyzed patient. When a particular defense is removed, another one is likely to take its place.

> A 64-year-old withdrawn woman had not walked for several years. Neurological examinations showed no abnormalities. Through a

concerted effort by the ward team, the patient was taken out of her wheelchair at regular intervals and taken for brief walks, supported by two attendants. After initial resistance, the patient began to go along with the walks. But soon she began to have outbursts of rage, when anybody came close to her. Thus, both the "inability" to walk and the display of rage served to keep others away. When one behavior pattern was removed, another emerged to take its place. In this patient, the rage attacks were less maladaptive than the inability to walk because, after all, she had begun to interact with other people. After a few months, the rage attacks subsided while progress in walking continued.

A specific form of correcting maladaptive behavior is *behavior modification*. Its theory and practice are based on the assumption that maladaptive behavior patterns are response habits which have been learned and become part of the character. The therapeutic goal is to modify such behavior and reverse the learning process by selected techniques, including extinction procedures, counterconditioning, desensitization, negative reinforcement, and operant conditioning by token rewards. Clinical experience with these techniques in geropsychiatric management is still limited. It seems however, that even in cases of moderate or severe organic brain syndrome the patient's behavior still can be modified, provided the reinforcement is specifically suited to the individual patient.[17, 18]

HOPE AND SECURITY

Reassurance

The wish for reassurance reflects the universal human need for emotional security. The effectiveness of reassurance depends on whether it is true or false. False reassurance is not effective because it is prompted by the wrong motive, e.g., the need to protect one's own self. False reassurance has a reactive quality; it is an automatic, reflex-like response, rather than consciously thought through. True reassurance, on the other hand, is deliberate and thought through. It acknowledges the personal meaning of a problem to the individual, the probability that emotional distress will arise and his need for help in coping with it. True reassurance is also conveyed to a patient by emotional security and lack of alarm in the therapist. For example, discussing an emotionally charged topic in a tone that combines calm and lack of alarm can have a detoxifying effect on the patient's inner turmoil.

The Use of Regression

Optimal regression permits the patient to accept his dependency, and therefore, care from others. When a "positive transference" (trust) exists, the patient looks forward to contacts with his physician, nurse, etc. If possible, visits should be scheduled at regular intervals so that the patient has something definite to look forward to, and the element of uncertainty is removed. In a hospital setting, optimal regression can be quickly established by means of frequent, brief visits (e.g., 5 minutes, three times a day, at the same appointed times).

Maintaining Hope

An essential part of regression is an alteration in the time sense and temporal perspective. By taking on the different time scale, the patient does not look ahead as far into the future (e.g., days instead of weeks or months). This may relieve anxiety and create a situation in which hope can be maintained or reactivated. Through living day by day, good prospects become real possibilities. When the future offers few, if any, good prospects, one may attempt to draw the patient's attention to what is presently at hand or immediately ahead. The same principle applies to patients dwelling on a past which contained few shares of happiness. A sense of disillusionment or despair may be prevented by focusing on whatever satisfactory experiences are available in the immediate here and now. On the other hand, when a person's past does contain many shares of happiness, it is useful to encourage the patient to reminisce about them. Through memory he has access to gratifying retrospects.

PRESERVING DIGNITY

Dignity involves a special type of self-esteem: to be regarded well in the eyes of others. This element of being "regarded" is also essential to its counterpart, shame. *Dignity and shame* are possible only when one is seen by another. One does not lose dignity in privacy, but in public. To protect dignity, it is necessary to provide the older person with the essentials of privacy: a space he can call his own, a place where he feels he belongs and can keep his belongings. In addition to lack of privacy, dignity can be lost in other ways and situations.

The elderly patient, his body, his self, and self-image, often is in a fragile condition, or a state of crisis. In view of this, it is all the more important to *foster his sense of identity*, his self-image as a person. Thus, it would be traumatic for a person who sees himself as courageous to break down with fear and trembling; for an optimist, to express pessimism; for a friendly person, to admit vindictiveness; for a generous person, to express envy. The risk to be avoided is that of "loss of face." The injudicious puncturing of a social facade would leave the patient feeling helpless and embarrassed.

Feelings of inadequacy and shame may occur for various reasons, for example, embarrassing disfigurements. To protect himself against possible ridicule and disgust from others, the patient withdraws. The price of intact dignity is isolation and loneliness; also, once the patient himself feels ashamed, the people around him will feel embarrassed, too. The best management is to prevent such vicious circles from developing. In the case of a disfigurement, for example, we would do well to be especially aware of the need to show the patient respect, transcending the phenomenon of the pathological alterations we are facing and relating to the whole person with respect. Instilling in the patient a foundation of *self-respect* may enable him, in turn, to face others without shame.

What may also be embarrassing is a physical state of helplessness, a sense of loss of mastery, or the experience of being treated as a "case." It follows that all those efforts aimed at reducing helplessness and *promoting a sense of control* will also enhance the patient's dignity. In protecting the patient's dignity, we protect his person, his self-image, his image to others, and, in the final analysis, our own dignity. Our esteem for the old is based not only on how they appear to us now, but also on what they once were in the past, as a historically unique entity.

References

1. Zinberg, N. E.: Special problems of gerontologic psychiatry. In: *Geriatric Psychiatry*, edited by M.A. Berezin and S. Cath, International Universities Press, New York, 1965. pp. 147–149.
2. Gaitz, C. M.: Barriers to the delivery of psychiatric services to the elderly. *Gerontologist 14*:210–214, 1974.
3. Silverman, A., Kahn, B. H., and Anderson, G.: A model for working with multigenerational families. *Social Casework 58*:131–135, 1977.
4. Bunzel, J. H.: Recognition, relevance and de-activation of gerontophobia. *J. Am. Geriatr. Soc. 21*:77–80, 1973.
5. Butler, R. N.: *Why Survive? Being Old in America.* Harper & Row, New York City, 1975.
6. Spence, D. L., Feigenbaum, E. M., Fitzgerald, Jr. et al: Medical student attitudes toward the geriatric patient. *J. Am. Geriatr. Soc. 16*:967–983, 1968.
7. Lawton, M. P.: Geropsychological knowledge as a background for psychotherapy with older people. *J. Geriatr. Psychiatry 9*:221–233, 1976.
8. Lewis, M. I., and Butler, R. N.: Life review therapy: putting memories to work in individual and group psychotherapy. *Geriatrics 29*:165–173, 1974.
9. Linden, M. E.: Group psychotherapy with institutionalized senile women, II. Study in gerontologic human relations. *Int. J. Group Psychother. 3*:150–170, 1953.
10. Berger, L. F.: Activating a psychogeriatric group. *Psychiatr. Q. 50*:63–66, 1978.
11. Deutsch, C. B., and Kramer, N.: Outpatient group psychotherapy for the elderly: an alternative to institutionalization. *Hosp. Community Psychiatry 28*:440–442, 1977.
12. Gottesman, L. E.: The response of long-hospitalized aged psychiatric patients to milieu treatment. *Gerontologist 7*:47–48, 1967.
13. Folsom, J. C.: Reality orientation for the elderly mental patient. *J. Geriatric Psychiatry 1*:291–307, 1968.
14. Brook, P., Degun, G., and Mather, M.: Reality orientation, a therapy for psychogeriatric patients: a controlled study. *Br. J. Psychiatry 127*:42–45, 1975.
15. Treatment Team, V. A. Hospital, Tuscaloosa, Alabama: Attitude therapy and the team approach. *Mental Hospitals 16*:307–323, 1965.
16. Ginzberg, R.: Attitude therapy in geriatric ward psychiatry. *J. Am. Geriatr. Soc. 3*:445–462, 1952.
17. Mueller, D. J., and Atlas, L.: Resocialization of regressed elderly residents: a behavioral management approach. *J. Gerontol. 27*:390–392, 1972.
18. Ankus, M., and Quarrington, B.: Operant behavior in the memory-disordered. *J. Gerontol. 27*:500–510, 1972.

12

management of anxiety*

INTRODUCTION

There are many obscurities in the clinical management of anxiety and the affective disorders, witness the fact that some psychotropic drugs can have paradoxical effects; that some antidepressants and antipsychotics are useful to treat anxiety; that many anxiety states have depressive features, and vice versa; etc. There are several reasons why certain drugs and psychotherapeutic interventions are often unpredictable. First, it is not always clear what the dominant affect is. One affect may cover another one; e.g., defensive anger covering an underlying feeling of shame, guilt, or grief. Secondly, while some affects are "free-floating" and become clinically manifest, others may be latent, being held in check by specific defense mechanisms. In this case, the affect is not manifest, but covert; its presence is in terms of a predisposition, or a potential to react emotionally in a certain way. Finally, a person does not simply have only one affect, but usually a spectrum of feelings; e.g., the cluster of depression, envy, and vindictiveness.

An affect (or cluster or affects) is the result of at least two sets of factors: the psychobiological state of the interior, and one's present perspective which encompasses prospects ahead in the future and retrospective antecedents in past history. A position in the present implies a prospect, an outlook into the future. Anxiety results when a perspective in the present necessitates the anticipation of pain or danger, while hope prevails with the prospect of pleasure or joy. Thus, both anxiety and hope are affects oriented to the future. Any decrease of hope (any lessening of the probability of good prospects) results in anxiety. Thus, anxiety is the emotion produced as one moves from a hopeful perspective toward a less hopeful one, along a line that eventually terminates in hopelessness. At this terminal point, where one no longer has anything to lose, anxiety ceases.

At the other extreme of the continuum, where hope is in a maximal configuration, the opportunity for anxiety is likewise the greatest: it is at this point, where I have everything to gain, that I can lose the most.

* In collaboration with Alan D. Whanger, M. D.

When the perspective has actually changed in the direction from hope toward hopelessness, grief occurs as a response to this loss. The existence of grief does not mean that I cannot continue to feel anxiety about a subsequent, pending loss. Thus, at any given point, between the two extremes of the hope-despair continuum, anxiety (or fear) and depression (or grief) are merely two sides of the coin, being separated only by the difference of "not yet" and "no longer." Moving along the trajectory, then, anxiety will be the dominating feature; at the midpoint, anxiety and depression will be about equal; during the last phase, depression will progressively eclipse anxiety, until the latter ceases at the end point of despair.

The position of hope being associated with high energy potential allows for the use of high energy coping mechanisms to brace against the slide toward less hopeful positions. (The effect of anxiety is activation and arousal; the physiological pathways involved are especially the pituitary-adrenal axis and the endocrine systems. The metabolical effects are, by and large, catabolic.) Adaptive coping mechanisms will restore the hopeful perspective. Maladaptive defenses will cause progressive deterioration of the position and increasing momentum in the downward slide. Somewhere, a point of no return may be reached, which involves the realization that not enough energy is available to stop and reverse the downward course. When efforts to stop the slide are abandoned, surrender and giving up occur, and low energy defenses take over (regression, letting go, retreat). This change may subjectively be experienced as the "bottom dropping out." (The physiological state associated with depression, in contrast to anxiety, is mostly one of retardation and suppression of neurovegetative and endocrine functions and may include anabolic processes).

MANAGEMENT OF ANXIETY

Clinical management of anxiety, affective disorders, and other mental illness, especially in aged patients, does not rely on just one therapeutic modality, e.g., drugs or psychotherapy. Rather, it involves a comprehensive approach in which drugs, psychotherapy, medical treatment, socioeconomical measures, and environmental manipulation are fitted into a therapeutic program which will suit the needs of the individual patient.

PSYCHOPHARMACOLOGY

Antianxiety Drugs

The *antianxiety drugs* include the benzodiazepines, propanediols, and diphenylmethanes. There is clinical evidence that these drugs are safe and effective in treating anxiety in the elderly. They lessen anxiety and tension related to situational stresses or physical illness, but do not modify psychotic symptomatology.[1–3] Certain tricyclic antidepressants and phenothiazines are also occasionally used to treat anxiety and agitation in elderly patients.

Benzodiazepines. The *benzodiazepines* include many popular drugs, such as diazepam (Valium), chlordiazepoxide (Librium), oxazepam (Serax), flurazepam (Dalmane), chlorazepate (Tranxene), lorazepam (Ativan), and prazepam (Verstran). Chlordiazepoxide, diazepam, and oxazepam are similar in their sedative, muscle relaxant, and anticonvulsant properties. They do differ with regard to dosage and duration of action. Diazepam is somewhat more potent than chlordiazepoxide, which is the longest-acting. Oxazepam has a shorter half-life, and requires larger doses.[4] Lorazepam has the shortest half-life, which is helpful in older patients because it reduces the problem of accumulation of plasma levels which contribute to oversedation or ataxia. Actually, the half-life of diazepam is increased about 3-fold in the elderly, making its use much more hazardous. The benzodiazepines are primarily used for treatment of anxiety, and have largely replaced older drugs; e.g., meprobamate, phenobarbital, or bromides. Many physical symptoms associated with anxiety (e.g., headaches, gastrointestinal distress, fatigue) respond well. Chlorazepate presents a special problem in the elderly, as it requires stomach acid for proper utilization, and the relative achlorhydria of some older persons makes its effect unpredictable.

Propanediol Derivatives. Propanediol derivatives include meprobamate (Miltown, Equanil) and tybamate (Tybatran). While these drugs have both sedative and relaxant properties, they are not used in the elderly because of the ease of overuse and addictions with serious withdrawal problems.[5]

Diphenylmethane Derivatives. The *diphenylmethane derivatives* include diphenhydramine (Benadryl) and hydroxyzine (Atarax, Vistaril).[6] Diphenhydramine is a widely used antihistamine, with sedative qualities. It is often useful in inducing sleep with few side effects and has no addiction potential, but its value for treating anxiety is limited. Hydroxyzine, chiefly sedative, is also antihistaminic. Its effectiveness in the elderly seems variable.

Tricyclic Antidepressants and Phenothiazines. Other drugs used in the treatment of anxiety include certain *tricyclic antidepressants* and *phenothiazines*. Amitriptyline, doxepin, imipramine, desipramine, and nortriptyline can be anxiolytic, in addition to their antidepressant effect.[7] Some phenothiazines in small doses, such as thioridazine (Mellaril) or trifluoperazine (Stelazine), are useful for anxiety and tension, but have the disadvantage of lowering the blood pressure and other side effects more often, compared with the benzodiazepines. They also may cause feelings of lassitude or unreality.

Ethyl Alcohol. Ethyl alcohol is the oldest and the most widely used anxiolytic drug, having been called "the nurse of old age" by Galen. The beneficial effect of about 3 ounces of wine, or a glass of beer, late in the afternoon, on morale, tension, communications, and sleep has been noted in the elderly.[8, 9] It has its hazards, however, as many elderly have a decreased tolerance for alcohol, and it may potentiate the effects and the side-effects of many other psychoactive drugs.[10]

Barbiturates. The *barbiturates* are infrequently used in the elderly now because of their dulling of cortical function, their stimulation of and interference with various enzyme systems, and their potential for addiction. Stotsky and Borozne found low doses of butabarbital (Butisol) to be effective, however.[11]

Propanolol. The drug propanolol (Inderal) has been used elsewhere for the relief of anxiety and panic attacks, although its use for such in the United States has still not received official FDA approval.[12]

Treatment Considerations

The minor tranquilizers are relatively *safe* in comparison to barbiturates. Unlike the latter, they do not seem to activate liver enzyme systems. Also, the benzodiazepines decrease the possibility of suicide in the depressed patient, since large amounts can be taken without fatal results, in contrast to barbiturates and meprobamate.

Some patients react to minor tranquilizers in a *paradoxical* way. They seem to resist the drug action, and become agitated rather than calm. Clearly, age-related pathology, e.g., an organic brain syndrome may modify the clinical effects of these drugs by making the person more prone to confusion, in addition to many other variables. In the elderly, chlordiazepoxide (Librium) has been observed to lead particularly to the paradoxical increase in irritability and hostility.[13]

Individual *susceptibility* to the sedative effect of these drugs varies, so that it is difficult to set general standards for dosage, although a generally safe rule is to use about one-third of the regular adult dose, and to increase it slowly if necessary. Side-effects may occur even with small doses, and some people experience drowsiness and unsteadiness of gait. Ataxia, nystagmus, and uncoordination are clinical signs suggesting chronic overdosage. At very high dosage levels, benzodiazepines produce severe unsteadiness of gait, drowsiness, orthostatic hypotension, and coma. The muscle relaxant properties of these drugs may be deleterious in old persons who have already lost some of their physical strength.[14]

Addiction and habituation can occur, usually when large doses have been taken for a long time. This is a greater risk than with the major tranquilizers, because the pleasure potential of minor tranquilizers can be similar to that of barbiturates and alcohol. Abrupt withdrawal from large doses of meprobamate, chlordiazepoxide, or diazepam results in a syndrome similar to barbiturate withdrawal. The use of any anxiolytic agent may cause a secondary clinical depression, especially in the elderly who have a history of affective illness.[15]

While taking antianxiety drugs, the same *precautions* as for other psychotropic drugs are applicable: no alcohol, and special care in situations where drowsiness and impaired coordination would be hazardous.

It is advisable to *discontinue periodically* the minor tranquilizers, to avoid habituation and drug dependency, and to determine to what extent the placebo effect may play a role.

Patients often take minor tranquilizers, along with *other drugs* with sedative effects. Many alcoholics become habituated to minor tranquilizers without stopping drinking. On a short term basis, alcohol can potentiate the effect of tranquilizers and antidepressants, so that the dosage must be reduced to avoid toxic effects. Chronic alcohol use, however, induces changes in liver enzyme activity, resulting in more rapid metabolism and reducing the effect of drugs detoxified by the liver, e.g., the benzodiazepines. The latter are metabolized more rapidly in the alcoholic, so that larger doses are required for therapeutic effect.

Sedatives and Hypnotics

Sleep in the Old. Old people tend to have less total sleep time compared with normal young adults, even though they may need more, rather than less, sleep.[16] The percentage of rapid eye movement (REM) sleep is slightly less; but stage 4 sleep (deep sleep) tends to be considerably less, or sometimes even absent. Stage 4 sleep is considered to be the most effective for fulfilling biological needs.[17] In addition, it takes longer for older people to fall asleep, and once they are asleep, they tend to awaken more readily.[18] It is probably no exaggeration to state that of all signs, symptoms, and complaints in the field of medicine and psychiatry, disturbed sleep is the most common. It is important to keep in mind that from a physiological point of view, sleep is not at all the passive state it once was thought to be; and that, psychologically speaking, sleep is an art which many people never master. In conditions of anxiety, depression, and other mental illness, sleep disturbances are often first to appear and last to disappear.

Complex Management Problems. In addition to the high frequency of sleep disorders, older people usually also present complex problems in management. Some psychotropic agents, for example, are effective in inducing sleep, but happen to suppress REM sleep. Some tricyclic antidepressants have the effect of increasing REM latency, decreasing REM sleep time, and increasing stages 3 and 4 non-REM sleep. Certain CNS stimulants, such as phenmetrazine (Preludin), tranylcypromine (Parnate), and methylphenidate (Ritalin) also decrease REM time. Since dreaming activity is associated with REM sleep, one needs to remain alert to the possible effects of such drug-induced dream deprivation. Two other drugs deserve mention because of their widespread use: caffein and alcohol. It appears that, for many, caffein does not begin to exert its sleep-interfering effect until middle age. REM sleep is not appreciably affected by caffeine. Alcohol, being a CNS depressant, tends to facilitate the process of falling asleep, but not infrequently this is followed by awakening earlier than usual. REM sleep time is decreased by the use of alcohol.[4]

The ideal hypnotic would have the effect of rapid sleep induction, without changing the normal phases of sleep, and ensuring a full night's sleep without a daytime hangover. It should present no risks of habituation, tolerance, or suicide if taken in overdosage. The currently available hypnotics meet the above criteria in varying degrees, but none of them completely.

Hypnotics. Hypnotics should be used judiciously in the treatment of elderly patients. An appropriate indication would be for the relief of simple insomnia; i.e., insomnia not associated with depression, anxiety, or pain. Most of the hypnotics, such as secobarbital (Seconal), pentobarbital (Nembutal), methyprylon (Noludar), ethchlorvynol (Placidyl), methaqualone (Quaalude), and glutethimide (Doriden) suppress REM sleep and are easily toxic or habit-forming in the aged, and are best avoided.[19] Paraldehyde is relatively safe, but highly unpleasant to use. The best present hypnotic is chloralhydrate (Noctec), which does not significantly suppress REM sleep, leaves little hangover or ataxia, and has a fairly low risk of habituation. It can be given in 0.5- or 1.0-g doses at bedtime. Its main drawback is occasional gastric irritation, and rarely a paradoxical excitement reaction may occur.

The next most useful hypnotic in the elderly probably is flurazepam (Dalmane) which has little effect on REM. It does tend to have a long plasma half-life in the elderly, however, and this accumulation may tend to lead to significant CNS depressant activity.[2] If used, it is probably best taken not more often than twice weekly.

Bromides are available in some over-the-counter hypnotics. Gradually increasing abuse of bromides results in bromide intoxication, which resembles an acute organic brain syndrome in its symptomatology. In suspected cases, serum bromide level should be tested. Treatment involves discontinuation of bromides, and, if necessary, administering 2–4 g of sodium chloride every 4 hours, or ammonium chloride, which provides a chloride for displacing the bromide and has a diuretic effect.

Mild Anxiety and Tension. For insomnia due to *mild anxiety and tension* one may give oxazepam (Serax), diazepam (Valium), or flurazepam (Dalmane). When pain complicates the problem, it is often helpful to give a bedtime analgesic, such as acetaminophen (Tylenol) or enteric coated aspirin.

Severe Anxiety or Depression. Sedatives and hypnotics have little effect in cases of *severe anxiety or depression.* In the case of anxiety-depression of severe degree, antidepressants and/or phenathiazines should be used, rather than sedatives or antianxiety drugs. In cases of mild to moderate severity, antianxiety drugs can be given, distributed throughout the day. A larger evening dose may eliminate the need for a hypnotic at bedtime.

Organic Brain Syndromes. In patients with *organic brain syndromes* who are anxious and agitated, such as in "sundowner's syndrome," it is almost always necessary to administer a low dose of a major tranquilizer such as haloperidol (Haldol), thioridazine (Mellaril), or thiothixene (Navane). In addition, environmental supports such as better lighting, the family close by, and reality orientation help to calm the individual.

Antihistamines. The *antihistamines* will often help to improve sleep in anxiety states because of their sedative side-effects. The two most used are diphenhydramine (Benadryl) and promethazine (Phenergan) in doses of 12.5 or 25 mg at bedtime.

L-Tryptophan. The substance L-tryptophan has been noted to have sedative properties, and has been used as a mild hypnotic drug recently.

CLINICAL MANAGEMENT

Anxiety states in the elderly may be grouped depending on the origin of the anxiety: *depletion anxiety* refers to insecurity about loss of external supplies, and the possibility of isolation and loneliness. *Helplessness* pertains to fears of loss of control and mastery, with feelings of shame. *Chronic neurotic anxiety* is usually a carry-over from earlier years, with physiological tension, motor agitation, and depressive admixtures. *Acute anxiety* may develop as an acute stress reaction, or adjustment reaction of late life; or it may represent acute traumatic anxiety, resulting from a weakening of the ego's capacity to screen and ward off unwanted stimuli, as in catastrophic reactions of brain-damaged patients, or due to informational overload. *Anxiety associated with psychoses* may be secondary to schizophrenic delusions, associated with paranoid states (persecutory anxiety), or associated with chronic brain syndrome and senile dementia.

Generally speaking, to allay anxiety, all the therapeutic principles underlying optimal therapist-patient relationship must be observed. The promotion of appropriate dependency in the patient is therapeutically useful because it takes his attention away from anxiety-provoking concerns. Optimal regression, possible only in a firmly established therapist-patient relationship, is an effective antidote against anxiety; and when the motive of anxiety is absent, maladaptive defenses may be prevented from developing. An attempt should be made to prevent, eliminate, or treat anxiety-provoking factors which, in the aged, often pertain to loss of external supplies, role uncertainty, intrafamilial strife, borderline economic resources, relentless progress of physical disability, drastic changes in the body image, etc. Antianxiety agents or sedatives should be employed promptly and decisively to interrupt any vicious cycle of anxiety-depression, physical illness, and other stresses.

Depletion Anxiety

In elderly individuals, the nature of anxiety is not primarily in terms of a danger signal pertaining to unacceptable impulses from within, but to object losses and loss of external supplies. Developmentally, this corresponds with separation anxiety; the apathetic depressions in old persons may be the clinical counterpart of anaclitic depressions in infants. Depressive anxiety may be precipitated or exacerbated by a loss or an environmental change. The patient himself may not always be aware of the source of his anxiety, and therefore a careful, thorough exploration of his life situation is in order. For example, it is possible that the patient's anxiety is based on the assumption that others will not be available or accessible when he will be in need of help. Frequently, this is expressed as anxiety about becoming a burden on others and as fears of abandonment.

The effect of anxiety is to increase the workload on a body whose homeostatic capacity is already diminished. In heart disease, for example, anxiety may make the difference between compensation and decompensation; the anxious patient overburdens his heart by becoming unduly restless. Hence, there is the need for antianxiety drugs that will diminish the subjective experience of apprehension and protect the patient from the physiological stress associated with anxiety. Antianxiety agents, in the context of an optimal therapist-patient relationship, may also facilitate the process of gathering information about the patient's life situation. One should quickly explore the possible causes of the anxiety, before it becomes chronic.

In addition to these immediate goals, there is the long-term therapeutic goal to re-establish the patient's equilibrium on a lasting basis. This will involve several procedures.

Make sure that necessary support is provided in the areas of concern; e.g., financial assistance, homemaker services, legal aid, providing social contacts to prevent undue isolation, etc.

In some cases, it is necessary to establish a permanent relationship with the patient. At the very minimum, the patient should be told that he should feel free to return whenever he feels the need for this. If the patient is continued on antianxiety medications, this represents an implicit contract to follow him at regular intervals.

If proper support has been provided, it may be useful to take the patient off the medications and to observe how he is doing. When he comes back, still feeling anxious, after the alleged deficiencies in his life situation have been corrected, obviously there is more than meets the eye. Chances are then that the anxiety has multiple origins, and that the original complaint was only the tip of the iceberg.

Anxiety Associated with Helplessness

Anxiety also may be generated by a move from a perspective of self-confidence in the direction of helplessness. Anxiety pertaining to loss of control and mastery may be acute (as in sudden physical illness) or slowly progressive (due to slowly accumulating losses in the area of personal competence and autonomy). The anxious feelings associated with this are in terms of loss of self-confidence and shame.

The initial goals in therapy are to develop an optimal physician-patient relationship and to reduce some of the anxiety by way of medication. Once the patient has begun to feel more secure in the relationship with the therapist, specific concerns can be identified. Usually it is more difficult to obtain this type of information than in depletion-anxiety (where the patient can simply point his finger to an external problem). In the case of helplessness, however, the deficiency is more personal, and may be embarrassing for the patient to verbalize. It may pertain to any neuromuscular, mental, and social capacities that represent basic instrumentalities in the areas of love, play, and work.

Under the protective aegis of the therapist-patient relationship, the patient is gently but firmly advised to get whatever medical examinations are in order. It is surprising how often elderly patients will resist having their alleged physical or mental defects examined. They may express fear about getting lost in the labyrinth of the modern hospital, or finding out that theirs is a hopeless case. It may be necessary to provide arrangements to make sure that the patient does go through channels and will not get lost in the maze of the hospital. After medical evaluation, it is frequently also a problem to get the patient to accept the recommended treatment. Here again, the "positive transference" element in the relationship can serve its purpose.

In spite of appropriate medical evaluations and treatment, a residue of decreased physical, mental, or social competence may remain, enough to keep the anxiety going. In this case, supportive therapy should be maintained for an indefinite period of time. The goals of therapy include helping the patient adjust to the appropriate level of functioning, and simultaneously making efforts to provide for corresponding changes in the environment. The latter are the reciprocal of the changes in the patient's status; the more helpless the patient, the more helpful the environment must become.

A few points with regard to psychotherapeutic techniques are as follows.

Generally, for the purpose of reducing helplessness and enhancing a sense of control, an obsessive-compulsive behavioral style may be encouraged: preference for closure and predictability, avoidance of risks and uncertainty, and emphasis on schemas and schedules. One can emphasize the importance of regular routines and rhythmically patterning the patient's life activities.

The relatives can be advised that feelings of helplessness in the aged family member can be alleviated by anticipating some of his needs. Such anticipation of needs before they arise fosters a subjective sense of control and thus may prevent angry frustration, depression, or shame. Patients who are handicapped by varying degrees of memory loss often have a relationship with one or more relatives in which the latter serve as an extracorporeal, prosthetic memory device. In contacts with such patients and their relatives, one can observe that whenever the patient's memory fails him, he sends out a nonverbal signal (a quick look) toward the relative, who then responds by filling in the necessary details. Typically, neither the patient nor the relative is aware of the extent to which this goes on.

It is essential, however, to remind the patient of remaining assets, and to encourage mobilization and diversions consistent with his remaining potential. Premature care or undue amount of support has an adverse effect, by promoting regression. Thus, it is often difficult to stay on an intermediate course, avoiding on the one hand the extreme of insufficient support (which would create more anxiety) and on the other hand, too much support (which would promote regression). The importance of sustaining patterns of activity is emphasized by the fact that decreased physical activity and bed rest can cause significant changes in the distribution, metabolism, and excretion of drugs.[20]

Motivation for activity must include a goal that seems worth the effort. A patient may learn to walk following a stroke, but unless he has a motive for walking, he may soon abandon the attempt. The milieu of the average institution frequently offers little incentive to activity, thus fostering regression and deterioration. Self care and independence have appeal only to the extent that there is something to live for. Whether in an outpatient or inpatient setting, the therapist and other members of the treatment team can become sources of incentive, by appropriately rewarding the patient's efforts.

Chronic Neurotic Anxiety

This may be a carry-over from earlier adult years. By now, the psychodynamics of the anxiety neurosis are less important than they might have been when the patient was young. After a lifetime of behavioral patterns based on neurotic anxiety, an etiologically-based therapy (insight therapy) is not indicated. The behavioral patterns and symptoms have become ingrained in the character although they are usually not egosyntonic. The patient suffers from tension and agitation, but is unable to explain why. Varying degrees of depression are usually present as well.

The *physiological concomitants* of anxiety (muscular tension, insomnia, cardiovascular distress, stomach upsets, urinary frequency, etc.) are usually more prominent than the subjective feelings of anxiety. Generally, such patients do not respond well to therapeutic attempts aimed at insight, counseling, or guidance, without drug therapy. To most of them, the physical symptoms or agitation are sufficiently real to convince them that their problem is physical. They may intellectually agree that their symptoms have an emotional origin, but this acknowledgment usually comes about only after one has begun to aim therapy at the physical symptoms.

Although antianxiety drugs can be used for the symptomatic treatment of anxiety, agitation, insomnia, and tension, these symptoms often can also be alleviated by *increasing the patient's level of activity*. The expenditure of energy must be channeled toward constructive activities; aimless agitation will aggravate the patient's anxiety because of the lack of structure and meaningful fit. In drawing up a planned program of activities, some basic points must be kept in mind.

The need for an individualized approach to the elderly patient is pointed up by the fact that for each individual, sick or healthy, the pattern of age decrements is characteristic and the rate of decline varies from one function to another.

Activity is to be more than passive participation in time-filling work. Therapeutic activity has purpose; the more completely it absorbs the patient's energies, the more beneficial it will be. When activities bring about contacts with other people, isolation is reduced.

In designing an activity program for the patient, the following steps are required: find out patient's interests, make a list of potential activities (indoors, outdoors) appropriate for the season, determine patient's attention span for each of the activities, preferred time of the day, and preferred sequence of activities, arrive at a mutually agreed regimen of daily activities, which should cover about 1 month at the time, have patient come back to report on regimen, review, and make changes as needed. These patients frequently like simple, mechanical work, which does not require problem-solving or a deadline; e.g., gardening.

Various relaxation techniques may be helpful with the elderly, such as autohypnosis, biofeedback, yoga exercises, or music therapy.[21]

If insomnia remains significant inspite of increased activities during the day, one may cluster the doses of antianxiety drugs toward the evening to obtain maximum benefit from them during the night. During a period of interruption of the minor tranquilizers, it will be necessary to use a sedative or hypnotic to ensure adequate sleep. When the antianxiety drugs are started again, the sedatives should be discontinued. In this manner, the risk of habituation to either type of drug can be reduced, even though the patient may maintain a psychological dependency on medication.

In many cases, *maintenance drug therapy* is needed to alleviate the discomfort that could interfere with the patient's optimal participation in the therapeutic relationship. One of the benzodiazepines may be used for patients with mild tension and agitation and whose ego strength is good. For more severe anxiety, especially associated with diffuse somatic complaints, one of the major tranquilizers in small doses may be necessary.

Depression with agitation: if tension continues despite the use of minor tranquilizers, one should consider the diagnosis of depression instead of anxiety. Depression shares many symptoms with anxiety, but its pathogenesis and therapy are different. In mild depression, one can start with small doses of a tricyclic antidepressant, especially if insomnia is present. If there is no improvement in a few days, a gradually increasing dose may be needed. Tricyclic antidepressants may relieve the depression, but occasionally cause agitation instead. A benzodiazepine may control mild agitation, but more severe agitation requires a phenothiazine. Doxepin (Sinequan, Adapin) and thioridazine are antidepressant agents that do not cause as much agitation. The antianxiety effect of these drugs is prompt, but, as with other antidepressants, relief of the depression may not become manifest for 2–3 weeks. Other medications used for mixed anxiety-depression are combinations such as the proprietary mixture of perphenazine and amitriptyline (Triavil or Etrafon) or tailored combinations such as doxepin and haloperidol, or thiothixene.

The restlessness and agitation due to chronic anxiety should be differentiated from akathisia, a side-effect of antipsychotic drugs; from muscular quiverings, which can be a side effect of lithium; and from agitated depression. Therefore, prior to starting minor tranquilizers, it is useful to have a drug-free baseline.

Acute Anxiety Reactions

Acute stress reactions or *acute adjustment reactions of late life* are not uncommon. Such reactive anxiety may occur as a response to any stress or trauma, including retirement, acute physical illness, loss of a loved one, and so on. The treatment approach will depend on the patient's ego strength and general resources vis-à-vis the magnitude of the stress. It is in the nature of an adjustment reaction to be rather short in duration, transitory, and responsive to counseling or guidance. Psychotherapy should focus on the patient's reactions to the precipitating event or on resolving the environmental stress. Medication should be limited to a few weeks, since chronic reliance on drugs may provide just enough relief to keep the patient from seeking a decisive solution. Often nighttime sedation is sufficient.

Acute traumatic anxiety may develop in older patients due to weakening of a specific ego function: the so-called stimulus barrier. Normally, the ego is able to screen and ward off unwanted stimuli through various mechanisms; e.g., selective inattention, increased inner activity of the self, or turning to external diversions so as to create a "white noise" that drowns out unwanted stimuli. In conditions of moderate to severe regression (due to psychological factors or physical illness), the ego boundary becomes more penetrable, and the patient is more vulnerable to a barrage of unwanted stimuli. Such a barrage may attain the quality of a bombardment. Even minor stimuli (e.g., a dripping faucet) are capable of producing such traumatic anxiety. This type of anxiety arises automatically when the psyche is overwhelmed by an influx of external or internal stimuli too great to be mastered. It is characteristic of infancy when the ego is immature, but may occur whenever the ego is relatively weak, for example, in old age. Clinically, it may be manifested not primarily in terms of anxiety in the usual sense of the word, but by a diffuse, primitive response of intense, painful displeasure. Milder cases show restlessness, tension, and irritability. More severe cases are characterized by outbursts of anger and rage, or defensive attempts to re-establish a stimulus barrier by way of withdrawal.[22]

Clinical management is supportive and includes drug therapy and environmental procedures. For milder cases, the benzodiazepines can be used first; if the symptoms persist, or in more severe cases, phenothiazines or other antipsychotic agents should be tried.

Supportive measures pertaining to environmental structuring essentially involve the providing of an "ego prosthesis." When the combined impact of the illness and regression breaks down ego organization, leading to diminished resistance to external stimuli (noise, procedures, and changes in the environment), a regimen can be provided that serves as an "ego prosthesis." Such an artificial ego implies organizing the patient's environment for him, with the spatiotemporal relations of his milieu kept constant. The principle is that of "sameness"; by keeping the milieu constant, the sense of loss of mastery in the patient is minimized. Constancy can also be applied to arrangement of furniture, temperature, light, procedural methods, etc. Temporal constancy pertains to times of visits by the physician, nurses, relatives, etc.

Anxiety Associated with Psychoses

Delusional phobias, persecutory anxieties, and paranoid fears may occur in the context of chronic paranoid schizophrenia, late life paraphrenia, paranoid states, or at some point along the final common path toward dementia. Clinical management includes the use of antipsychotic agents, in addition to whatever medical, social, and environmental intervention is indicated. In many such patients, the anxiety and helpless panic respond well to an approach which consists of providing a structured relationship or environment and being generously supportive, while at the same time firmly insisting on suppression of psychotic thoughts and focusing on the realities of the here-and-now.

References

1. Gershon, S.: Antianxiety agents. In: *Advances in Behavioral Biology, Psychopharmacology and Aging*, edited by C. Eisdorfer and W. E. Fann, vol. 6, Plenum Press, New York, 1973. pp. 183–187.
2. Piland, B.: The aging process and psychoactive drug use in clinical treatment. In: *The Aging Process and Psychoactive Drug Use*, Services Research Monograph Series, No. 79–813, U. S. Department of Health, Education and Welfare, Washington, D.C., 1979. pp. 1–16.

3. Prien, R. F., and Cole, J. O.: The use of psychopharmacological drugs in the aged. In: *Principles of Psychopharmacology*, edited by W. G. Clark and J. del Guidice, ed. 2, Academic Press, New York, 1978. pp. 593–605.
4. Hollister, L. E.: Psychiatric and neurologic disorders. In: *Clinical Pharmacology*, edited by K. L. Melmon and H. F. Morrelli, chap. 11, The MacMillan Company, New York, 1972. pp. 455–459.
5. Kapnick, P. L.: Organic treatment of the elderly. In: *The Clinical Psychology of Aging*, edited by M. Storandt, I. C. Siegler, and M. F. Elias, Plenum Press, New York, 1978. pp. 225–251.
6. Gulevich, G.: Psychopharmacological treatment of the aged. In: *Psychopharmacology from Theory to Practice*, edited by J. D. Barchas, P. A. Berger, R. D. Ciaranello, and G. R. Elliott, Oxford University Press, New York, 1977. pp. 448–465.
7. Prange, A. J.: The use of antidepressant drugs in the elderly patient. In: *Advances in Behavioral Biology, Psychopharmacology and Aging*, edited by C. Eisdorfer and W. E. Fann, vol. 6, Plenum Press, New York, 1973. pp. 225–237.
8. Kastenbaum, R., and Slater, P. E.: Effects of wine on the interpersonal behavior of geriatric patients: an exploratory study. In: *New Thoughts on Old Age*, edited by R. Kastenbaum, Springer Publishing Company, Inc., New York, 1964. pp. 191–204.
9. Chien, C. P.: Psychiatric treatment for geriatric patients: pub or drug? *Am. J. Psychiatry 127(2)*:1070–1074, 1971.
10. Whanger, A. D., and Busse E. W.: Geriatrics. In: *The Therapist's Handbook: Treatment Methods of Mental Disorders*, edited by B. B. Wolman, van Nostrand Reinhold Company, New York, 1976. pp. 287–324.
11. Stotsky, B. A., and Borozne, J.: Butisol sodium vs. librium among geriatric and younger outpatients and nursing home patients. *Diseases of the Nervous System 33*:254–267, 1972.
12. Denber, H. C. B.: *Textbook of Clinical Psychopharmacology*. Stratton Intercontinental Medical Book Corporation, New York, 1979.
13. Lenhart, D. G.: The use of medications in the elderly population. *Nursing Clinics of North America 11*:135–143, 1976.
14. Linnoila, M., and Viukari, M.: Efficacy and side effects of Nitrazepam and Thioridazine as sleeping aids in psychogeriatric in-patients. *Br. J. Psychiatry 128*:566–569, 1976.
15. Fann, W. E., Wheless, J. C., and Richmann, B. W.: Treating the aged with psychotropic drugs. *The Gerontologist 16*:322–328, 1976.
16. Goldfarb, A. I.: Geriatric psychiatry. In: *Comprehensive Textbook of Psychiatry*, edited by A. M. Freedman and H. I. Kaplan, chap. 47, The Williams and Wilkins Company, Baltimore, 1967. pp. 1564–1587.
17. Agnew, H. W., Webb, W. W., and Williams, R. L.: Sleep patterns in late middle aged males: an EEG study. *Electroencephalography Clinical Neurophysiology 23*:168–171, 1967.
18. Kahn, E., and Fisher, C.: The sleep characteristics of the normal aged male. *J. Nervous Mental Dis. 148*:477–494, 1969.
19. Pattison, J. H., and Allen, R. P.: Comparison of the hypnotic effectiveness of Secobarbital, Pentobarbital, Methyprylon, and Ethchlorvynol. *J. Am. Geriat. Soc. 20*:398–412, 1972.
20. Levy, G.: Effect of bed rest on distribution and elimination of drugs. *J. Pharmaceutical Sci. 56*:928, 1967.
21. Whanger, A. D.: Nutrition, diet and exercise. In: *Handbook of Geriatric Psychiatry*, edited by E. W. Busse and D. G. Blazer, van Nostrand Reinhold Company, New York, 1979.
22. Nehrke, M. F., Belluci, G., and Gabriel, S. J.: Death anxiety, locus of control and life satisfaction in the elderly: toward a definition of ego-integrity. *Omega 8(4)*:359–368, 1978.

13

management of affective disorders*

DEPRESSION

PSYCHOPHARMACOLOGY

Antidepressant Drugs

The *antidepressant drugs* include the monamine oxidase (MAO) inhibitors, the tricyclic group, and other agents with occasional antidepressant effects (certain phenothiazines, stimulants, and antianxiety drugs).

MAO Inhibitors. They inhibit the deamination breakdown of catecholamines and indoleamines which results in increased amounts of the neurotransmitters norepinephrine, dopamine, and serotonin at the central receptor sites in the brain. There are a number of drugs with MAO inhibitor activity, but many of these are not available for psychiatric use in the United States. Those available belong to one of two chemical groups: the hydrazides, represented by phenelzine (Nardil), and the nonhydrazides represented by tranylcypromine (Parnate).[1,2] While theoretically MAO inhibitors should be very useful in treating the elderly because of their increased levels of MAO in various areas of the brain, in reality they should generally be used infrequently.[3] They have hazardous interactive toxicity with other drugs, and with certain foodstuffs. The general indications for their use are a past history of responding well to MAO inhibitors, and a poor response to other antidepressants.[4] Ordinarily, these drugs should be given in a hospital or other tightly controlled setting because of the risk of serious side effects (hallucinations, hyperreflexia, and sometimes fatal hypertensive crises) precipitated by the ingestion of foods rich in tyramine such as chicken livers or aged cheese, or of various medications containing pressor amines, such as cold remedies.

Tricyclic Antidepressants. The *tricyclic antidepressants* are phenothiazine analogs, but have a different pharmacological action, being useful against depression. Their mode of action is thought to be in terms of increasing the amounts of biogenic amines at central receptor sites.

* In collaboration with Alan D. Whanger, M.D.

The general effects of the tricyclics are adrenergic or anticholinergic, and may involve the cardiovascular, gastrointestinal, hematogenic, endocrine, and central nervous systems, as well as the liver. The tricyclics can be grouped according to their sedating properties. Those that are nonsedating are imipramine (Tofranil), desipramine (Pertofran, Norpramin), nortriptyline (Pamelor, Aventyl), and protriptyline (Vivactil). Sedating tricyclics include amitriptyline (Elavil) and doxepin (Sinequan). Amitriptyline, doxepin, imipramine, and desipramine also can relieve anxiety in the context of depression. Protriptyline, on the other hand, as a stimulating drug.[5]

Dosage: Generally, the tricyclics are similar in potency of action and dosage range, except for nortriptyline (Pamelor, Aventyl) and protriptyline (Vivactil) which are more potent. The dosage level for out-patient maintenance usually is about one-half or two-thirds of that in the hospital setting. Dose levels for elderly patients are generally lower than for younger adults; the initial dose is smaller and increments are made at a slower rate. Salzman recommends a test dose of 10–25 mg orally, repeating the sitting and standing blood pressure in 45 minutes to check for a potentially serious orthostatic hypotensive reaction.[6] The starting doses should be about 30 mg/day, and the amount increased in small amounts at about 3-day intervals. Using this approach, with regular monitoring for side-effects, the dosage ceiling for an individual elderly patient is established, which may take up to three weeks. Total dosage for the elderly is often about one-third of that used for a younger person.

Tricyclics have more *side-effects* in old patients than in younger patients (Table 13.1). *Psychological-behavioral* side-effects include mild hypomanic excitement, exacerbation of schizophrenic symptoms, and exacerbation of manic conditions. Adding a phenothiazine helps in manic shifts or when a latent schizophrenic reaction is activated by the antidepressant. *Physical* side-effects often are related to anticholinergic actions: e.g., dry mouth, lowered threshold for toxic confusion, glaucoma, urinary retention, constipation, and cardiovascular problems. Some of these can be potentially serious.[7] The central anticholinergic syndrome, in combination with the peripheral signs of anticholinergic toxicity, resembles the symptomatology of atropine or scopolamine toxicity.[8] The exact mechanism of another infrequent side effect, i.e., extrapyramidal symptoms, is obscure. It should not be treated with antiparkinson drugs, because they can cause toxic confusion, like the tricyclics. When this side-effect occurs, it is best to lower the dose of the tricyclic drug.

Other Antidepressants. *Phenothiazines* have been used with success in treatment of agitated and hostile depression. Thioridazine (Mellaril) has been most used for this, although it does have significant anticholinergic and hypotensive effects in many elderly.[9] In order to minimize these side-effects, it seems better to start at low doses such as 10 mg twice

Table 13.1
Important Side-Effects of Tricyclic Antidepressants

Clinical signs	Causative factors	Prevention and treatment
Behavioral		
Excitement, "manic shift"	Stimulating effect	Lower dose or change drug
Exacerbation of psychotic symptoms	Underlying paranoid or schizophrenic disorder	Use antipsychotics in combination or alone
CNS		
Electroencephalogram changes	Large doses; parenteral administration	Lower dose; avoid parenteral administration
Seizures	Family history of epilepsy; history of CNS injury	Don't combine with MAOI
	Combination with MAOI	Wait 2 weeks after one drug before starting another
Parkinsonism; tremors	Unclear; rare	Lower dose or change drug; don't use antiparkinson drugs
Central anticholinergic syndrome: acute confusion hallucinations agitation short term memory loss	Anticholinergic effects Combination with antipsychotics or antiparkinson drugs	*differential diagnosis*: Korsakoff; transient ischemic attacks; etc. Check peripheral anticholinergic signs *treatment*: physostigmine; stop drugs
Neurological		
Hypertonus Hyperreflexia	Anticholinergic or adrenergic effects; combination with MAOI	Lower dose or stop drug
Ataxia Neuropathies		Avoid polypharmacy
Tremors, fasciculations	Old age; vitamin deficiencies	Give vitamins
Cardiovascular		
EKG changes Hypotension	Pre-existing CVD	Do pretreatment EKG
Myocardial infarcts (→ CVA)	Adrenergic & anticholinergic effects	Monitor cardiovascular indices
Increased blood pressure in hypertensive patients	Blocking of guanethedine	Stop drug or use other antihypertensive, e.g., hydralazine
Eyes		
Glaucoma Blurred vision Accomodation paralysis	Anticholinergic effects	Lower dose or stop drug; treat glaucoma
Genitourinary		
Urinary retention Delayed ejaculation	Prostate hypertrophy	Lower dose or stop drug
Gastrointestinal		
Dry mouth, constipation		Lower dose or stop drug; stool softeners
Fecal impaction		Stop drug

daily, and slowly build up at 3-day intervals, watching carefully for orthostatic blood pressure changes.[10]

When anxiety and agitation coexist with depression, antipsychotics can be combined with tricyclics. A combination of perphenazine (Trilafon) and amitriptyline (Triavil, Etrafon) is frequently used for treatment of agitated depressions of mild or moderate degree. A variety of mixtures have been used, but there is no clear-cut answer yet as to which is best.[11]

Antianxiety drugs are sometimes beneficial to reduce mild or moderate depression associated with anxiety. The combination meprobamate and benactyzine (Deprol) has also been used for this purpose. Recently, a combination of amitriptyline and chlordiazepoxide (Librium) has been marketed as an antidepressant (Limbitrol), but there is little experience with it in the elderly. Diazepam (Valium) seems to have mild antidepressant properties in some older patients, but there are risks of side-effects, habituation, and even possible secondary depression.[12] Schatzberg and Cole observed the improvement of some patients with depression on benzodiazepines, but felt this was related to the reduction of anxiety symptoms rather than to the drug having a true antidepressant effect.[13]

Gerovital H3 has been studied with regard to its antidepressant effects.[14–16] The evidence so far suggests that Gerovital H3 (GH3) has mild antidepressant qualities and can be effective and safe in treating depression in the elderly. GH3 is a weak, reversible, and competitive inhibitor of MAO, which selectively inhibits the deamination of certain important brain monoamines. There is no risk of the hypertensive crisis so typical of other MAO inhibitors.

Treatment Considerations

It is advisable to get pretreatment baseline medical data, and to monitor the following physiological functions during drug therapy as indicated: heart (electrocardiogram), neurological (sensory and motor function, coordination), eyes (intraocular pressure), genitourinary (prostate, libido), metabolism (blood sugar), and liver tests.

Drug therapy ordinarily begins with one of the tricyclic drugs. A general rule of thumb is to use one of the activating drugs in retarded depression, and one of the sedating drugs in anxious or agitated depression. The greatest experience has been with imipramine (Tofranil) and amitriptyline (Elavil) as representatives of the activating and sedating groups of drugs, respectively. Both of these agents have rather potent anticholinergic effects, especially amitriptyline, and so may not prove to be the best choice.[17] Desipramine (Norpramine) has the least anticholinergic side-effects, and doxepin (Sinequan, Adapin) is probably least stressful on the cardivascular system, although possibly also the weakest antidepressant.[18] Nortriptyline (Pamelor, Aventyl) may have some advantages in that, while it is a somewhat more potent agent, it is rather effective in both agitated and retarded depressions, and in both norepinephrine and serotonin depletion states.[19] Since multiple factors play a role in producing therapeutic or toxic effects, there is considerable variability among patients with regard to optimal dose and maximum dose tolerated. Different therapists approach the problem in different ways, but starting slowly is generally safer. A typical approach would be to start at 10 mg, three times a day, and increase the dose by about 25 mg/day every 3rd day until there is improvement or significant side-effects.[10] It is probably safer to split the dose in the elderly rather than giving it all at one time. Those who are going to respond to a particular drug will usually do so within the first 2 weeks.[20] If there is not significant improvement in 3 weeks, the drug should be changed, or a shift made to electroconvulsive therapy (ECT).

In *acute* depressions, drug therapy is continued for 4–6 weeks beyond the point of maximum therapeutic benefit, then in gradually diminishing doses. The patient needs to be followed up for at least several months, depending on the duration of the episode and the speed of recovery. In patients with *recurrent* or *chronic* depression, antidepressant drugs may need to be continued indefinitely at a low dose.[21] There are significant cardiovascular side-effects of the tricyclics in the aged, especially those with prior organic heart disease. Therefore, it is prudent frequently to monitor the cardiac states during therapy.[22]

Side-effects, like *placebo effects,* may become part of the overall symptomatology. One means of preventing such a complication is a good therapist-patient relationship, which will have the effect of "detoxifying" or neutralizing some unwanted drug effects. The patient may be advised to consider mild side-effects, such as dry mouth, as evidence of favorable drug action.[2] Drowsiness usually disappears soon in patients who will favorably respond to tricyclic drugs; if it continues, another drug may be tried. Blurred vision and dry mouth often do persist.

Despite close chemical resemblance to the phenothiazines, the tricyclics are not as safe when taken in high doses. *Overdosage* produces coma, clonic movements or seizures, respiratory depression, hyperpyrexia, and disturbances of cardiac rhythm.

It is not sound clinical practice to treat every depression with drugs. When there is marked loss of weight, serious risk of suicide, or other self-destructive behavior, *ECT* is indicated and can be life-saving. Delay for trial of drugs leads to greater risk of suicide, chronicity, and more expense and socioeconomic disruption.

Tricyclics should not be combined with MAO inhibitors in older patients. Such a combination may lead to a *synergistic* effect manifested by intense central nervous system sympathetic stimulation: restlessness, muscle twitching, hypertension, convulsions, and hyperpyrexia, followed by death. There must be a waiting period of about 2 weeks between one type of drug and the other.

Assessment of *treatment effectiveness* and *clinical improvement* may be hampered by several factors. First, there is no clear-cut nosology of depression. Second, affective disorders are usually self-limited in duration, with remissions being followed by recurrent episodes. Third, some depressed patients hate to admit that they feel better. Consequently, it is essential to evaluate improvement (or lack thereof), as much as possible, by way of *objective* criteria. The latter pertain mostly to the physiological concomitants. Thus, clinical improvement can be assessed by observing the degree to which patterns of sleep, appetite, weight, bowel function, psychomotor activity, and sexual activities are being restored to normal. *Subjective* criteria include the patient's mood statement, reports about decreasing physical malaise, the ability to concentrate, and the return of initiative and interests.

The danger of *suicide* should always be kept in mind, particularly when the seriously depressed patient seems to be getting better. During an intermediate phase of recovery from depression, the patient may have regained enough energy to carry out an earlier plan for suicide.

As the depression improves, the patient may begin to show more *anger and hostility*. Usually these negative feelings were present all along, but suppressed by the patient. The development of *paranoid features*, however, may indicate that the depression is worsening. It is, therefore, important to differentiate between anger, irascibility, querulousness, etc., on the one hand, and suspiciousness, ideas of reference, and paranoid ideation, on the other hand.

CLINICAL MANAGEMENT

Reactive Depressions

Reactive depressions (adjustment disorder with depressed mood) in which a specific event is the precipitating factor usually last for 1–3 months. Such a grief reaction, with its lowered mood, sense of emptiness, and physical distress, is a natural response to the loss of a loved one. Grief of more than a year's duration, however, is pathological, suggesting an ambivalent relationship with the lost object, or circumstances which otherwise inhibited emotional expression. Psychotherapy of a prolonged grief reaction should focus on mobilizing and expressing the emotions, and on exploring the role of ambivalence. Medications generally should be limited to nighttime sedation. Antidepressants are usually ineffective and, in fact, may obfuscate the process of working through the loss.

Acute Grief Reactions

Management of *acute grief reactions* (uncomplicated bereavement) involves promoting a realistic awareness on the part of the patient of the loss which he suffered, and encouraging open expression of his bereavement. Ventilation of grief and sadness affords the patient a sense of relief that is both physiological and psychological, and also enables him to feel closer to the therapist who is present to share the experience. Sometimes, an individual needs the reassurance that grief and sadness are natural and that mourning represents a period which must be entered, traversed, and completed. But at the same time, he can be advised that, while thoughts concerning the lost object will be frequently on his mind, it is wise to seek new activities and contacts to avoid excessive preoccupation with the loss. Thus, one attempts to guide the patient down an intermediate path which, on the one hand, avoids premature closure (suppression of grief) and, on the other, steers away from excessive melancholic involvement, by venturing into new activities which will eventually engage the energy previously invested in the lost object. Frequently, simple counseling techniques are sufficient.

> A 67-year-old unmarried woman continued to mourn her mother's death for many months. She had lived with her mother for many years and filled her time by taking care of her. Since the mother had had a serious heart condition, the patient had been well aware that death could come at any time. Yet, in spite of this anticipatory grief work, she remained painfully preoccupied with the loss. Her unresolved grief was illustrated by an unrealistic plan to become a nurse's aid, an attempt to perpetuate the role she had played vis-à-vis her mother. She said she was not even able to go into the room which her mother had occupied for so many years. "There would be too many painful memories if I go in that room." The suggestion was made that she rearrange the furniture in her house, remove her mother's bed, and buy some new furniture. The patient expressed surprise that she herself had not thought of this solution.

Defenses aimed at avoiding awareness of grief and loss (denial, suppression, rationalization) can become maladaptive and require clinical intervention for several reasons. Hyperactivity, inherent in being diversion-prone, may exhaust the patient. Although mild forms of denial can be conducive to good adjustment, extreme denial (often coupled with rebellious protest) is self-destructive, since the patient tends to reject appropriate assistance. Finally, the longer one holds on to an illusion, the more painful the disillusionment will be.

In dealing with denial, it is necessary to proceed with caution. One should never try to break through the denial by forcefully uncovering the underlying emotions and confronting the patient with them. Ventilation of concerns is useful for specific therapeutical goals. Certain emotions lying just below the surface (grief about loss of an organ, anger at medical personnel, guilt about dependency imposed by illness) can be alleviated by expressing them. It is also useful to bring out into the open unrealistic assumptions or magical notions, such as guilt feelings about having done something wrong in the past, or even having lived the wrong kind of life, and now being punished for that in terms of having a physical affliction or having suffered other losses.

In many aged persons, however, the self is in a state of transition or crisis. So, it is not always prudent to probe for deeper thoughts and emotions, especially those which do not contribute to the patient's sense of closure, such as past disillusionments.[23] The tendency of many older people to make the best of it, to count one's blessings, to retouch life's pictures stored in the memory by highlighting the bright and obscuring the dark, all this is not just a denial of some piece of reality. Rather, the attempt to seek out the sunny side of things in the here and now and, in retrospect, to beautify the past is nothing else but the work of that vital principle, hope.

Chronic Neurotic Depression

Chronic neurotic depressions (chronic depressive disorder) are quite common and may be manifested by a diversity of clinical symptomatology. Frequently, anxiety is a relatively prominent feature. Clinical management of these conditions can be most difficult. It is often easier to deal with a frankly psychotic depression, in which ECT or other antidepressant treatment is quickly effective. In contrast, chronic neurotic depressions may drag on, with minor ups and downs, not unlike the fate of Sisyphus. The vexing problem with many neurotic depressions, at any age, is the masochistic core of needing to suffer, and often for an ulterior (i.e., vindictive) purpose. This tendency is clinically demonstrated by the so-called negative therapeutic reaction; that is, at the very moment we have every reason to believe that the patient should improve, the opposite happens and he gets worse. This also presents problems for the therapist who must come to grips with his own frustration and countertransference. Not infrequently the combination of a few negative therapeutic reactions on the patient's part and a steady build up of countertransference feelings in the therapist add up to a termination of the relationship after a few months or years.

By the time a patient with a history of chronic depression has reached middle age and moved into sensecence, the emotional and behavioral patterns are usually well-established. Depending on multiple factors (See Chapters 3 and 6), these patients may hold their own, gradually change for the better, or slowly decompensate. For some individuals, a chronic depression becomes a way of life (depressive personality disorder).

> A chronically depressed woman had managed to remain the center of the family by her stubborn silence, withdrawal, and asceticism. She found the energy to maintain this painful existence in one source: she cherished, with a vengeance, the memory of a thoughtless remark from her husband, 20 years ago. Even though he and their three children cared a good deal for her, she had become increasingly withdrawn and depressed. More and more

often, she found herself at the edge of suicide. In the therapeutic contacts with this patient, she first would adamantly refuse any medications. After she had finally, in desperation, agreed to take antidepressant drugs, she indicated there was "a most important problem," but stubbornly declined to talk about it. Likewise, various suggestions and recommendations in the course of therapy were dismissed. Yet, she would continuously complain of the agony she was in. After she eventually verbalized her "most important problem" (i.e., her husband's slighting her), there was no let up in her savage depression. After several years of psychotherapy and numerous antidepressants, she still was not willing or able to let go of the depression; the secondary gains (controlling her family) were of such a magnitude that she was willing to pay the high price of continuous suffering. This case also illustrates the role of narcissism and vindictiveness in depression and her inability to forgive and forget.

Mild Depressions of Recent Onset

Depressions of a *mild* degree and relatively *recent* onset can be treated with guidance type of psychotherapy, often in combination with antidepressant drugs. The psychotherapy focuses on exploring the factors that produce the lowered self-esteem which is central to the depression, as well as clarifying environmental influences. Quite often such depressions occur in the beginning of the *involutional* period, which again points out that most depressions of the involutional type are not psychotic.

Many of these patients are female, in their late 40's and 50's. One of the major goals in therapy is to prevent decompensation toward hypochondriasis, or a fixation of the patient's withdrawal. It will be necessary to focus on the need for developing new interests, contacts, and activities. Tricyclic antidepressants may be useful adjuncts for the treatment of menopausal depressions. The benzodiazepines are effective when anxiety and mild agitation are present.

Occasionally, the patient's spouse will be seen as well, in conjoint sessions. Marital counseling and sexual advice is probably more often needed than carried out. Handling sexual and other highly personal matters in joint sessions requires special discretion and judgment to prevent further disruption of an interpersonal balance, which is often already tenuous.

In the case of female patients, the past history often reveals gynecological problems and surgery, including a hysterectomy. Surprisingly, some patients are not certain whether the ovaries were removed or left in. At any rate, endocrinological factors may play a role in these depressions, and estrogen replacement therapy should be considered for possible inclusion in the management of postmenopausal depressions.[24–26]

The involutional depressions in men tend to occur at a later age, and are less distinct in symptomatology. When sexual involution coincides with retirement, it may be difficult to sort out which factor is more important. Some men develop an involutional depression in their 50's; and when the depressive episode is rather prolonged, and includes many physical complaints, early retirement is a risk. This may permanently lower their self-esteem. The depression is complicated by increased anxiety, which may require indefinite supportive psychotherapy and drug therapy (antidepressants and antianxiety drugs in milder cases, combinations of antidepressants and phenothiazines in more serious cases). Again, the focus in therapy is on utilizing the patient's remaining assets; limiting one's commiseration with the patient in favor of an attitude of firm insistence, while directing him toward new interests. A program of activities may need to be developed as described above.

Depressive Equivalents

Depressive equivalents are common, in both female and male patients, during senescence.[27] The first problem one has to deal with may be the patient's resentment toward the medical profession. Such patients may have seen many physicians for their physical complaints, some of whom may already have informed them that the underlying cause is "psychological." During the initial contacts, it is important to tune in on the patient's feelings of resentment and futility, and to convey through empathetic responses a sense of understanding. Having established rapport with the patient, the next goal is to get the patient in touch with his real feelings. This means one has to get behind the surface layer of physical symptoms, and explore, together with the patient, what feelings might exist on that deeper level. At this stage in therapy, it would theoretically be better to withhold antidepressant drugs, and this is possible in cases of mild-to-moderate severity.

> An attractive, middle-aged woman had complained for many years of a swollen sensation in her arms, constant sleepiness, a feeling that other people seemed to be far away, and a persistent craving for chocolate. Her mood was one of mild tension and apprehension about the physical sensations. In psychotherapy, it was possible to interpret these as a defense against her becoming aware of an underlying depression. Only after she had stopped focusing on the physical sensations did the depression emerge and was the patient in a position to explore why she was depressed. While she had been taking various antidepressant drugs, prior to psychotherapy, none of these appeared to be effective. On the other hand, once she realized what the source of her misery was, she was able to go ahead with appropriate, corrective action. This, in turn, resulted in a disappearance of the depression.

Because insight alone is not always enough to bring about corrective action and improvement of the depression, antidepressants or anxiolytics may need to be used, depending on the patient's reactions to various life events.[28] In the case of antianxiety drugs, the patient himself can often decide when he needs them and then they can be prescribed on a p.r.n. basis, but one does need to indicate what the maximum daily dose is. With antidepressants, the patient should not be the judge of when or how much to take. These are taken regularly, in specified amounts, until the physician decides to change the regimen.

Further Comments on Psychotherapy

When unconscious hostility appears to play a major role in the development of guilt feelings, the therapist may carefully probe for such negative feelings. The hostile, vengeful thoughts and feelings may have been thoroughly walled off, and caution is needed when inserting one's probe through this defensive wall into the interior of the emotional abscess. The evacuation of its contents, i.e., the expression of hostile feelings, must be done in a low key manner, and only after a positive relationship has been established. The therapeutical quality of the procedure depends on the suppressed hostility being brought out in the open, wherein the light of reality there usually is a way for its detoxification.

Also important in the psychotherapeutical management of guilt feelings is to remove fantasies, views, or conclusions which the patient has developed on the basis of magical thinking. One type of patient may hold himself responsible for something that, in fact, was beyond his control. Another patient ascribes his current misery, or its cause, to alleged misdeeds or failures in the past. A third type of situation involves the guilt feelings in persons who have been taking care of a chronically ill relative. After the latter's death, the survivor is painfully preoccupied with the question: "Did I do all that I could or should have done?" In most cases, one can reassure the patient with a statement to the effect that "from what we know about you and what you have done, it is clear that you did everything you were capable of: to give the best you have is all that can be humanly expected."

Other psychotherapeutic techniques which may be useful in dealing with neurotic guilt include: encouraging the patient to suppress self-depreciating fantasies and to abandon excessive introspection in favor of an orientation toward present realities; trying to liberate the depressed patient from the prison of the past (where he dwells on his sins, transgressions, shortcomings) by siding with him as he faces the discomforting openness of the future; demonstrating to the patient that such gratifications as affection, approval, etc. do not require prepayment in the form of self-derogation, guilt feelings, or other misery; that it is all right to receive gifts without strings attached; unmasking the patient's continuous preoccupation with his shortcomings, guilt feelings, or sense of rejection as a means of coercion or expression of hostility (especially for patients who obtain sizeable fringe benefits from their depression in terms of making their family miserable, or coercing them into giving special favors by effective display of depressive misery); and pointing out to the patient who constantly complains about his worthlessness and sinfulness the existence of an underlying layer of self-aggrandizement. In effect, such patients are "playing God," in as much as they have set themselves up as the sole judge, as if the judgment of others no longer matters.

Psychotic Depressions

Psychotic depressions (major depressive disorder) may be an involutional melancholia, the depressive phase of manic-depressive illness, a retarded psychotic depression, or an agitated depression. Hospitalization is indicated to ensure vigorous treatment. Antidepressant therapy is usually started with drugs rather than ECT; but there are exceptions, especially psychotic depressions in elderly male patients, because of the high suicidal risk. Patients who are going to get good responses to antidepressants will achieve them within 2–3 weeks. If there is no response within this time, electroconvulsive therapy should be considered. Properly given, ECT remains the safest, most effective treatment for depressive psychoses.

Electroconvulsive Therapy

Indications. In general, old age is not a contraindiction against ECT. If properly administered, ECT tends to be safer than many psychotropic drugs because of their many side effects. The *indications* for ECT include the major depressive and manic disorders. ECT is effective in more than three-fourths of patients with such disorders.[29] Although ECT can be given in conjunction with antianxiety, antipsychotic, and antidepressant drugs, it is wise to give only one type of treatment at the time in order to be able to assess the efficacy of each form of treatment, as well as to make the treatment safer.

Organic Brain Syndrome. ECT may be used for the treatment of moderate to severe depression, in the presence of mild *organic brain syndrome*. In view of the frequently difficult differential diagnosis between depression and organicity, the administration of ECT in these cases will have the element of a therapeutical trial. If the patient improves, the diagnosis of depression is justified in retrospect.

Complications. The risk of serious *complications* can be reduced by hospitalization (outpatient ECT for elderly patients generally is contraindicated), ruling out serious systemic illnesses (recent myocardial infarct, cardiorespiratory decompensation, uremia, hepatic failure, severe organic brain syndrome), use of muscle relaxants (succinylcholine) to avoid bone fractures, adequate oxygenation before each ECT to counteract the interference with respiration caused by muscle relaxants, and even omission of short-acting barbiturates if there are not good anesthesia facilities and personnel available.[30]

Schedule. ECT in the elderly is often given at 2- or 3-day intervals for the first three treatments, and then the frequency is reduced to every 4 or 5 days. Improvement will usually become manifest after the first few treatments, but there is no set number of treatments that should be given. A useful guide is to treat to the point of good improvement, and then give two additional ECT treatments to consolidate the gain.[10]

Pseudodementia. Some depressed patients may show cognitive deficits, incontinence, and confusion, rather than overt depression. When they are successfully treated with antidepressants or ECT, these symptoms disappear.[31] If not properly treated, however, these *pseudodemented* patients may remain institutionalized until they die.[8] Older patients who appear confused and depressed may respond well to tricyclic antidepressants, with an improvement of cognitive function and mood, but ECT remains the most effective form of treatment for severe depression.

Quick Response. A *quick response* to ECT should be viewed with some reservation. The improvement of the affective disorder may be related to the effect of ECT on memory function, rather than on the basis of a real alleviation of the underlying disorder. Due to the effect on memory, and as part of the post-ECT confusion, the patient becomes less alert and less capable of emotional expression. Thus, premature interruption of ECT may cause a relapse, upon recovery of memory function. Since many elderly patients have marginal cerebral resources, and tend to become confused by ECT, early improvement is not alway genuine.[2]

Post-ECT Confusion. It usually becomes detectable after three or four treatments. If confusion is relatively severe, the frequency of the treatments should be diminished. The confusion itself is not a serious side-effect provided the patient receives adequate supervision and protection during this time. After several weeks, it usually clears up, and the patient's mental capacities return to the pre-ECT level of functioning. If severe disabling confusion persists for more than 1 or 2 days after a treatment, it may be necessary to terminate the ECT.

Technical Points. In giving ECT to the elderly, several *technical points* should be kept in mind; namely, give an adequate dose of atropine (e.g., 0.8 mg) prior to treatment, use a generous dose of succinylcholine (Anectine) (e.g., 60 mg) to ensure adequate muscle relaxation to prevent fractures, use a high dose of current as the skin resistance and seizure threshold are high in the elderly, and keep the patient well oxygenated.

Memory deficits may be minimized by proper choice of electrode placement and optimal spacing of the treatments. Experience has shown that memory deficits can be reduced by an approach which combines adequate oxygenation, minimal currents for induction, unilateral nondominant placement of electrodes, minimal barbiturate anesthesia, and as wide a spacing of treatments as therapeutically feasible.[32]

APATHY

Apathy (literally "absence of emotion") refers to a condition of emotional exhaustion (as in severe physical illness) or a state of profound emotional withdrawal (as in schizophrenia and senility).

Depletion of Narcissistic Supplies

In the *depressions of late life*, the affective manifestations may not be as prominent, and the patient may appear to be apathetic. Such types of depression are often comparable to the so-called anaclitic depressions. The primary etiological factor in these is object loss and depletion of narcissistic supplies. In addition, some late life depressions involve the psychodynamics of withdrawal and regression, rather than the "typical" depressive mechanisms of introjection, hostile identification, etc. Clinical management will be aimed at correcting the factor of depletion and insufficiency of narcissistic supplies (e.g., supportive measures such as increasing social contacts, decreasing relative sensory deprivation, reestablishing a hopeful perspective, etc.). In addition, antidepressant drugs may be given but their role is secondary to the importance of a broad, comprehensive, supportive approach.

Emotional Exhaustion

Apathy, in the sense of *emotional exhaustion*, should not be treated by an approach of stimulation but by intensive supportive treatment. The principle involved is to nurture and restore an organism whose inner resources and adaptive capacity are critically diminished. This involves adequate treatment of any physiological disturbance; ensuring adequate sleep, rest, food intake, and promotion of anabolical-metabolical processes in general; and elimination of emotional insecurity by establishing a firm rapport and permitting the patient to become dependent on the parental figure of the therapist (anaclitic therapy). Upon return of emotional responsiveness and interest in the external world, one should not withdraw his support, but maintain contact with the patient allowing him to set his own tempo of emotional recovery. To withdraw from the patient when he improves is to encourage relapse in apathy. Important during this recovery phase is exploring with the patient toward which persons and activities his reawakened interests can be directed.

Withdrawal and Seclusiveness

Apathy, in the sense of *withdrawal and seclusiveness*, may respond to an approach of appropriate stimulation. Many such patients are apathetic, not because of exhaustion, but because they prefer the gratifications of their inner fantasy world over those provided by the real world. The treatment approach includes: eliminating possible iatrogenic apathy, e.g., a chemical straightjacket due to excessive tranquilization; eliminating undue social isolation and relative sensory deprivation; remotivation, resocialization, and other group experiences; auxiliary therapies (OT, RT, IT, and PT); and appropriate stimulation involving a clinical trial of antipsychotics or antidepressants. In the apathy of some chronic "burned out" schizophrenics, there may be a depressive element. In view of this possibility, tricyclic antidepressants may be given a trial, perhaps in combination with the antipsychotic drugs which the patient already is receiving. However, if the apathy is due to prolonged withdrawal and seclusiveness, antidepressant drugs are not likely to be effective. A syndrome called Poor Motivation Syndrome has been identified in which the individuals show no depression nor dementia, but are extremely dependent, and demanding, complain of fatigue and weakness, sag to the floor or bed, and have little concern for the burden they put on others. A 3-week course of *d*-amphetamine (Dexedrine) was found helpful with many of these.[33]

Giving Up

Apathy, in the sense of hopelessness, involves the mechanism of *giving up*. Regression carried to its extreme ends in surrender to the threat. Clinically, a pattern of giving up may manifest itself in apathy. When apathy is a reflection of underlying anxiety of overwhelming intensity, antianxiety medications may produce what seems to be a paradoxical response: instead of becoming more tranquil, the patient becomes more active, more alive.

MANIC CONDITIONS

Manic grandiosity and hyperactivity require treatment especially when the patient's behavior is self-destructive, causes serious disruptions in his milieu, or when his overconfidence and lack of judgment prompt him to make unwise decisions or engage in inappropriate actions. ECT may be considered when psychotropic drugs fail to produce clinical improvement, or when the patient's manic behavior has resulted in physiological exhaustion.

BIPOLAR DISORDERS

Lithium

Lithium is effective in the treatment and prevention of bipolar affective disorder, including the manic and the depressive types. In contrast to its effectiveness in bipolar affective disorders, lithium does not appear to be as useful in unipolar affective disorders.[34] Lithium inhibits the enzyme tyrosine hydroxylase, and increases the deamination of norepinephrine, which results in decreased amounts of norepinephrine at the receptor sites in the brain. It also has a marked effect on sodium and potassium metabolism. In view of the toxicity and frequent complications of this drug, lithium therapy for the elderly should be initiated in the hospital generally.

In an acute or *severe manic attack*, it is best to bring the episode under control with a sedating antipsychotic drug such as chlorpromazine (Thorazine) or haloperidol (Haldol), either orally or intramuscularly. The drug of choice is haloperidol.[35] When the attack is under control, then the patient can be started on lithium carbonate. The effect of lithium occurs in several days, and by 3 weeks the episode should be under control.[36] When there is no urgent need to achieve quick remission, as for example, in *hypomanic* conditions, lithium can be given without the antipsychotics. Since lithium is useful in preventing recurrence of manic-depressive illness, many patients are continued on it. Antidepressant drugs may be used in combination with lithium.

In hypomanic and manic patients, the prognosis for remission is good, but occasionally such patients present a clinical picture of *pseudosenility* (compare Chapter 5, p. 85). A thorough mental status examination will show that the "cognitive deficits" are, in fact, due to functional deficits in concentration and attention span, with distractibility and so on. Thus, the differential diagnosis is crucial, because if these (essentially manic) patients do not receive specific treatment, their condition may quickly worsen due to physical exhaustion, and by then they will appear more "senile," a self-fulfilling prophecy.

Dosage Schedule

Start with 300 mg of lithium carbonate daily and do serum levels two or three times a week. Increase dose slowly after serum level has become stable, and until therapeutic effects are achieved. Continue to monitor for side-effects and toxicity. While in younger patients the half-life of lithium is about 24 hours, in elderly patients it is prolonged to 36–48 hours. Hence, smaller doses of lithium will result in a therapeutic blood level. Since elderly patients excrete lithium more slowly, they can build up the desired blood level with lower doses. For example, to achieve a therapeutic level of 1.2 to 1.5 mEq/l, one might give a younger patient a daily dose of 1500 mg, but an elderly patient 600–900 mg.[8] In many cases, however, an older manic may get a good therapeutic response in the range of 0.7 to 0.9 mEq/l. Since the serum lithium level tends to fluctuate somewhat unpredictably in older persons, it must be monitored rather closely, and checked when there is any unusual alteration in the clinical course.

Side-Effects

Lithium produces CNS, gastrointestinal, and neuromuscular toxicity;

and aged patients are more susceptible to these, especially confusion. Side effects may develop at lower blood levels (even as low as 0.7 mEq/l) and this necessitates close monitoring of the blood levels. Mild side-effects are anorexia, nausea, vomiting, diarrhea, and mild tremors. Serious side-effects include dystonia and dysarthria; polydipsia and polyuria; ataxia, hyperreflexia, and muscle spasms; confusion and coma.[7] Unsupervised use of lithium may cause electrolyte imbalance, especially low salt and potassium levels. Discontinuation of lithium, giving fluids, and supplementary NaCl and KCl will correct the toxic state. Special caution is required in the presence of cardiac or renal disease.

Toxicity

Increasing confusion, a major sign of lithium *toxicity*, usually occurs when an out-patient is maintained on lithium without close medical supervision. The family may ascribe this to "senility" and delay medical help until the patient is near coma. Therefore, patients and relatives should be instructed about side-effects and toxicity. Lithium toxicity may develop insidiously. It is manifested by a worsening of the tremor, fasciculations, slurred speech, drowsiness and confusion, ataxia and choreoathetoid movements, and a diabetes insipidus-like syndrome (increased water intake and urine output).[8]

EXPANSIVENESS

Expansive behavior occurs not only in manic disorders, but also in certain paranoid conditions, and in some cases of organic brain syndrome.

Paranoid Conditions; Organic Brain Syndromes

In *paranoid* conditions, the patient's thought contents may be grandiose, and his behavior expansive or aggressive, but the affect of euphoria or elation is lacking. On the other hand, superficial cheerfulness may be present in certain *organic brain syndromes*, such as the amnestic syndrome and organic affective syndrome. Paranoid grandiosity preferably is treated with antipsychotic drugs, ECT rarely being indicated. The same holds true for grandiose and expansive behavior associated with chronic brain syndrome. Hyperactivity in patients with chronic brain syndrome may be treated with one of the antipsychotic agents.

Hyperactivity; Acute Brain Syndrome

Hyperactive or expansive behavior in *acute brain syndrome*, such as caused by alcoholism, requires that primary attention be given to eliminating the cause of the organic brain syndrome, along with symptomatic treatment with benzodiazepine derivatives, if the cause is alcohol abuse. Otherwise one of the major tranquilizers such as haloperidol or chlorpromazine intramuscularly or orally will help to control agitation and other symptoms better. Phenothiazines (e.g., chlorpromazine, promazine, perphenazine, or prochlorperazine) also control gastrointestinal disturbances in the alcoholic.

Psychotic Manic Disorder

When the manic disorder is not part of a manic-depressive illness, but appears to be an isolated instance, the diagnosis *psychotic manic disorder* (manic disorder, single episode) is appropriate. Treatment of such cases would involve the use of antipsychotics or ECT rather than lithium. All of these patients should be suspected of having an early serious systemic illness; medical and neurological evaluation and treatment is an essential part of the clinical management of psychotic manic reactions. When the psychodynamic configuration in these patients is what one would expect for a psychotic depression, antidepressant drugs may be given a therapeutical trial.

References

1. Quitkin, F., Rifkin, A., and Klein, D. F.: Monoamine oxidase inhibitors. *Arch. Gen. Psychiatry 36*(*7*):749–760, 1979.
2. Goldfarb, A. I.: Geriatric psychiatry. In: *Comprehensive Textbook of Psychiatry,* edited by A. M. Freedman and H. I. Kaplan, chap. 47, The Williams and Wilkins Company, Baltimore, 1967. pp. 1564–1587.
3. Epstein, L. J.: Anxiolytics, antidepressants, and neuroleptics in the treatment of geriatric patients. In: *Psychopharmacology: A Generation of Progress,* edited by M. A. Lipton, A. Dimascio, and K. F. Killam, Raven Press, New York, 1978.
4. Hollister, L. E.: Psychotherapeutic drugs. In: *Neuropsychiatric Side Effects of Drugs in the Elderly,* edited by A. J. Levenson, Raven Press, New York, 1979.
5. Prange, A. J.: The use of antidepressant drugs in the elderly patient. In: *Advances in Behavioral Biology,* edited by C. Eisdorfer and W. E. Fann, vol. 6, Plenum Press, New York, 1973. pp. 225–237.
6. Salzman, C., van der Kolk, B., and Shader, R. I.: Psychopharmacology and the geriatric patient. In: *Manual of Psychiatric Therapeutics Practical Psychopharmacology and Psychiatry,* edited by Richard I. Shader, Little, Brown and Company, Boston, 1975. pp. 171–184.
7. Janowsky, D., El-Yousef, M. D., and Davis, J. M.: Side effects associated with psychotropic drugs. In: *Drug Issues in Geropsychiatry,* edited by W. E. Fann and G. L. Maddox, The Williams and Wilkins Company, Baltimore, 1974. pp. 19–28.
8. Davis, J. M., Fann, W. E., El-Yousef, M. K., and Janowsky, D. S.: Clinical problems in treating the aged with psychotropic drugs. In: *Advances in Behavioral Biology,* edited by C. Eisdorfer and W. E. Fann, vol. 6, Plenum Press, New York, 1973. pp. 111–125.
9. Fann, W. E.: Pharmacotherapy in older depressed patients. *J. Gerontol. 31:*304–310, 1976.
10. Whanger, A. D., and Busse, E. W.: Geriatrics. In: *The Therapist's Handbook, Treatment Methods of Mental Disorders,* edited by Benjamin B. Wolman, van Nostrand Reinhold Company, New York, 1976. pp. 287–324.
11. Fracchia, J., Sheppard, C., and Merlis, S.: Treatment patterns in psychiatry: relationships to symptoms and aging. *J. Am. Geriatr. Soc. 21:*34–38, 1973.
12. Fann, W. E., Wheless, J. C., and Richman, B. W.: Treating the aged with psychotropic drugs. *The Gerontologist 16:*322–328, 1976.
13. Schatzberg, A. F., and Cole, J. O.: Benzodiazepines in depressive disorders. *Arch. Gen. Psychiatry 35:*1359–1365, 1978.
14. MacFarlane, M. D.: Possible rationale for procaine (Gerovital H3) therapy in geriatrics: inhibition of monoamine oxidase. *J. Am. Geriatr. Soc. 21:*414–418, 1973.
15. Zung, W. W. K., Gianturco, D., Pfeiffer, E., Wang, H. S., Whanger, A., Bridge, T. P., and Potkin, S. G.: Evaluation of Gerovital H3 as an antidepressant drug. *Psychosomatics 15:* 127–131, 1974.

16. Cohen, S. and Ditman, K.: Gerovital H3 in the treatment of the depressed aging patient. *Psychosomatics 15:*15–19, 1974.
17. Piland, B.: The aging process and psychoactive drug use in clinical treatment. In: *National Institute on Drug Abuse, Services Research Monography Series. Publication No. 79-813,* United States Department of Health, Education and Welfare, Washington, D. C., 1979.
18. Gulevich, G.: Psychopharmacological treatment of the aged. In: *Psychopharmacology,* edited by J. D. Barchas, P. A. Berger, R. D. Ciarenello, and G. R. Elliott, Oxford University Press, New York, 1977. pp. 448–465.
19. Maas, J. W.: Biogenic amines and depression. *Arch. Gen. Psychiatry 32:*1357–1361, 1975.
20. Butler, R. N., and Lewis, M. I.: *Aging and Mental Health Positive Psychosocial Approaches,* ed. 2, The C. V. Mosby Company, St. Louis, 1977.
21. Post, F.: The functional psychoses. In: *Studies in Geriatric Psychiatry,* edited by A. D. Isaacs and F. Post, chap. 4, John Wiley and Sons, Ltd., New York, 1978. pp. 77–94.
22. Rodstein, M., and Oei, L. S.: Cardiovascular side effects of long-term therapy with tricyclic antidepressants in the aged. *J. Am. Geriatr. Soc. 27:*231–234, 1979.
23. Brink, T. L.: Geriatric rigidity and its psychotherapeutic implications. *J. Am. Geriatr. Soc. 26:*274–277, 1978.
24. Wilson, R. A., and Wilson, T. A.: The basic philosophy of estrogen maintenance. *J. Am. Geriatr. Soc. 26:*521–523, 1972.
25. Meema, H. E., and Meema, S.: Involutional bone loss in women and the feasibility of preventing structural failure. *J. Am. Geriatr. Soc. 22:*443–451, 1974.
26. Rhoads, F. P.: Continuous cyclic hormonal therapy. *J. Am. Geriatr. Soc. 22:*183–185, 1974.
27. Salzman, C., and Shader, R. I.: Depression in the elderly. I. Relationship between depression, psychologic defense mechanisms and physical illness. *J. Am. Geriatr. Soc. 26:*253–260, 1978.
28. Goldstein, S. E.: Depression in the elderly. *J. Am. Geriatr. Soc. 27:*38–42, 1979.
29. Wilson, W. P., and Major, L. F.: Electroshock and the aged patient. In: *Advances in Behavioral Biology,* edited by C. Eisdorfer and W. E. Fann, vol. 6, Plenum Press, New York, 1973. pp. 239–244.
30. Lowenbach, H.: How well does electroshock treatment work in depression in the elderly? In: *Mental Illness in Later Life,* edited by E. W. Busse and E. Pfeiffer, American Psychiatric Association, Washington, D. C., 1973. pp. 246–248.
31. Salzman, C., and Shader, R. I.: Clinical evaluation of depression in the elderly. In: *Psychiatric Symptoms and Cognitive Loss in the Elderly,* edited by A. Raskin and L. F. Jarvik, John Wiley and Sons, New York, 1979. pp. 39–72.
32. Fink, M.: Neuropsychology of electroconvulsive therapy. In: *Convulsive Therapy, Theory and Practice,* chap. 9, Raven Press, New York, 1979. pp. 107–129.
33. Clark, A. N. G., and Mankikar: d-Amphetamine in elderly patients refractory to rehabilitation procedures. *J. Am. Geriatr. Soc. 27:*174–177, 1979.
34. Coppen, A., Noguera, R., Bailey, J., Burns, B. H., Swani, M. S., Hare, E. H., Gardner, R., and Maggs, R.: Prophylactic lithium in affective disorders. *Lancet 2:*275, 1971.
35. Gershon, S.: The treatment of manic-depressive states. In: *Manual of Psychiatric Therapeutics, Practical Psychopharmacology and Psychiatry,* edited by Richard I. Shader, Little, Brown, and Company, Boston, 1975. pp. 101–114.
36. Kral, V. A.: An overview of psychopharmacology of old age. *Psychopharm. Bull. 12:*51–52, 1976.

14

hypochondriasis and related states

INTRODUCTION

The clinical management of hypochondriasis depends on the degree of self-absorption and the context in which it has developed. We can distinguish between types that are relatively mild, transitory, benign and those that are of a chronic, progressive, malignant nature. The degree of self-absorption corresponds with the extent of withdrawal, and depends on whether the patient considers his state of stagnation as still reversible or a permanent impasse.

In the early, milder forms, the echoes of the disillusionment and depression that anteceded the hypochondriasis can still be heard.[1–3] Since withdrawal from others has not extended over a long distance, the process is still reversible; external objects have not suffered significant depreciation.

During the intermediate phase, a greater distance separates the patient from others; there has been more devaluation of external objects by the patient. He has not yet reached the point of no return and his perspective still permits him to believe that the process is reversible. Along with his increased alienation, however, he views life with more skepticism and bitterness. Feelings of ambivalence toward others are prominent; three sets of wishes are in a tug of war: to move back toward people, further away from them, or move against them. In the wake of bitterness follows envy toward those who appear to be more fortunate; increased disappointments in those who did not try to entice him back and convince him that his skepticism was not justified; and hostility toward those who did not help him when he came to them in his search for hope. The patient may stagnate in bitter resignation, or decide to do something about it.

When such a psychodynamic constellation receives a charge of energy, the result may be aggressive vindictiveness. Part of the patient's goal is to vindicate himself, as if he has a score to settle. But the struggle is often futile, or even conducive to further deterioration of his position. His vindictiveness (manifested by chronic complaints, fault finding, obstinate refusal to collaborate with others, subtle, vengeful sabotage of therapeutic programs, etc.) has the effect of confirming what the patient suspected all along: that people are no good. At this point, ideas of reference, feelings of being singled out for neglect or mistreatment, and related paranoid elements may enter the picture.

It is also possible that, rather than taking vindictive action, the patient continues in his move away from others. Along this pathway, a point of no return is reached, when the distance to go back has become too great; the patient feels that the process is irreversible. External objects become less visible, then out of sight, and, finally, out of mind. Other people do not matter anymore, and the patient does not care anymore. His anger and hate being replaced by indifference, there is no more ambivalence. Resignation makes place for fatalism, a perspective closely related to that of hopelessness.

MANAGEMENT OF HYPOCHONDRIASIS

The hypochondriacal patient presents many difficulties in therapeutic management.[4–8] The enthusiastic therapist who sets out actively to do something about the patient's complaint may find to his surprise that the symptoms do not respond; or that when they do respond they are replaced by other symptoms; or even that the patient may get more depressed as the physical symptoms improve. The first requirement in management is a formulation of the specific psychodynamic factors playing a role. The physician's understanding and formulation, however, are not to be communicated to the patient, as in insight-oriented therapy. Any interpretation of the dynamics tends to be dismissed by the patient, and may, in fact, cause an exacerbation of the symptoms. To explain to the patient, in more general terms that he has no real physical illness and that the symptoms are related to emotional conflict, is of no help either. Sometimes, the patient may intellectually agree that the mind can affect the body, but he is sure this does not apply to his case, nor would it do any good to advise him to stop worrying. At first sight, this may seem quite rational and reassuring, but it fails because to the patient, such reassurance is "false." The patient's reaction to such advice usually is paradoxical: an increase in his complaints. Because he needs to maintain his only defense, he must now convince the therapist that the latter was wrong in his diagnosis.

Rather, it would be wise to treat the symptoms without expecting that they will disappear. This is not therapeutic hypocrisy or cynicism, but involves a dual communication, on two levels. On the superficial level, the patient and therapist are engaged in a traditional contract: to do something about the complaint. On a deeper level, however, there is a tacit understanding that in order to function the patient needs his symptoms; that they are a form of coping with personal problems and life situations, perhaps the only coping technique available right now; and that the therapist is prepared to do the best he can to treat these symptoms, no matter how long it will take.

VICISSITUDES

Giving a Particular Diagnosis

Some clinicians may decide to go along with the patient's contention that he is physically ill, *giving him a particular diagnosis* and a specific medication. Again, from a rational point of view, one would expect that such an accepting approach (taking the patient on his word, recognizing the legitimacy of his symptoms) would give the patient what he wants. And, indeed, there now may follow a period of quiescence of complaints. But sooner or later the patient returns, either with the old symptoms or with new complaints. The patient's first triumph was a pseudovictory. Winning the therapist over to his side was only a victory-in-defeat. The real winner was the physician who had maneuvered to set the stage for a traditional medical contract (the patient has an "illness," he gets medicine, and is "supposed to get better"). But meanwhile, the physician had gotten the patient out of his office, so he was the winner in this game. He had responded to the patient by implying: "O.K., we will do it your way, so you will be satisfied—and if not, don't blame me."

The patient's symptoms will return, because the hypochondriasis represents his only major defense.[9] From this point on, several vicissitudes may develop in the doctor-patient relationship. The patient may go back to the same physician for round two, with a new set of complaints, or with the original symptoms. (The fact that he returns to the same physician is prognostically a good sign which should not be overlooked.)

New Complaints

If the patient comes back with a *new set of complaints*, there are several risks and traps. One would be to give a new diagnosis, thereby sending the patient on his way to becoming an ambulatory nomenclature. He'll collect one diagnosis after another using them as needed in his contacts with physicians and other caretaking personnel, to explain his behavior, to justify his requests for medications, and so on.

> One "professional" hypochondriac, a postmenopausal woman had been making rounds on innumerable physicians. In the course of a decade, she had developed an awesome collection of diagnoses, each of which symbolized an injustice done to her. She was capable of nonstop talkathons, using all the diagnoses and treatments given to her as points of departure into righteous indignation. The soliloquy would start off as a quiet lament, then become a litany with the ever-recurring refrain of nobody caring, ending in a crescendo of accusations.

By presenting new complaints, the patient (usually without consciously realizing this) puts the physician on the spot. The patient is implying that the first medication he received was not good enough to prevent new symptoms, or that the initial diagnosis was not accurate. During this "round two" of the relationship, the physician has the option of changing the medication or the diagnosis. If only the medication is changed, the patient will wonder how the old diagnosis can be maintained vis-à-vis the new symptoms, or how the new medication can be justified vis-à-vis the old diagnosis. If the physician maintains his original diagnosis, he is put on the spot in terms of explaining the failure of the treatment, searching for a justification to continue its use, or having to decide on another medicine. If the physician changes the diagnosis, he has little choice but to change the medication as well. By changing the diagnosis, however, he has simply added a new one to the patient's nomenclature. The first diagnosis is kept in reserve by the patient, as a standby, for handy reference or p.r.n. manipulation.

In this manner, round two appears to end, in the same way as in the first contact. But the fact that the patient has a new diagnosis will only reinforce his hypochondriacal self-image; and, in addition, he has probably lost some confidence in the physician, whom he can bend to his will. Moreover, with the new diagnosis and new medication, the patient is now again supposed to be "a good patient," in terms of responding favorably to the doctor's diagnosis and therapeutic skills. It is obvious that such an approach eventually ends in failure and in termination of the doctor-patient relationship. Thus, a second round may be followed by several more rounds, but after some time both participants begin to see the futility of their efforts.

Same Complaints

If the patient returns with the *same complaints* as in round one, he is coming on more strongly. In effect, he gives the physician a "dare"; the refractory symptoms acquire an element of obstinacy or defiance. The physician has now the option of changing the diagnosis or the treatment. A change in diagnosis is tantamount to the physician's admission that he no longer has a grasp on the situation. The patient may achieve a small victory in the context of his coercion and gamesmanship, but his confidence in the physician will be diminished. The risk of adding more diagnoses is compounded by the danger of having to give medication for each of these "illnesses." What also frequently happens somewhere along the line, is that the patient has succeeded in convincing a surgeon that an operation is indicated. The irrevocable fact of a surgical procedure and the visible trophy of a surgical scar can be used by the hypochondriac to prove that the problem was really physical or that he was mistreated (because of the surgical "attack").[2, 3]

One way or the other, the therapist's tact and patience are sorely tried.

The temptation is strong to fall into one of the patient's traps, and surrender to a coercive ploy, for example, by saying something like: "Well, since my treatment was no success, maybe you'd prefer to see someone else—I'll be glad to give you a good referral."

Changing Physicians

The timid patient who prefers to shy away from confrontation may go to a *different physician* with his original complaints. The first physician may never know it, and conclude that the patient had been treated successfully. In reality, however, our patient is making rounds on the physicians in the area.

EFFECTIVE APPROACH

The vicissitudes, then, that may develop after one has given the hypochondriac a real diagnosis, make it clear that this approach is not effective.

Accept Hypochondriacal Defense

The first step toward effective management is the recognition that the hypochondriac *needs his physical complaints* to maintain adequate self esteem and object relationships. When a physician tells his patient that his symptoms are not real, but emotional, or imaginary, he merely increases the patient's adjustment problems. Even more damaging would be to give such information to the relatives. This is tantamount to pulling the rug from underneath the patient. The relatives will inform the hypochondriac that the doctor has told them he has no basis for his complaints. The hypochondriac then is forced to become more defensive and prove he is really sick; he also feels he has been betrayed by the physician, who has now become an enemy. This is one of the ways in which hypochondriacal patients develop a sense of being treated unfairly, or victimized. This may even proceed to the point where feelings of persecution and paranoid ideas develop.

The therapist who accepts the fact that the patient needs his hypochondriacal defense, thereby accepts the patient as well. If he listens attentively and avoids confronting the patient with medical facts, the latter will feel secure rather than threatened by somebody intent on taking his defense away.

Circumvent Diagnosis

When the patient *asks for a diagnosis*, it is prudent to circumvent this ploy, and respond to the effect that "it is obvious that you have trouble—there is a problem—at this point I am not certain about the real cause—but I am glad to do whatever I can to help you." Usually, the hypochondriac will accept such a statement, which at face value seems noncommittal but at a deeper level is actually a statement of the physician's commitment.

Drug Prescription

Meanwhile, the therapist has to do something. Without some form of treatment, the patient may feel rejected because his symptoms are not taken seriously, or because his illness is not real enough to necessitate medication. Of course, many hypochondriacs do have actual somatic symptomatology which would respond to appropriate medication. *Drugs* may be prescribed provided one does not further contribute to polypharmacy and provided the drug has not already been used and become contaminated by the patient's negative fantasies. It is better not to convey that this drug will be 100 percent effective, but that "it will help take the edge off the problem—and we'll have to see how much relief you'll get from it." The latter phrase implies that the patient is to come back to tell the physician how he is doing. By following this approach, one creates a "no lose" situation: neither the doctor nor the patient will be forced into a position of defeat. The element of "no lose" is essential to prevent the manipulative ploys and coercive games which would otherwise destroy the therapeutic alliance.

Testing Therapist

During the next phase, the patient will *test out* the therapist's truthfulness. He will do so in several ways. He may ask "When do you want me to come back?" The answer depends on several variables, such as the therapist's schedule, the amount of support needed by the patient, etc. A practical compromise is that return visits be scheduled no more than once a week, and no less than once a month; that each visit last from 20–30 minutes; and, that the patient be told that "if anything comes up before the next visit, be sure to call me."

The next test may be the patient's question: "How long will it take? How long will I need to take this medication? How long will I need to see you?" Giving an optimistic answer, to the effect that the patient may soon recover or improve, is tantamount to failing the patient's test. The latter knows full well that things won't happen this way—He can't see himself that soon without the security of his illness. Giving a pessimistic answer, to the effect that the patient's condition is permanent, is also wrong, because the patient will wonder about the physician's professional motives of having him come back for follow-up visits. If the situation is that bleak, why bother with any treatment?

The correct response to the question is based on the recognition that the patient is not trying to find an objective piece of truth from the physician, but rather some evidence that the latter is "true" to him. The patient frequently makes the test of truthfulness even more difficult, e.g., by complaining that the time schedule for the follow-up visit is inconvenient. (The patient's thoughts would run something like: "Doctor, I am giving you a chance to get out of this appointment with me—all you have to say to me now is: 'Gee, that is too bad—why don't you give me a call when you have some convenient time'—and if that's what you are going to say, I'll know you are like all the rest, the other ones who did not care, and just were polite, going through the motions to make me think they cared"). So, to avoid this trap, the therapist needs to face the situation with honesty, decide on the "trueness" of his commitment to the patient, and reiterate with firmness: "It is important for you to come, and I expect to see you, even if it is inconvenient." The tacit message here is: "Look, in this relationship, we aren't going to duck inconveniences, and you can expect the same on my part." The point is implicitly made that the importance of the relationship transcends the magnitude of inconvenience. Thus, one introduces a basic therapeutic ingredient: for the patient to carry on in spite of his problems.

Follow-up

When the hypochondriacal patient returns for *follow-up* appointments, he finds that the physician's attitude has not changed. When he expresses hostility against previous physicians, one must refrain himself from defending his colleagues, confining his remarks to recognition of the patient's previous experiences as disappointing. Again, no diagnosis or prognosis is ventured. During the interview, the therapist does not try to select the topics but there may be opportunities to guide the patient toward areas of conflict.

When the patient begins to improve, this should not become a basis for declaring him to be "cured," or to have had "maximum benefits" from the treatment, and then terminating the treatment program. Rather, the opposite view should be taken: the patient's improvement indicates that the treatment regime is sound and must be continued. By the same token, one would not stop giving insulin to a diabetic because he is responding well. Thus, the fact that the patient improves on a particular treatment regime may be a reason for continuing, rather than stopping it.

(Incidentally, the same applies to another situation, that is, some cases where a patient improves during hospitalization. Many patients with chronic physical or mental problems improve once they are in the supportive setting of a hospital. The hospital staff may then decide to discharge the patient, "back into the community." Soon after release from the hospital, we find this same patient being readmitted. The point is that the decision to discharge the patient did not consider the fact that the improvement was due precisely to his being in the hospital.)

Outward-oriented Activities

As the patient returns for future appointments, the physician will easily detect any tendency on the patient's part to shift away from his self-absorption. More emphasis may be directed toward problems related to people, external interests or *outward-oriented activities.* Thus, the patient may gradually become less preoccupied with his imaginary ills. He may have an exacerbation of his symptoms when his problems increase but at least he is able to return to reasonable efficiency in his living habits. Having established a secure relationship with the physician, he knows he will not be attacked, and the energy which he has been using to ward off such attacks can be directed toward more rewarding endeavors. He has gained some confidence because even if he falters in some way, he can return to this one person who will not accuse him of being a failure, but will accept him without the need for an alibi.

SOME COMMENTS ON PLACEBOS AND DRUGS

Negative and Positive Placebo Effects

The *placebo effect* can be defined as any effect from a substance or procedure *not* caused by its pharmacodynamic properties. The placebo effect is derived from the meaning to the patient of the whole situation surrounding the therapeutic effort. Placebo effects are not imaginary, but can actually cause measurable physiological changes. The type of medication given to the hypochondriac may come close to being a placebo, e.g., vitamins. Such a placebo-like drug is justifiable if it does not interfere with the primary goal in treatment. The Latin derivation of placebo (= "I will please") implies getting involved with the patient rather than getting rid of him. Thus, giving placebos is not a simple procedure, but presupposes an optimal doctor-patient relationship; the placebo effect is an effect of the doctor-patient relationship. The patient takes his prescription with the feeling of "he is taking care of me." This is the *meaning* of the therapeutic effort to him.

It is also important to keep in mind that placebo effects can be either negative or positive, a phenomenon related to positive and negative transference. Thus, the existence of positive and negative placebo effects will be a source of information to the physician, about the degree of ambivalence in the relationship. Some patients with a high degree of ambivalence toward the therapist may lose the prescription on their way home; others just keep it and don't have it filled; again, other patients will disregard the prescription and secretly buy their own favorite patent drugs. In some cases, the negative placebo effect consists of an alleged inability to swallow the drug; or it may cause nausea and vomiting; or if the drug remains inside, it causes various types of idiosyncratic discomfort.

> A unique rare type of placebo effect was seen in a patient who had longstanding physical symptoms, but refused to take medications. She finally was persuaded that it would be safe to take the medication (an antidepressant). At the next visit, she looked much

better. The therapist remarked on her improved appearance, the reduction of physical symptoms, etc., and the patient was in full agreement. So, it seemed that both therapist and patient were resonating on the same wavelength, until, by the end of the interview, she casually remarked: "By the way, I did not take any of the medication you prescribed." Essentially, this illustrates a negative transference, manifested in terms of a "flight into health." The patient was, in effect, saying: "Look, I do not really need you—I can do it on my own."

The other extreme is illustrated by the case of an obese, elderly woman who used to frequent the hospital emergency room (ER) complaining of pain "all over" in her stomach. The ER nurse had become well acquainted with her and had, by way of serendipity, arrived at an effective treatment: injecting a few cc's of saline subcutaneously in the abdominal region. Within a few minutes, the patient would get up, state how much better she felt, and leave contentedly. The patient had become emotionally dependent on the accessibility of the nurse whenever she was in distress. The availability of the procedure had become a symbol for the availability of a person.

Pain

Management of *pain* in the hypochondriacal patient should involve a consideration of the intimate connections between anxiety, depression, tension, and pain.[10, 11] Organic pain conforms in a characteristic manner to what one would expect on the basis of anatomical lesions. The fact that perception of pain and reaction to pain-inducing stimuli decreases with age may be a complicating factor. Compared with younger people, the aged person may not readily perceive the early onset of pathological changes and this presents a handicap in diagnosis and treatment. Pain which is more or less psychogenic, however, is related to anxious fantasies about an illness, to mental conceptions of progressions of pathology, and to body image disturbances. Painful distress which has significant psychogenic components is usually reported by way of idiosyncratic phrases that do not conform to anatomical facts but are related to the body image. The regressed or hypochondriacal patient may be so preoccupied with bodily overconcern, that almost any sensation or distress can be perceived as painful.

It should not be forgotten, however, that many older persons do suffer from one or more chronic illnesses, which may cause a variety of distressing symptoms. A longstanding pattern of psychogenic pain should not tempt the clinician to be less alert to the development of an authentic organic illness: even a hypochondriac can get physically sick.

Persistent physical complaints are common in many psychiatric disorders, such as schizophrenia and organic brain syndrome.[12] The physical complaints of the schizophrenic patient, often strange or bizarre, may represent his attempt to give expression to his chaotic inner world. To some extent, the same is true of the patient with organic brain syndrome. Psychiatric treatment of these cases usually involves antipsychotic drugs.

While usually it is true, that idiosyncratic descriptions of pain suggest a "psychic signature,"[13] in the case of patients with organic brain syndrome or dementia, this rule does not apply. The complaint of physical pain may be expressed by these patients in a highly idiosyncratic form, involving delusions, hallucinations, or bizarre behavior. The mechanism responsible for this, was described earlier and revolves around the loss of abstract thinking (see case of patient whose feces were stones, p. 82, and the case of patient complaining of ants crawling over her skin, p. 56). In cases of fecal impaction, for example, patients may express their distress, nonverbally, through changes in posture and gait.

Pain may give rise to fear and disorganization of thought and behavior. In addition to specific treatment, relief from pain is indicated as a means of controlling the emergence of florid psychopathology in frightened persons with reduced or marginal cerebral competence.[7]

MANAGEMENT OF RELATED STATES

VINDICTIVENESS

Psychotherapeutic management can be more complex and demanding in cases of hypochondriasis, where the patient has become chronically embittered, and acts this out by way of *vindictive behavior*. These hostile behavior patterns are frequent problems in nursing homes and rest homes. Characteristically, the pattern of hostility has become more prominent over a period of several years. The clinical phenomena correspond with a regression to an oral-sadistic or anal-sadistic phase of development, in which ambivalence is a prominent feature.

The clinical manifestations include refusal to accept assistance deemed appropriate by concerned others; being "mean, ugly, cantankerous, obstreperous"; excessive complaining about medical, social, or material needs, but recalcitrance in cooperating with corrective intervention; nearly total lack of appreciation for what is done in their behalf; blaming others for their plight; cursing, fussing, and arguing; hitting persons too close for comfort (relatives, roommates in a rest home, hospital attendants); spiteful acts (e.g., soiling themselves, just after having been cleaned up); refusing to tend to personal hygiene (occasionally to scare others away and create a no-man's land around them); and so on.

Management of these behavior patterns requires an exploration of the role played by the premorbid personality and recent stresses; and a recognition that the hostile behavior patterns are clinical *manifestations of regression* to an early ambivalent phase of development. The orally aggressive patient "bites the hand that feeds him," but yet feels dependent on that same person. In cases of anal-sadistic regression, the typical features are stubbornness, obstructionism, oppositional behavior, and "making a mess" out of things; such a patient does not appear to be as dependent. In both categories, the common denominator is the patient's ambivalence toward the significant persons around him, with the negative, hateful feelings being in the foreground. It is essential to recognize that one is dealing with the behavioral expressions of ambivalence and to keep reminding oneself of the psychodynamic forces producing the patient's disagreeable behavior, to avoid countertransference feelings.

The next step is, from a position of neutral objectivity and with an attitude of *detached concern*, to address oneself to the underlying concern, and try to alleviate the stress. This may be a feeling of exasperating helplessness, shameful loss of dignity, bitterness about having been betrayed, fighting against letting go for fear of being let down, etc. In offering the needed support, it is often necessary to use a special form of tact: the supplies are given to the patient in a surreptitious manner; they are being slipped over to him, as it were. The giving is not openly done, not explicitly or formally, but tacitly and casually. This matter-of-fact method makes it possible for the patient to have his cake and eat it: he is receiving the needed narcissistic supplies, and can still have his kicks by indulging in various protestations.

Once the patient has accepted the supplies, the stage for a *collaborative relationship* has been set. For a period of time, the main focus is on getting the patient to accept, digest, and assimilate what is being offered to him, and the hostile behavior is left alone, for the time being. This phase reaches its goal when the patient appears to have a sense of certainty that the provider (the feeding hand) is reliable; that his own hostility will not destroy the giver, and that his own illwill cannot contaminate the other's goodwill. Essentially, the patient learns during this phase that there is indeed love with no strings attached, the gift is not a bait, and if he swallowed it, he'd be painfully hooked.

During the last phase, one may attempt to deal with the regression and the associated disagreeable behavior by *setting limits*. One method would be simply to convey to the patient one's own disapproval for the way he sometimes acts, but without the threat of "shape up or ship out." More effective probably is the approach of conveying to the patient the recognition that he is making some good progress, and that this attests to his strength or courage, an admirable achievement. Again, the fact, that the patient's strength, so to speak, has been borrowed from the therapist is left unspoken, covered by the tacit pact. At this point, one might bring up a question to the effect of: Would the patient now be strong or courageous enough to do something that goes against his grain, like showing some appreciation to this person, or kindness to that one? In this manner, one might try to change the patient's "false pride" into authentic pride. But even during a moment of warmth, or an act of kindness, the patient may still show his barbs, e.g., in the form of the rationalization: "I am only nice and kind for your benefit—because you want me to."

REVERSAL OF AUTISM

While in most cases, hypochondriasis is the consequence of disengagement, in some instances, the reverse is true. It then represents a favorable development which actually may be encouraged. This happens when a very withdrawn, autistic, or schizophrenic patient begins to turn his attention toward the real world. The first object encountered is his own body, which is, as mentioned before, something like a bridge between the inner self and the outer world. Two cases were presented earlier (See Chapter 8, p. 136, and Chapter 9, p. 155) illustrating the appearance of somatic self-absorption in schizophrenic patients as a favorable development. The presence of physical complaints sets the stage for contact and interaction between the patient and another person.[14]

MAINTAINING CLOSENESS

Hypochondriacal complaints may also represent a primitive, nonverbal cry for help, or a means of *maintaining closeness.* This happens in situations, where isolation has been imposed from without, rather than developed from within. In some children, we see that the very anticipation of loneliness can set in motion a hypochondriacal process which serves the purpose of preventing the possibility of isolation from becoming a reality. Such children may complain of aches and pains when they face relative loneliness at bedtime. The physical complaint serves as an expedient medium to express a nameless dread, and to keep in touch with the protective parental figure. The element of vagueness in these physical complaints provides a useful clue. If a parent consistently disregards such clues, but responds to the physical complaints at face value, the foundations for hypochondriacal reaction patterns are being laid. Such responses to anxiety situations, especially separation anxiety, may persist from childhood, through the adult years, into late life.

> An elderly female patient had been for many years on the geropsychiatric unit of a mental hospital because of senile dementia. Her ability to communicate had progressively deteriorated, but she still was agile in her walking and daily living activities. During ward rounds, this patient would come to the physician and express a vague complaint about her neck. When asked to repeat the complaint, the second version would differ from the first. While the patient's hands would be gesticulating all over the afflicted zone,

there was an intent gaze in her eyes, trying to lock into the physician's eyes. After a brief on-the-spot examination, the physician would tell what seemed to be the trouble, and promise something would be done about it. The effect of this on the patient was rather striking: her complaint seemed gone, and she appeared pleased, as though this was all there was to it with nothing further to be expected. This state of closure lasted until the next ward round, when the interaction would be repeated.

References

1. Lesse, S.: Behavioral problems masking depression—cultural and clinical survey. *Am. J. Psychotherapy 33*:41–53, 1979.
2. Lesse, S.: Hypochondriasis and psychosomatic disorders masking depression. In: *Masked Depression*, edited by S. Lesse, chapter 4, Jason Aronson, Inc., New York, 1974.
3. Charatan, F. B.: Depression in old age. *New York State Journal of Medicine 75*:2505–2509, 1975.
4. Brink, T. L., Belanger, J., Bryant, J., Capri, D., Janakes, C., Jasculca, S., and Oliveira, C.: Hypochondriasis in an institutional geriatric population: construction of a scale (HSIG). *J. Am. Geriatr. Soc. 26*:557–559, 1978.
5. Busse, E. W.: Hypochondriasis in the elderly: a reaction to social stress. *J. Am. Geriatr. Society 24*(4):145–149, 1976.
6. Goldstein, S. E., and Birnbom, F.: Hypochondriasis and the elderly. *J. Am. Geriatr. Soc. 24*:150–154, 1976.
7. Salzman, C., and Shader, R. I.: Depression in the elderly. I. Relationship between depression, psychologic defense mechanisms and physical illness. *J. Am. Geriatr. Soc. 26*:253–260, 1978.
8. Walsh, A. C.: Hypochondriasis associated with organic brain syndrome: a new approach to therapy. *J. Am. Geriatr. Soc. 24*(9):430–431, 1976.
9. Busse, E. W., and Pfeiffer, E.: Functional psychiatric disorders in old age. In: *Behavior and Adaptation in Late Life*, edited by E. W. Busse and E. Pfeiffer, chap. 10, Little, Brown and Company, 1970. pp. 183–235.
10. Byrne, D. G.: Neuroticism, illness behavior and coronary heart disease. *Psychother. Psychosom. 26*:317–321, 1975.
11. Busse, E. W., and Blazer, D.: Disorders related to biological functioning. In: *Handbook of Geriatric Psychiatry*, edited by E. W. Busse and D. G. Blazer, chapter 18, Van Nostrand Reinhold Company, New York. pp. 403–405.
12. Munro, A.: Monosymptomatic hypochondriacal psychosis manifesting as delusions of parasitosis. A description of four cases successfully treated with Pimozide. *Arch. Dermatol. 114*:940–943, 1978.
13. Engel, G. L.: Psychogenic pain and the pain-prone patient. *Am. J. Med. 26*:899, 1959.
14. Kast, E. C.: On being old and on dying. *J. Am. Geriatr. Soc. 20*:524–530, 1972.

15

schizophrenic and senile psychoses*

PSYCHOPHARMACOLOGY

ANTIPSYCHOTIC DRUGS

This group of drugs includes the phenothiazines, butyrophenones, thioxanthene derivatives, as well as the newer dibenzoxazepine (Loxitane) and indole (Moban), and the now little used Rauwolfia compounds.[1–4] The *mode of action* of the commonly used drugs includes an inhibition of critical noradrenergic and dopaminergic receptor sites in the CNS; possibly, desensitization of the reticular activating system to impulses transmitted from the primary sensory pathway collaterals; and an anticholinergic effect. Much of the emotional response to external or internal stimuli would be reduced by such actions.[5] The development of extrapyramidal reactions, a frequent and unique concomitant effect of antipsychotics, may be mediated by the dopaminergic blockade.

In contrast to sedatives, these agents calm the excited or agitated patient without induction of sleep. Their main characteristic effects are: 1) the relief of agitation, violent and irrational behavior, and perceptual disturbances; and 2) the extrapyramidal side effects. They tend to increase muscle tone, lower the convulsive threshold, and have a negligible risk of drug dependence. Many psychotic manifestations, such as disturbed thinking, paranoid symptoms, delusions, emotional and social withdrawal, and personal neglect, may improve. Amelioration of such psychotic symptoms justifies the name: antipsychotic.

Phenothiazine Derivatives

Phenothiazines, the most frequently used antipsychotic agents, comprise three subgroups: aliphatics, piperidyls, and piperazines. The piperazines congeners with a halogen (especially fluorine), attached to the main nucleus, have an increased potency, but extrapyramidal syndromes are more common and controlling dosage is more difficult. Compounds with an *aliphatic* side chain (e.g., chlorpromazine) are relatively low in potency and high in sedative effects. The *piperidyl* group includes thioridazine (Mellaril). Variants of the *piperazine* side chain, along with

* In collaboration with Alan D. Whanger, M.D.

variations of the ring substituent, create a large class of piperazinyl phenothiazines, e.g., prochlorperazine (Compazine), perphenazine (Trifalon), trifluoperazine (Stelazine), fluphenazine (Prolixin, Permitil). These compounds are more potent than the aliphatic series. They possess less sedative effects than the other two classes, but are more likely to produce extrapyramidal reactions at equivalent therapeutical doses.

Thioxanthene Derivatives

Substitution of a carbon atom for the nitrogen in the central ring of the phenothiazine nucleus produces the *thioxanthene* nucleus. Chlorprothixine (Taractan) and thiothixene (Navane) are thioxanthene derivatives.

Butyrophenone Derivatives

Haloperidol (Haldol), a butyrophenone derivative, resembles the phenothiazines in antipsychotic action and evoking extrapyramidal syndromes. It is an effective antipsychotic, but can produce muscular rigidity and extrapyramidal symptoms at dosages of more than 1.5 mg daily.

TREATMENT CONSIDERATIONS

Indications

Phenothiazines and other antipsychotics can be used to treat schizophrenia, paranoid states, organic psychoses, agitated depressions, or severe anxiety states in the elderly.[6] Relative *contraindications* include central nervous system (CNS) depression due to drugs such as alcohol or barbiturates; Parkinson's disease, organic brain syndrome with lethargy and clouded sensorium, hypertensive patients taking guanethidine, or glaucoma.

Selection of Drug

The great number of drugs available creates practical problems in choosing drugs. It is probably best, on the whole, to start with one of the less sedative, less hypotensive drugs (e.g., haloperidol or thiothixene).[7] If undue extrapyramidal signs develop, the dose can be reduced or a change made to thioridazine or chlorpromazine. The rationale is to avoid extrapyramidal symptoms, since the latter would require an additional drug, i.e., antiparkinson agents.[8] The choice of the proper drug involves an individualized approach, because there is much overlap of side-effects among drugs, and aged patients usually require smaller doses.[9] Most antipsychotic drugs are equally efficacious, although individual patients respond differently to different drugs. Therefore, the choice of drug is often empirical. A rational way to narrow the choice of antipsychotics is to master the pharmacology and use of one of each of the three types of phenothiazines, one of the two thioxanthenes, and a butyrophenone.[10]

Dosage

In contrast to younger patients, massive doses of antipsychotic drugs are not indicated for geropsychiatric patients. This is particularly relevant in view of the risk of long-term toxicity of a permanent nature, e.g., tardive dyskinesia, an extrapyramidal syndrome involving various dystonic movements, especially of the face and tongue. By avoiding unduly prolonged use of antipsychotics whenever clinically feasible, the risk of tardive dyskinesia is reduced.[11] Likewise, other side effects (e.g., postural hypotension which, in turn, may cause strokes, heart attacks, falls, and fractures) may be prevented by maintaining patients on a low dosage or, if possible, stopping the drug altogether.

Phenothiazines in liquid preparations are useful for patients who cannot or will not swallow tablets. Many drugs are available for intramuscular administration, but this increases the risk of hypotensive reactions. One phenothiazine is available in a long-acting intramuscular form which may occasionally be helpful, especially in elderly schizophrenics. This drug, fluphenazine (Prolixin), is available either as the enanthate compound with effects lasting about 2 weeks, or as the decanoate compound lasting about 4 weeks. Oral medications should be substituted as soon as possible.[12]

Drug Combinations

Antipsychotic drugs have been used with other drugs as well as other psychiatric therapies. A frequent combination is with tricyclic antidepressants, but this has the likelihood of increased side effects.[13] They may be combined with low dose of antianxiety drugs. They have been used simultaneously with electroconvulsive therapy (ECT), but it is generally better to stop them prior to ECT, especially to avoid cardiac complications.[14]

Side-Effects (Tables 15.1 and 15.2)

Hypotension may manifest itself as progressive confusion, or transient ischemic attacks. Every aged patient should have his blood pressure taken supine, and sitting or standing. Postural hypotension, once occurring, can last for many days and may even require bed rest to prevent stressing the cardiovascular system.[15]

Extrapyramidal effects apparently are produced due to the blocking of dopaminergic receptor sites in the corpus striatum. Haloperidol, in daily amounts of more than 1.5–2.0 mg tends to cause extrapyramidal symptoms and muscular rigidity. Acute extrapyramidal signs, the most common effects of antipsychotics, respond well to antiparkinson drugs. *Anticholinergic* agents for treating parkinsonism due to antipsychotics include benztropin mesylate (Cogentin); trihexyphenidyl (Artane); biperiden (Akineton); procyclidine (Kemadrin); and diphenhydramine

Table 15.1
Side-Effects of Antipsychotics

Clinical signs	Causative factors	Prevention & treatment
Behavioral		
Oversedation	Dose, age, especially aliphatics & thioridazine	Avoid other CNS depressants, lower dose or change drug
Aggravation of psychiatric symptoms	Premorbid personality; patients with insight; depersonalization	Lower dose or change drug, use anti-anxiety drug
Cardiovascular		
Postural hypotension → syncope, CVA, or heart attack	Adrenergic blocking & anticholinergic effect (especially chlorpromazine & thioridazine)	Lower dose or change drug, check electrolytes, do not use epinephrine
Cardiac arrhythmia, palpitations, tachycardia	Age, dose, parenteral administration, drug-drug toxicity, existing cardiovascular disease	Lower dose, avoid intravenous administration & polypharmacy, pretreatment cardiac evaluation, monitor cardiovascular factors
EKG changes (Q and T wave distortions)	Especially with thioridazine	Do pretreatment base-line EKG
EEG		
EEG slowing, lowered seizure threshold, convulsions	Dose level, individual susceptibility, organic brain syndrome	Lower dose, consider anticonvulsants (after proper evaluation)
Autonomic nervous system		
Nasal congestion, dry mouth, constipation, urinary retention, inhibition of ejaculation	Adrenergic-blocking & anticholinergic effects Combination with tricylics & antiparkinson drugs	Explanation & reassurance, lower dose, or stop drug if symptoms are severe or continue, review need for tricyclics and antiparkinson drugs
Weight gain, edema	Hypothalamic effect (especially thioridazine)	Lower dose or change drug if symptoms are severe
Ocular		
Blurred vision, pigmentary retinopathy	Anticholinergic effects, prolonged high dose	Keep thioridazine under 800 mg daily
Melanin pigmentation, corneal and lens deposits	Long-term treatment, high doses	Switch to "low dose" piperazine derivative
Skin		
Dermatoses photosensitivity	Allergic or toxic reaction	Stop or change drug, avoid exposure to sun
Blood		
Agranulocytosis, purpura, hemolytic anemia, pancytopenia	Rare, elderly women, usually first 3 months	Stop drug, medical treatment
Cholestatic jaundice	Rare, usually early in treatment	Stop drug, medical treatment

Table 15.2
Extrapyramidal Side-Effects of Antipsychotics

Parkinsonism	Dyskinesias: early or tardive			
	Akathisia	Dystonia	Facial-bucco-lingual	Choreoathetosis
Clinical manifestations				
Rigidity, bradykinesia, pill-rolling tremors, resting tremors, salivation and seborrhea, shuffling gait	Uncontrollable restlessness, feelings of muscular quivering	Posturing of face, neck and tongue: retrocollis and torticollis, oculogyric crises	Chewing & mouthing movement, aimless writhing of tongue, lip-smacking	Choreiform and athetoid movements of neck, trunk, and extremities
Early in treatment	Days-months after treatment	Early or late in treatment	Early or late in treatment	Late (tardive)
Generally reversible	Usually reversible	Acute = reversible	Usually irreversible	Usually irreversible
Causative or predisposing factors				
More in old age and women	Middle-age, more in women	Younger, more in men	Older patients, more in women	
Current dose level		Current dose level in acute dystonia	Sum total of drug amount over the years	
Individual susceptibility to dopamine blocking effects		Individual susceptibility to anticholinergic effects		
↙ Activity of dopamine or ↗ activity of cholinergic system in striatum	↗ Activity of dopamine system or ↙ activity of cholinergic system in striatum (relative imbalance)			
Prevention or treatment				
Differential diagnosis: agitated depression	Differential diagnosis: early Huntington	Differential diagnosis: dystónia due to lithium	Differential diagnosis: spontaneous facial-bucco-lingual dyskinesia	
Antihistamines, antiparkinson drugs	Lower dose or change drug, no L-Dopa, try thioridazine, antiparkinson drugs	Avoid long term use of antipsychotics (especially piperazines), use lowest possible doses, periodic drug-free intervals, don't use antiparkinson drugs routinely		
		Benadryl for acute dystonia	Increasing doses of antipsychotics give transient relief, but probably worsen basic neuropathology	

(Benadryl). Their side effects are essentially similar to those of the tricyclic antidepressants. These drugs should not be given routinely, because some patients will not develop significant extrapyramidal side-effects to begin with. Since antiparkinson drugs have anticholinergic effects, they may contribute to the risks of polypharmacy and drug-drug toxicity.[16]

Tardive dyskinesia is associated with long-term use of phenothiazines and appears in many older patients, particularly brain-damaged women. It is associated with buccal-facial-lingual movements and involuntary movements of the limbs and trunk. Although an increase in the amount of phenothiazine can reverse the signs, this is only a temporary effect and the pattern reappears.[17] Therefore, authorities recommend the use of drug-free intervals, reduced dosages, and drug withdrawal, with the rationale that a reduction in the total amount given over the years will lessen the risk of dyskinesia.[18]

Akathisia may appear after rather short periods of treatment with antipsychotics. It consists of uncontrollable restlessness and agitation which are not typical of the original psychotic disorder.[19] The differentiation from severe anxiety states and agitated depression may be difficult, especially when a reliable record or past history is not available. Akathisia may respond well to diphenhydramine (Benadryl) and other antiparkinson agents.

Other side-effects secondary to the *anticholinergic* action include constipation, urinary retention, and an increased risk of glaucoma.

Additional side-effects may include alterations in the electrocardiogram, reduced drive and libido, liver toxicity, leukopenia, dermatitis, and endocrine disturbances.

OTHER COMPOUNDS AND DRUGS

A number of other compounds, which are not psychotropic in the strict sense of the word, need to be briefly reviewed, because of their effects on cerebral functioning. Included here are certain vitamins and hormones, vasodilators, and anticoagulants, stimulants, and so-called nootropic compounds.

Vitamins

According to Libow, more than 10 percent of the elderly have deficiencies of several important vitamins.[20] Deficiency of *vitamin* B_1 (thiamine) causes beriberi, part of which is the Wernicke-Korsakoff syndrome. Thiamine is a mild appetite stimulant and under stress tends to be depleted in the adrenal cortex, where it has essential metabolical action. *Ascorbic acid* also appears to be essential to adrenal cortical function. It is rapidly depleted with stress and poor nutrition. Since toxicity of vitamin B and C is very low, the use of these vitamins in large amounts is frequently recommended.[21] However, the usefulness of preventive vitamin therapy in the aged has not been sufficiently verified by double-blind studies.[22] *Niacin* (nicotinic acid) deficiency produces pellagra, which may be manifested by various CNS disturbances such as impaired memory and orientation, confabulations, cogwheel rigidity, and primitive grasping and sucking reflexes. *Vitamin* B_{12} is used for the treatment of pernicious anemia, a chronic macrocytic anemia, in which CNS symptoms occur in 40 percent of the patients.[20] Deficiencies in *folic acid* may be due to inadequate diet, chronic alcoholism, intestinal malabsorption, or antagonism between folic acid and diphenylhydantoin. A deficiency in folic acid may result in a macrocytic anemia. Folic acid without vitamin B_{12} is contraindicated in the treatment of pernicious anemia since it may aggravate the neurocerebral symptomatology.

Hormones

Estrogen replacement therapy for postmenopausal women may be effective in preventing or slowing down the development of osteoporosis. In some postmenopausal depressions in which headaches, generalized aches and pains (due to osteoporosis), and chronic fatigue are major complaints, estrogen therapy can be effective. Since estrogens are known to increase the incidence of endometrial carcinoma, such therapy is not routinely indicated for postmenopausal women, but only on the basis of significant estrogen deficiency.[6, 23]

As anabolical agents, *testosterone* or androgen derivatives may be useful in terms of improving appetite and weight. There has been some suggestion that androgen therapy may improve memory function, but it may also produce liver toxicity.[24] There appears to be no beneficial effects from the use of estrogen on the mental functions of elderly male patients with cerebral arteriosclerosis or senile psychosis.[25]

Hypothyroidism can be mistakenly diagnosed as senile dementia (See case on p. 64). There is probably no justification for the practice, occasionally encountered, of giving thyroid preparations to older persons who complain of apathy, weakness, or fatigue. The proper indication for thyroid preparation is hypothroidism verified by laboratory tests. *Hyperthyroidism* may cause a thyrotoxic psychoses, but in the elderly it may be manifested by apathy and depression. This condition has been termed "apathetic hyperthyroidism." [20]

Changes in the *blood sugar level* also may cause CNS symptoms. *Hyperglycemia:* The more easily detectable hyperglycemia is the ketoacidotic state. Less common is the lactic acidosis syndrome seen in diabetic patients taking phenformin (DBI). Less easily detectable but more common, is the nonketotic hyperosmolarity syndrome (hyperglycemia and confusion without ketosis). This syndrome and hypoinsulinemia may also be induced by drugs such as diphenylhydantoin. *Hypoglycemia* may occur during treatment with insulin or the sulfonylureas (tolbutamide, chlorpropamide). Predisposing factors include diminished caloric intake, with physical or mental illness, and reduced hepatic or renal function.[20]

Corticosteroid hormones suppress the body's immune defenses. Their usual psychological effect is an initial euphoria, and then depression. Recent studies have shown that fragments of the adrenocorticotropic hormone (ACTH 4–10) have a positive effect in affect states, improving the electroencephalogram, and even improving memory retrieval in elderly with organic brain syndromes.[26]

Vasodilators

The many claims that *vasodilating* and related agents are useful have generally not been supported by well-controlled studies. On the other hand, it may be wise to give some of these drugs the benefit of the doubt, for the time being. *Nicotinic acid* is supposedly a vasodilator, but its value for producing lasting therapeutic benefits in elderly patients is probably negligible. *Cyclandelate* (Cyclospasmol) has been shown to produce small, but significant, improvement of several mental functions as has the vasodilator papaverine (Pavabid). It is likely, however, that the effects are due to metabolical effects such as dopamine receptor blockade rather than to the dilation of the cerebral arteries.[27, 28] There actually may be difficulty produced by peripheral vasodilation shunting blood away from the brain.

Hydergine. A combination of the hydrogenated derivatives of three alkaloids of ergotoxin, has been tried in the treatment of geropsychiatric patients. Various authors report beneficial effects, such as lessening of emotional withdrawal, conceptual disorganization, depressive mood, motor retardation, blunted affect, and disorientation.[29–32]

Nootropics. There are a variety of drugs being investigated that supposedly improve neuronal functioning. One of these is called Peracetan, but is not yet available in the United States.[33]

CLINICAL MANAGEMENT

CONFUSION AND DISORIENTATION

Physical Etiological Factors

The presence of confusion and disorientation, especially when acute, requires first a search for *physical etiological* factors (see Table 15.3). Effective treatment of such factors causing an acute secondary organic brain syndrome is of paramount importance.[34]

Medications

In addition to the treatment of somatic factors, the following measures should be considered, pertaining to *medications*.

Eliminate unnecessary medications; prevent polypharmacy. Drugs that

Table 15.3
Causes of Pseudosenility*

Medications: errors in self-administration; L-dopa, steroids; diuretics; drugs with CNS action, e.g., phenothiazines, barbiturates.

Metabolic Factors:

1. *Hypercalcemia* due to lung or breast cancer, multiple myeloma, hyperparathyroidism, Paget's disease, or thiazide.
2. *Hyperglycemia* involving ketoacidosis or lactic acidosis.
3. *Hypoglycemia* secondary to insulin or sulfonylureas.
4. *Hypothyroidism* and *hyperthyroidism.*
5. *Hypernatremia* due to inadequate fluid intake, intravenous hypertonic saline, tube feeding of high protein mixtures.
6. *Hyponatremia* due to bronchogenic carcinoma, C.V.A., postoperative.
7. *Azotemia* due to nephritis, dehydration, prostatic hypertrophy, neurogenic uropathy (diabetes, anticholinergics, adrenergics), potent diuretics causing bladder overload (e.g., furosemide).
8. *Febrile* conditions.

Nutrition: deficiencies in vitamins C, B_{12}, thiamine, riboflavin.

CNS tumors: gliomas (50–60%); metastatic (20–50%).

Hepatic: cirrhosis, hepatitis.

Cardiac failure: due to arrhythmia, congestive heart failure, pulmonary emboli, or acute myocardial infarction.

Cerebrovascular: transient ischemic attacks, C.V.A., subdural hematoma (20% of all intracranial masses).

Pulmonary: emphysema with hypoxia or hypercapnea.

Acute emotional stress or depression.

* Modified from: Libow, L. S.: Pseudo-Senility: Acute and Reversible Organic Brain Syndromes. *J. Am. Geriatr. Soc. 21:* 112–120, 1973.

are slow acting or metabolized slowly may be contraindicated.

Remain alert to CNS side-effects of lithium (causing confusion) and the possibility of a central anticholinergic syndrome (see p. 164).

If the patient is already receiving other medications (for pre-existing physical illness), be aware of possible interactional effects between these drugs, and also between the latter and the drug to be selected for sedating the confused patient.

In acute confusion and disorientation, the major tranquilizers such as haloperidol (Haldol), thiothixene (Navane), or chlorpromazine (Thorazine) should be used in appropriate dose orally or parenterally.[35, 36]

Environmental Aspects

Therapeutic measures that are not pharmacodynamic are primarily *environmental* in nature and are aimed at preventing decompensation of a brain which has marginal reserve. Cerebral decompensation due to environmental factors has been reviewed in terms of a functional brain syndrome (see p. 62).

Maintenance of spatial and temporal constancy, such as keeping the external environment the same, reducing the frequency of strangers and new personnel, and avoiding transfers and alterations in routine.

Regular explanations of procedures in simple terms, and mentioning one's name and function at regular intervals.

Alleviating nocturnal confusion by preventing the relative isolation and sensory deprivation which may occur during the night.

Alleviating psychogenic factors which may contribute to confusion and disorientation, e.g., extreme withdrawal (as in depressive stupor), severe agitation, panic, etc.

Promoting contact with reality by way of visitors, familiar newspapers, calendars, clocks, pictures of spouse, children, etc. (reality orientation).[37]

Structuring a time perspective: within each day, meaningful events should be arranged, and the days of the week should become distinguishable from each other by virtue of noticeable day-to-day differences in the routine. Otherwise, the hours and days become undifferentiated time, and it would be useless to try reorienting the patient with clocks and calendars, as they would only indicate empty, meaningless time.

Specific group experiences, such as remotivation and resocialization. This category of therapeutical measures becomes more relevant as the acute confusion subsides and the patient is reaching the base-line level of his cerebral status, e.g., a chronic brain syndrome of mild to moderate degree.[15]

Nocturnal Confusions

Nocturnal confusion is common in organic brain syndromes, and frequently is a major complaint on the part of the family. Nocturnal restlessness also may occur after an environmental change, such as hospitalization or an intrahospital transfer. It may take from several days up to a few weeks for the patient to readjust himself to the new environment. These types of nocturnal restlessness and disorientation can sometimes be alleviated by leaving a nightlight on in the patient's room. Physical restraints should be avoided if at all possible. A family member staying in the room is often a calming influence.

An example illustrating the multifaceted aspects of confusion and disorientation is the following case.

> An 82-year-old widow arrived by bus at the local bus terminal. She drew attention from the bus station personnel because she kept aimlessly wandering around. When questioned, she stated that she "did not know where she was, nor where she had come from." She was then taken to a local hospital. Physical and mental status examinations revealed an organic brain syndrome, arteriosclerotic cardiovascular disease, and nutritional anemia, all of mild degree. The history, as it unfolded over a period of weeks, revealed that the patient had been moving, for many years, between the homes of her five children. They lived in different states, so the patient did a good

bit of travel. Reportedly, she never stayed with one child for more than a few months, and "she would unexpectedly leave." Significantly, the patient would not get along well with the family during a particular stay. Most likely, the patient received subtle messages to the effect that she was not all that welcome. Thus, soon after arrival in one of her children's homes, she would more and more "draw away" until she "unexpectedly" (sic!) left. In the more remote history, it is of interest that the patient was the youngest of ten children. She had not been "planned" by her parents. One of the basic themes of her existence had been that there was "no place for her." She married, had five children, and after her husband died (when she was 36 years old), she raised them by herself, staying in the home where the children had been born. After the last child left home, the patient did likewise. Thus, her caring for the children had represented an attempt to establish the home she never had herself when young. In the light of this past history, the original presenting symptom ("I don't know where I am, and where I came from") is not just the concrete manifestation of an organic brain syndrome. It is overdetermined in that it also is the figurative expression of an existential theme. This patient was placed in a rest home; she has been taking thioridazine (Mellaril) 25 mg three times daily, and there have been no more confusional episodes.

DETERIORATION OF NEUROMUSCULAR SKILLS

Deterioration of neuromuscular skills includes regressive changes in coordination, locomotion, and control of the urinary and anal sphincters. Locomotor skills and sphincter control are acquired during the anal development phase. The equivalent term "autonomy" points up that sphincter control is not the only developmental issue, but that the acts of standing up and moving about vertically in a gravitational field are also important.

Loss of Locomotor Skills

During the process of senile regression, a point may be reached where the patient no longer seems to have the energy to push himself up against the force of gravity. He prefers to give in to the pull of gravity and seek the horizontal position, in bed or anywhere. This is a milestone in the path of regression, because the *loss of locomotor skills* sets the stage for loss of sphincter control, for decubitus and flexion contractures. In view of this, efforts should be made to maintain the patient's locomotor skills as long as possible by way of physical therapy and other activity programs. Oversedation and chemical straight jackets should be avoided. Walking can be done by the patient himself, with the help of a cane or a walker, or with the assistance of relatives, ward personnel, or other patients.[38]

Physical therapy, in general, has an important place in the spectrum of comprehensive management. Specific rehabilitation is indicated for neuromuscular malfunctions following a stroke or hip fracture, for preventing regressed patients from becoming bedridden and incontinent, and for preventing decubitus and contractures when patients are relatively immobilized in wheelchair or bed. Almost all patients benefit from appropriate physical exercise programs (passive or active). Needless to say that these physical procedures cannot fail to have a beneficial effect on the entire person.[39]

Geriatric prosthetics: the increasing array of prosthetic devices is one of the exciting developments of modern medicine. We already take for granted prosthetics such as glasses, hearing aids, dentures, artificial limbs, cardiac pacemakers, crutches, canes, and walkers, etc. Less known are other prosthetics such as the artificial hip joint and devices compensating for loss of sphincter control. Obviously, there are limits to the extent that prostheses can be used, in particular the constraints of the "host" characteristics. There comes a point at which even an ideal prosthesis no longer can fit, because the infirmity of the prospective recipient does not provide a support basis for the prosthesis. Nevertheless, it is hoped that further research will produce more prosthetic devices, refine the quality of those already in use, and that timely application of these devices will permit them to be utilized effectively by aging individuals.[40] For example, it should be possible to develop safe and effective mechanical devices which would enable the patient to maintain and exercise his locomotor skills. From a utopian point of view, it is conceivable that almost all organs and parts of the body can be replaced by a prosthetic device, the one exception being the brain.

Incontinence

Incontinence is a problem of major concern, both for the mental and physical effects on the individual, and also the demands on personnel time.

Causes of *fecal incontinence* include:

1. Local pathology (infections, prolapse of rectum, weakness of the pelvic floor, malignancies, etc.).

2. Neuromuscular incoordination of central origin (organic brain syndrome).

3. Acute confusional states, e.g., due to "transplantation shock," or massive regression.

4. "Intentional" incontinence may be a symptom of spiteful behavior, or may be due to conditioning (e.g., when the person has learned to get attention by soiling himself).

5. Constipation may lead to fecal impaction, and this in turn to incontinence. Fecal impaction may be due to decreased activity and the anticholinergic effects of psychotropic drugs. Fecal impaction should be

suspected if the patient is vomiting, bending over to one side, and if there is any increasing agitation, lethargy, or confusions.[15] In such cases, a careful rectal examination should be done forthwith. Apparently there can be an age-related decline of rectal sensitivity to distention which may play a role in the development of constipation patterns.[41]

Causes of *urinary incontinence* include:

1. In women: stress incontinence, uterine prolapse, weakness of the pelvic floor; in men: prostate hypertrophy.
2. Infections and neoplasms.
3. Urinary retention with overflow incontinence, due to bladder outlet obstruction, or neurogenic bladder.
4. Neurogenic incontinence, e.g., due to spinal cord lesions or organic brain syndrome.
5. In confusional states, the bladder and its neuronal connections are essentially intact, but the patient may be confused about the purpose of a toilet, or he may keep forgetting where the bathroom is.
6. Environmental factors: the patient may be pulled into a regressive drift because of the constant proximity of other patients who are incontinent.

Most cases of incontinence can be treated with some degree of success. An evaluation of etiological factors is the first step, with proper medical and surgical treatment, as indicated. Transient incontinence due to acute confusion will improve with the clearing of the confusion itself. In chronic incontinence, it is important to establish the specific pattern of incontinence. An incontinence chart consists of the systematic recording, by the nursing personnel, of all instances of urinary and fecal incontinence for individual patients. Such a chart has both diagnostic and therapeutic value. By recording the type of incontinence, and the time and context, it may be possible to detect pattern. Knowledge about the incontinence pattern typical for an individual patient is essential in retraining efforts. Retraining may be effective when senility or regression is not advanced. Maintaining locomotion may be essential in preventing incontinence. The use of drugs is restricted to those necessary to treat local pathology. The use of drugs affecting the physiology of bladder and rectum is controversial. Psychotropic drugs with anticholinergic side effects may need to be discontinued. Specific prosthetic devices are available for patients with permanent incontinence.[42]

Having the toilet doors marked by a bright color, by name, and by a silhouette of a man or woman may help some confused patients find the right facility more quickly. Taking the patient to the toilet at regular intervals also may be useful, especially when his pattern of incontinence is known. In cases with a functional (psychogenic) component, there is often improvement as the patient begins to participate in an active therapeutic milieu.

PHASES OF SENILE REGRESSION

Senile dementia involves regression through a series of backward steps through the phases of personality development.[43] The early phase is marked by reliving of past experiences, but when the patient becomes a participant in the events recalled, he is "living in the past." Subsequently, there is an inability to place events in their proper time frame, associated with memory defects. Reality testing begins to fail, objects are misplaced or "lost" and then thought to be stolen. But the condition is not yet irreversible, depending on physical illness, lack of support or other stresses. During the next phase, there is increasing withdrawal into fantasy life, with weakening of behavioral controls. Primitive drives may be acted upon or acted out. Logical thought and the ability to cope with novel situations progressively decline. The combination of decreased impulse control and the awareness of failure results in periodical rage. Those mental functions learned late in development disappear first, while those acquired early are retained the longest (e.g., responsiveness to rhythm). People that used to be familiar are no longer recognized. With the increased need for care come accusations of neglect. The environment is interpreted as hostile or protective depending on intrapsychic processes rather than on reality testing.[43]

All of this evokes considerable feeling in those responsible for the patient's care. In spite of the feelings of "need to care for" generated by the increasing helplessness, doing too much in the early phases of this stage only results in the loss of initiative for self help.

> An 83-year-old woman had resided in a rest home for several years, and was regularly taken to an outpatient clinic by the manager of the home. The patient was in a fairly advanced stage of senile regression. She stated she was 63 years old and was still grieving about the recent death of her husband—"but at least I can talk to my mother every few days—she cannot visit me because she lives in another town and has no transportation—so I call her up over the phone—talking with her makes me feel better." (The patient's mother had been deceased for at least 30 years.) At the end of the brief interview, the manager of the rest home turned to the physician asking him, "Could you find out if she knows me?" The physician asked the patient about this. She blandly looked at the rest home manager and said: "She?—I do not know her—I have never seen her before."

The journey back into the past varies in terms of its duration and the extent of reversibility. During the early phases, the episodes of living in the past are transient and reversible. Such episodes are characterized by the onset of acute confusion and hallucinatory experiences. The voices and visions often pertain to people in the patient's past, people who have died since. But through the patient's living in the past, there is a resurrection of the dead. By observing which particular people are resurrected, we are able to estimate the depth of the patient's regression into the past. For example, it is one thing for a patient to hear the voice of her father who died when she was 30 years old, but another thing if she hears her mother who died when she, the patient, was 13.

During the early phases of senile regression, it is possible to retrieve the patient from his drift into the past, e.g., by appropriate sensory stimulation and alleviation of undue social isolation. During the intermediate stage, the episodes of living in the past (with concomitant disorientation vis-à-vis the present) become more frequent and extended. During the final phase, the episodes coalesce into a continuous existence of living in the past, and this is usually irreversible.

To predict the outcome of organic and functional illness for an individual patient on the basis of the clinical diagnosis, however, is extremely difficult. The prognosis for each elderly patient with whatever psychiatric disorder cannot be based on his age, the diagnostic classification, or any one single variable. Rather, it must be based on the patient's total condition, including his sociocultural background, premorbid personality, current environmental, psychological, and physical stresses; as well as the structural and functional status of his brain.[44] Among aged institutionalized patients, predictions that death would occur within a certain time after admission were correct in only one-third of the cases. Usually the prediction was more pessimistic than the actual outcome.[45]

PSYCHOTHERAPY

Therapeutic Communication

Our definition of "psychotherapy" (see Chapter 11) points up the unique difficulties of applying this to patients with dementia. The "application of psychological techniques" is based on the premise that there is a suitable medium for transmitting therapeutic information. In dementia, however, this very medium (the communicative channels) is impaired. Secondly, the target toward which psychological techniques are directed to "decrease or remove psychological disability" (the brain) is afflicted with permanent damage. To deal with these difficulties, it is necessary to view psychotherapy as therapeutic communication. And, when we speak of individual psychotherapy in senile dementia, it is more useful to think of this as: how to be psychotherapeutic with the individual dementia patient.[46]

Transference

In psychotherapy with dementia patients, *transference* is not interpreted as in insight-oriented therapy. Transference usually goes along with an observing ego capable of discerning the "as if" element in comparing a person in the present with one in the past. The dementia patient loses the ability to compare; there is an impairment of the observing ego: the ego can no longer detach itself from an experience, but becomes an active participant. Transference phenomena in these patients may develop instantaneously.

> A 78-year-old woman's first statement to me was: "Your wife has died." There were several levels of meaning to this; at that moment of getting acquainted, the relevant idea was that if my wife was dead, we would be "available" for each other; and that for this to be on her mind, she probably liked me: somebody to be with. She provided further evidence of this, saying: "And she over here (the nurse) is your daughter." Through this concrete transference, she expressed a specific feeling: that it was like a family here, that she felt at home.

Other transference distortions refer to the environment. When patients says that this place here is a hotel, school, courthouse, or jail, this is not just "disorientation for place and person"; rather, such a misidentification often is a concretized representation of an inner feeling state.

> Later the above patient stated "Now you and I are married"—ideas of permanence and closeness are expressed through the concept of marriage. Proceeding along her line of thought, I asked if she was going to be in the family way. "Oh, yes—We'll have children but not now—in a few years." In other words, the closeness between us will not end for quite a while.

Language and Communication

Frequently, taking the patient's statements at face value is not conducive to understanding. Yet, for these patients, the very existence of any "true" communication would be, in and of itself, therapeutic: it keeps in touch with reality. The question is: How do we make sense out of the patient's frequently chaotic thoughts, and how can we enter into his world and speak his language? The chaotic thinking in dementia is the result of an impaired abstract capacity (in psychodynamic terms, regression from secondary to primary process thinking). The thought processes are similar to those observed in dreams. The fact that all of us "share" this primary process thinking may be a basis for understanding the patient's thinking. For the actual clinical situation, some *practical guidelines* are suggested by the very nature of primary process and the consequences of impaired abstract capacity.

In *paleological thought*, a common predicate leads to the establishment of an identity of two nouns (subjects).[47] The above 78-year-old patient called her ward physician "a preacher." When asked what preachers do: "they preach about heaven—that is nice." That was also the way she saw her physician. Cognitively, she was unable to recognize him as a member of the general category of "physicians," but emotionally, she received from him "good feelings" and associated these with the preacher she had known so long. Technically then, the first step is to observe the concrete idea presented (preacher). Next, we obtain the relevant attributes of this subject (preacher = man in authority + nice). Third, we see if this key fits other locks: "Man in authority who is nice" also fits the patient's doctor.

The primary process does *not know of a negative, a possibility, or conditionals.* The most frequently asked question by patients on a geropsychiatric in-patient unit is: "When can I go home?" Trying to give a logical answer (in keeping with secondary process and reality orientation) often appears to leave the patient distressed. Further inquiry may reveal that he does not even know where his home is; or he talks about a home where he lived long ago. The point is that the question is a statement; the word "when" means "now"; and "home" stands for "at home." Thus, the translation produces: "I do not feel at home here"—or "I don't belong here—I don't belong—and I feel lost."

In the primary process, there is no *time sense.* In an interview, a patient may move back and forth through the time tunnel without constraints. To tell him that "Today is (day, month, year) and we are at (institution, city, state), etc." might not be meaningful because he does not have the temporal structure to fit this information into.

Since impaired abstract capacity leads to inability to *account to oneself for one's acts,* it is not fruitful to ask the patient why he did this or that. One patient, when asked why she kept having trouble with her wheelchair, responded: "I have not had lunch yet." This also illustrates projection and condensation: imbedded in her response is the accusation "You don't feed me—that's why I can't do things around here."

Dementia patients have *difficulty getting started* on a task, taking initiatives, or making decisions. Once they are put on the right track, though, they may keep going, sometimes to the point of perseveration. Open-ended questions confuse the patient. It is useful to make contact by focusing on a concrete item, e.g., dress, or physical symptoms. Of all the objects in the patient's world, his body remains the closest one to him.

Inability to keep in mind various aspects of a situation simultaneously. The patient can see the individual tree, but cannot conceptualize the forest as an idea. If the nurse gives him a shot, "she hurts me—hurting me is what my enemy does—so, she is my enemy."

Another phenomenon, relevant to this context, is that the patient will end up rambling. When he sets out, in a statement, to make a point, he can't allow himself to digress (e.g., by adding descriptive details), because during the moment of digressing, he loses sight of where he was heading. He never gets to the point, never makes his point. To prevent such derailments, the therapist should firmly but gently intervene in the rambling and keep the patient on the right tract. It is crucial to do this in a good natured, noncritical manner lest the patient should feel put on the spot and is forced to face his failure.

The patient falls back on the so-called *emotional attitude.*[48] He responds to stimuli on the basis of the pleasure principle: either pleasant (good) or unpleasant (bad). Example of dialog: Who is that person (a nurse)? "She is nice." What kind of things does she do? "She is nice to me." How? "She gives me baths and food." Such a patient can enumerate certain qualities of the nurse but cannot recognize her as a member of a conceptual category ("nurses"). Since the ability to express emotions remains relatively intact, it is a good technique to tune in on the patient's emotional channels, rather than something abstract.

During interviews, avoid "conceptual" questions which would put the patient on the spot and cause a catastrophic reaction, (see p. 258). Decrease fear of the unknown by focusing on body sensations and physical symptoms. Many patients start off an interview by presenting physical symptoms seemingly bizarre or inappropriate. These should not be dismissed as irrelevant because it may be the patient's only way he can still make contact.

References

1. Davis, J. M., and Casper, R. C.: General principles of the clinical use of neuroleptics. In: *Principles of Psychopharmacology*, edited by W. G. Clark and J. del Giudice, ed. 2, Academic Press, New York, 1978. pp. 511–536.
2. Usdin, E.: Classification of psychotropic drugs. In: *Principles of Psychopharmacology*, edited by W. C. Clark and J. del Giudice, ed. 2, Academic Press, New York, 1978. pp. 193–246.
3. Friedel, R. O.: Pharmacokinetics in the geropsychiatric patient. In: *Psychopharmacology, a Generation of Progress*, edited by M. A. Lipton, A. DiMascio, and K. F. Killam. Raven Press, New York, 1978. pp. 1499–1505.
4. Prentice, R.: Patterns of psychoactive drug use among the elderly. In: *The Aging Process and Psychoactive Drug Use*, Services Research Monograph Series, No. 79-813, United States Department of Health, Education and Welfare, Washington, D. C., 1979. pp. 17–41.
5. Friedel, R. O.: Biochemical basis of psychopharmacology. In: *Drug Issues in Geropsychiatry*, edited by W. E. Fann and G. L. Maddox, The Williams and Wilkins Company, Baltimore, 1974. pp. 9–17.
6. Whanger, A. D., and Buysse, E. W.: Geriatrics. In: *The Therapist's Handbook, Treatment Methods of Mental Disorders*, edited by B. B. Wolman, Van Nostrand Reinhold Company, New York, 1976. pp. 287–324.
7. Branchey, M. H., Lee, J. H., Amin, R., and Simpson, G. M.: High- and low-potency neuroleptics in elderly psychiatric patients. *J. Am. Med. Assoc. 239(18)*:1860–1862, 1978.
8. Janowsky, D., El-Yousef, M. K., and Davis, J. M.: Side effects associated with psychotropic drugs. In: *Drug Issues in Geropsychiatry*, edited by W. E. Fann and G. L. Maddox. The Williams and Wilkins Co., Baltimore, 1974. pp. 19–28.
9. Bressler, R., and Palmer, J.: Drug interactions in the aged. In: *Drug Issues in Geropsychiatry*, edited by W. E. Fann and G. L. Maddox, The Williams & Wilkins Company, Baltimore, 1974. pp. 49–59.
10. Hollister, L. E.: Psychiatric and neurologic disorders. In *Clinical Pharmacology*, edited by K. L. Melmon and H. F. Morrell, chap. 11, The MacMillan Company, New York, 1972. pp. 463–467.

11. Holliter, L. E.: Psychotherapeutic drugs. In: *Neuropsychiatric Side Effects of Drugs in the Elderly*, edited by A. J. Levenson, vol. 9, Raven Press, New York, 1979. pp. 79–88.
12. Epstein, L. J.: Anxiolytics, antidepressants, and neuroleptics in the treatment of geriatric patients. In: *Psychopharmacology: A generation of Progress*, edited by M. A. Lipton, A. Dimascio, and K. F. Killam, Raven Press, New York, 1978. pp. 1517–1523.
13. Kral, V. A.: An overview of psychopharmacology of old age. *Psychopharmacol. Bull. 12*:51–52, 1976.
14. Salzman, C.: Electroconvulsive therapy. In: *Manual of Psychiatric Therapeutics, Practical Psychopharmacology and Psychiatry*, edited by R. I. Shader, Little, Brown and Company, Boston, 1975. pp. 115–124.
15. Whanger, A. D., and Busse, E. W.: Care in hospital. In: *Modern Perspectives in the Psychiatry of Old Age*, edited by J. G. Howells, chap. 21, Brunner-Mazel, New York, 1975. pp. 450–485.
16. Piland, B.: The aging process and psychoactive drug use in clinical treatment. In: *National Institute on Drug Abuse, The Aging Process and Psychoactive Drug Use.* Services Research Monograph Series, Publication No. 79-813, United States Department of Health, Education and Welfare, Washington, D. C., 1979.
17. Rosin, A. J.: Treatment of dyskinetic and choreatic movement disorders in adults. *Gerontology 24(1)*:46–57, 1978.
18. Fann, W. E., and Lake, C. R.: Drug induced movement disorders in the elderly: an appraisal of treatment. In: *Drug Issues in Geropsychiatry*, edited by W. E. Fann and G. L. Maddox, The Williams and Wilkins Company, Baltimore, 1974. pp. 41–48.
19. Burch, J. G.: A brief review of drug related neurologic disorders in the elderly. In: *Drug Issues in Geropsychiatry*, edited by W. E. Fann and G. L. Maddox, The Williams and Wilkins Company, Baltimore, 1974. pp. 29–33.
20. Libow, L. S.: Pseudo-senility: acute and reversible organic brain syndromes. *J. Am. Geriatr. Soc. 21*:112–120, 1973.
21. Whanger, A. D.: Vitamins and vigor at 65 plus. *Postgrad. Med. 53*:167–172, 1973.
22. Whanger, A. D.: Nutrition, diet, and exercise. In: *Handbook of Geriatric Psychiatry*, edited by E. W. Busse and D. Blazer, Van Nostrand Reinhold Company, New York, 1979.
23. Jarvik, L. F., and Wilkins, J. N.: Aging, hormones and mental functioning. In: *Neuropsychopharmacology*, edited by P. Deniker, C. Radouco-Thomas, and A. Villeneuve, vol. 1, Pergamon Press, New York, 1978. pp. 49–57.
24. Silver, D., Lehmann, H. E., Kral, V. A., and Ban, T. A.: Experimental geriatrics—selection and prediction of therapeutic responsiveness in geriatric patients. *Can. Psychiatr. Assoc. J. 13*:561, 1968.
25. Lifshitz, K., and Kline, N. S.: Use of an estrogen in the treatment of psychosis with cerebral atherosclerosis. *J. Am. Med. Assoc. 177*:501, 1961.
26. Branconnier, R. J., Cole, J. O., and Gardos, G.: ACTH 4–10 in the amelioration of neuropsychological symptomatology associated with senile organic brain syndrome. *Psychopharmacol. Bull.14(1)*:27–30, 1978.
27. Ban, T. A.: Vasodilators, stimulants, and anabolic agents in the treatment of geropsychiatric patients. In: *Psychopharmacology: A Generation of Progress*, edited by M. A. Lipton, A. Dimascio, and K. F. Killam, Raven Press, New York, 1978. pp. 1525–1533.
28. Hyams, D. E.: Cerebral function and drug therapy: the use of cerebral vasodilators, vasorelaxants, haemokinators and activators. In: *Textbook of Geriatric Medicine and Gerontology*, edited by J. C. Brocklehurst, ed. 2, Churchill Livingstone, Edinburgh, 1978. pp. 670–711.
29. Ditch, M., Kelly, F. J., and Resnick, O.: An ergot preparation (hydergine) in the treatment of cerebrovascular disorders in the geriatric patient, double blind study. *J. Am. Geriatr. Soc. 19*:208–217, 1971.
30. Roubicek, J., Geige, C. H., and Abt. K.: An ergot alkaloid preparation (hydergine) in geriatric therapy. *J. Am. Geriatr. Soc. 20*:222–229, 1972.
31. Matejcek, M., Knor, K., Piguet, P-V., and Weil, C.: Electroencephalographic and clinical changes as correlated in geriatric patients treated three months with an ergot alkaloid preparation. *J. Am. Geriatr. Soc. 27(1)*:198–202, 1979.
32. Gaitz, C. M., Varner, R. V., and Overall, J. E.: Pharmacotherapy for organic brain syndrome in late life. *Arch. Gen. Psychiatry 34*:839–845, 1977.

33. Gershon, S.: Better living through chemistry. In: *Aging: Ourselves Tomorrow*, edited by R. S. Garber and A. A. Sugerman, The Eighteenth Carrier Foundation Symposium, Division of Hoffmann-La Roche Inc., Nutley, N. J., 1979. pp. 21–31.
34. Wells, C. E.: Psuedodementia. *Am. J. Psychiatry 136*:895–900, 1979.
35. Charatan, F. B.: Acute confusion and the elderly. *Hosp. Physician 12(5)*:8–10, 1976.
36. Salzman, C., van der Kolk, B., and Shader, R. I.: Psychopharmacology and the geriatric patient. In: *Manual of Psychiatric Therapeutics, Practical Psychopharmacology and Psychiatry*, edited by R. I. Shader, Little, Brown and Company, Boston, 1975. pp. 171–184.
37. Folsom, J. C.: Reality orientation for the elderly mental patient. *J. Geriatr. Psychiatry 1*:291–307, 1968.
38. Whanger, A. D., and Busse, E. W.: Rehabilitation and the mentally disabled geriatric patient. In: *Rehabilitation, Medicine and Psychiatry*, edited by J. Meislin, Charles C Thomas, Springfield, Ill. 1976. pp. 145–161.
39. Harris, R., and Frankel, eds, *Guide to Fitness After Fifty*. Plenum Press, New York, 1977.
40. Lindsley, O. R.: Geriatric behavior prosthetics. In: *New Thoughts on Old Age*, edited by R. Kastenbaum, Springer Publishing, New York, 1964. pp. 41–60.
41. Newman, H. F., and Freeman, J.: Physiologic factors affecting defecatory sensation: relation to aging. *J. Am. Geriatr. Soc. 22*:553–554, 1974.
42. Brocklehurst, J. C.: The treatment of incontinence. In: *Intensive Course in Geriatrics for General Practitioners*, edited by E. Woodford-Williams and A. N. Exton-Smith, S. Karger, Basel, 1967. pp. 298–308.
43. Leeds, M.: Senile recession—a clinical entity. *J. Am. Geriatr. Soc. 8*:122–131, 1960.
44. Wang, H. S., and Whanger, A. D.: Brain impairment and longevity. In: *Prediction of Life Span*, edited by E. Palmore and F. C. Jeffers, Heath Lexington Books, Lexington, 1971.
45. Goldfarb, A. I., Fisch, M., and Gerber, I. E.: Predictors of mortality in the institutionalized aged. *Dis. Nerv. Syst. 27*:21–29, 1966.
46. Verwoerdt, A.: Psychotherapy in senile dementia. In: *Proceedings of the Conference on Clinical Aspects of Alzheimer's Disease*, National Institute of Mental Health, Rockville, Md., December 1978, in press.
47. Von Domarus, E.: The specific laws of logic in schizophrenia. In: *Languge and Thought in Schizophrenia*, edited by J. S. Kasanin, University of California Press, Berkeley, 1944. pp. 104–113.
48. Goldstein, K.: Functional disturbances in brain damage. In: *American Handbook of Psychiatry*, edited by S. Arieti, vol. 1, chap. 39, Basic Books, Inc., New York, 1959. pp. 770–793.

16

an old man with dementia (detailed case example)

The following case is presented in detail to illustrate the diagnostic complexities of dementia, the influence of premorbid personality characteristics on the clinical symptomatology, and recommendations for a comprehensive therapeutic regime.

Mr. Joseph K., a 79-year-old man of great wealth was admitted as an emergency to a local hospital. Earlier that day he had become agitated, confused, and suspicious of what was going on at home. He ordered his secretary to drive him to the City Hall. On the way over there, he changed his mind, and ordered the secretary to go to the County Court House. Having arrived there, he gave instructions to go to the railroad station. Meanwhile, some concerned relatives were following from afar, not daring to interfere, because Mr. K. had always been an awe-inspiring figure. In the course of his life he had built up a vast business empire (oil, cattle, etc.). His many philanthropic activities and substantial donations to community projects had given him an almost legendary stature. No one had ever told him what to do, or had the audacity to stand up to him. When Mr. K. had arrived at the railroad station, however, got out of the car, and proceeded to walk by himself along the railroad tracks, the relatives decided to intervene. He was rushed to a nearby hospital for emergency admission.

RECENT ILLNESS

Mr. K. had been in fairly good health until 3 years ago, when he began to complain of recurrent, brief spells of dizziness. This was treated by the family physician with anticoagulants, in an attempt to counteract cerebrovascular ischemia, but without significant relief.

There also had been a noticeable decrement in recent memory: difficulties in recalling names, recent events, and dates, or sudden inability to remember what he was about to say.

Reportedly, Mr. K. was aware of these changes in his intellectual faculties, but apparently was able to continue functioning in his usual work patterns. At least, he would go to his office everyday, and engage in decisions about business transactions involving huge amounts of money. Any suggestions made by his family, business associates, and physician to slow down, and to delegate more to others, were summarily dismissed. His obstinate refusal to let go, combined with the manifest deterioration of his judgment, caused much apprehension among his family, friends, and business associates.

A few months prior to admission, the patient had fallen on the street and fractured one of the small bones in his left foot. Presumably, the fall was a result of an attack of dizziness. (During later psychiatric examination, Mr. K. denied there had been anything like a fracture, maintaining that "it was just a bruise.")

The relatives further reported that Mr. K. had become much more irascible during the last few weeks. On the day of hospitalization, in fact, he had used "some very strong language" toward his accountant and his secretary.

PHYSICAL AND MENTAL EXAMINATION ON ADMISSION

Physical examination was essentially within normal limits, except for a moderate hearing loss. Blood pressure was 145/85. The admission note stated that he had visual hallucinations, and delusional ideas of a paranoid nature. He felt persecuted by members of an "underground organization, left wing radicals, or communists, who were trying to kidnap him and hold him hostage, so they would get a huge ransom." During the acute confusional state, the patient actually believed he had been kidnapped and now was "underground."

The mental confusion, hallucinations, and delusions cleared up within several days after admission to the hospital.

The electroencephalogram (EEG) was abnormal, being characterized by generalized slowing and dysrhythmia. No definite focal changes were noted.

MEDICAL HISTORY

Mr. K. had been in good health until the age of 72 when he developed coronary insufficiency as indicated by an electrocardiogram (EKG). Since then, there have been no significant cardiac or respiratory problems; his blood pressure has always been within normal limits. The most recent EKG was normal. There is no evidence of orthostatic hypotension, or major fluctuations in the pulse pressure. There was no past history of episodes of paralysis, aphasia, or other neurological signs that would suggest a major cerebrovascular accident. There is no evidence of any major psychiatric disorder in the past history, prior to the present episode.

FAMILY HISTORY

This was obtained from Mr. K.'s brother. Mr. K.'s wife died ten years ago, from cancer of the uterus. Reportedly, Mr. K. "grieved for only a short while after her death. He lost himself again in his work. In fact, he never stopped working." Significantly, there was never any overt talk between Mr. K. and his wife that she had a terminal illness and was about to die. The brother feels certain, though, that Mr. K. did know about the nature of his wife's illness.

The same type of reaction was observed following the death of his only child, a son. He died of leukemia, when Mr. K. was in his late 50's. Although he knew about his son's terminal illness, he reportedly "went on with business as usual. He would never sit down and grieve about a loss. In fact, he actually scolded his son for not working hard enough."

Comments: these observations point to a central feature of Mr. K.'s personality. He has always seen himself as a winner, and in a way he has never experienced defeat. He has reacted to losses (death of son and wife) in terms of denial. He has been able to avoid the working through of these losses, by concentrating more intensely on his work. The significant point is that he has not learned to cope with the inevitable losses of late life. Now that his own physical and mental capacities are declining, he finds himself equally unprepared to deal with these personal losses and to accept them. The behavior patterns which, in the past, served him so well in building up a vast business empire, have now become maladaptive.

PSYCHIATRIC EXAMINATION

Mr. K.'s general behavior was characterized by attempts to maintain control. It was he who decided which persons would be present during the interview, what topics to talk about, and in which manner. *Orientation* for time, place, person, and situation was intact. The sensorium was clear, but the capacity for attention and concentration was decreased to a mild-moderate extent. (The impression was gained that this decreased attentiveness resulted from a combination of impaired cognition and general defensiveness.) *Perception:* there was no evidence that impaired vision and hearing interfered with the interview. Illusions, perceptual distortions, or hallucinations were not noted. *Affect:* overtly manifest were suspiciousness and irritability. The patient questioned the motives of the examiner and other persons present. He quickly expressed annoyance when some wishes were not immediately carried out, e.g., getting his attorney to sit in during the interview. He seemed to be unaware of the unreasonable nature of some of his demands. (This implies lack of good judgment.) Interestingly, he would smile whenever he had difficulty answering a particular question. (This is in keeping with his tendency to deny and rationalize his losses. Behind the facade of suspiciousness and irritability, there would seem to be a great deal of anxiety. Under certain stress, e.g., interference with his defenses, this anxiety may increase to the point of overt panic. The suspiciousness and irritability serve to keep his attention focused externally. His occasional jocular behavior has a similar aim: diversion away from his own problems.)

Thought processes: no delusions were observed, but there were several ideas of reference, e.g., asking suspiciously what people were talking about prior to coming in his room. To some extent, this is understandable in view of his present situation, but the intensity of his response was not appropriate. Likewise, he became suspicious and defensive when asked about retirement, the aging process, future plans, etc. He dealt with the issue of retirement by questioning the interviewer's motives; he talked about the question of how old age had affected him by presenting a detached semi-intellectual description of the process of arteriosclerosis. When it came to his future plans, he became defiant, explaining that he had rejected previous medical advice to slow down in his work, and that he would continue working as before.

There is evidence of some loss of the capacity for abstract thought and conceptual thinking. For example, when asked about the year of his son's death, he knew that "this was 20 years ago." But after repeated questions what year it actually had been, and after establishing what the present year was, he was not able to subtract 20 years from that. Instead, he added them on to the present year, which brought him close to the end of the 20th century. At this point, he revealed perplexion and profound anxiety. His next statement was spoken in a mumbled way: "or 2000?" (This illustrates the catastrophic reaction[1] of brain-damaged individuals: the patient gives a wrong answer, is aware of his inability to perform accurately, develops profound anxiety, and becomes totally unable to perform at all.) The patient's wrong answer does not illustrate an inability to calculate, but conceptual confusion about the difference between two fundamental arithmetical procedures, i.e., subtraction versus addition.

(The history provides other examples of such conceptual confusion. A few weeks ago, he called one of the nurses a "waitress." Likewise, his search for the city hall, the court house and the railroad station was a manifestation of conceptual confusion: he knew he had to go somewhere for help, but was unable to assess the nature of his troubles, and accurately match this need with the proper place for help, a hospital. The fact that he sought out the city hall and court house is in keeping with the observation that he felt persecuted by the "underground" organization. This conceptual misinterpretation is primarily the result of the organic brain syndrome, but from a psychodynamic point of view, this delusion served to reinforce the tendencies of denial of the real problem, and represented a last desperate effort to maintain the intactness of the self and the self-image.)

Memory: there was considerable difficulty remembering names of persons he had known for some time. Interestingly, he turns to his relatives immediately, who then supply the correct name. The same is true with regard to dates and recent events. (Because Mr. K. has been, and still is, getting this type of support from his environment, he has not had to come to grips with the real extent of his memory loss. The implication for management is that he should continue to have, as much as possible, such external agents that can serve as a memory prosthesis for him. A stranger would not be able to function in this role.)

Judgment: it is clear from the above that the capacity for judgment is impaired.

DIAGNOSTIC IMPRESSION

The clinical data suggest the co-existence of two types of organic brain syndrome: Alzheimer's disease and multi-infarct dementia. The latter is suggested by the longstanding history of dizziness, and the occasional fainting spells, the recent occurrence of acute, transient episodes of confusion and excitement, the EEG findings ("generalized slowing and dysrhythmia, consistent with cerebral arteriosclerosis"), and the fluctuations in the course of the illness. Alzheimer's disease is indicated by significant memory impairment, especially for names, recent dates, and events, impaired cognitive abilities, especially a deficit in the capacity for abstract thought and concept formation, gradual personality changes, including increased suspiciousness, irritability and self-centeredness, as well as the emergence of pathological defense mechanisms (marked denial, projection), and the patient's age and gender: organic brain syndrome in a male octogenarian is usually due to senile brain atrophy.

The signs and symptoms of organic brain syndrome do not only depend on the structural, pathological changes in the brain, but also on characteristics of the premorbid personality. Some reference to significant personality factors was already made: his aggressive ambitiousness, his tendency to see himself as strong and undefeated, the rigid pattern of being absorbed in work, at the expense of leisure and recreational activities, his inability to adequately work through personal losses to the point of resolution of the grief and acceptance of loss, his tendency to continue patterns of coping that used to be adaptive (with the emphasis on aggressive mastery) but have now become obsolete. In fact, what appears to emerge now is an intensification of these earlier patterns, rather than attempts to accommodate himself to the realities of late life.

The diagnosis includes a chronic brain syndrome manifested by dizziness, memory deficit, impaired cognitive capacities, and changes in personality, and a history of acute brain syndrome, manifested by acute episodes of disorientation, hallucinations, and paranoid delusions.

PROGNOSIS

Prognosis for chronic brain syndrome is poor. Chances for reversal of basic pathology or symptomatology are practically nil. The chances for arresting the progress of the disease process are very small. However, prognosis with regard to the acute brain syndrome is fair. With proper medical, psychiatrical, and nursing care management, the risks of further episodes of acute brain syndrome may be greatly diminished.

RECOMMENDATIONS

Rule out the possibility of occlusive disease of the extracranial cerebrovascular supply, e.g., atherosclerosis of the carotid arteries. Special studies, such as cerebral blood flow determinations, may be indicated. Rule out possible episodes of hypotension or decreased pulse pressure, from whatever sources, because these would interfere with adequate brain oxygenation, or aggravate an already existing deficiency in cerebral oxygenation.

Maintain optimal *physical health,* with special attention to cardiovascular, renal, and respiratory functions. Maintain adequate nutrition and dental care. Administer regular high potency multiple vitamins. Try to reduce hearing impairment by providing suitable hearing aid.

Specific medications and procedures aimed at *improving cerebral oxygenation* and functioning generally have doubtful value. In no instance is there a significant chance of clinical benefit, but some medications reportedly have been useful.

Medications that appear to be useless: monosodium glutamate, RNA therapy.

Medications or procedures that are experimental or controversial include hyperbaric oxygenation,[2] metrazol (alone or in combinations), procaine therapy, anabolic steroid hormones, special diets, such as low-cholesterol, low-fat, choline or inositol, etc.[3, 4]

Medications that are *possibly helpful* should be given a trial: hydergine; vasorelaxants; anticoagulants; and high potency multiple vitamins.[5, 6]

Hydergine (dihydrogenated alkaloids of ergotoxine, DHAE) has been found to be useful for the treatment of cerebrovascular insufficiency. Apparently, it is a safe drug, which may improve important aspects of cognitive function, mood, behavior, and the ability to perform daily living tasks.[7–9]

The effectiveness of *vasorelaxant agents,* such as papaverine, is less certain. In one double-blind study, hydergine was superior to papaverine in improving mental alertness, confusion, depression, and inertia.[10] Nicotinic acid, which supposedly is a vasodilator, does not appear to produce therapeutic benefits for patients with cerebrovascular ischemia.[11] Cyclandelate is another vasodilator, which may have possible usefulness, but its therapeutic efficacy has not been clearly demonstrated.[12]

Anticoagulants, e.g., Dicumarol, have been used in the treatment of cerebrovascular ischemia and senile dementia, on the assumption that anticoagulant therapy will improve the cerebral blood flow, or prevent further impairment. Several reports in the literature suggest that anticoagulant therapy can be beneficial, especially in elderly patients who have arteriosclerosis with thromboembolic complications. Although there may be some uncertainty about the degree of their therapeutic or preventive usefulness, there is general agreement that if anticoagulants are administered, careful control and follow up is essential, in view of the risk of hemorrhages.[13, 14]

The role of *nutritional* deficiencies in geropsychiatric disorders is still uncertain. Whanger and Wang found that more than 70 percent of elderly hospitalized patients had been on inadequate diets. Of these, 50 percent had borderline or low levels of folic acid, and 12 percent had borderline or low levels of vitamin B_{12}, both of which may be associated with dementia and other psychiatric disorders.[15] Classical vitamin deficiencies are now-a-days rare, but when vitamin deficiencies do exist, multiple deficiencies are the rule. It is not always easy to determine whether such deficiencies are the cause of the mental disorder, or the result. In view of the frequent malnutrition in aged patients, it is prudent to administer a daily multivitamin preparation. It may take up to 1 year of therapy to reverse deficiency problems in the elderly. Even in the hospital or nursing home, aged patients may maintain nutritional deficiencies because of deficient food habits, e.g., eating mostly carbohydrates, loss of vitamins (especially vitamin C and folic acid) in institutional food, failure to eat the food served, and factors interfering with vitamin utilization (decrease in digestive enzymes, altered intestinal flora, and the use of mineral oil and antivitamin drugs like phenobarbital).[16, 17]

Medications recommended for *psychiatric disturbances* include the following.

For *acute episodes* of restlessness, excitement, confusion or aggressive behavior: haloperidol (Haldol), 0.5 mg three times daily (t.i.d.), or one of the phenothiazines, such as trifluoperazine (Stelazine), 2 mg twice a day (b.i.d.), thioridazine (Mellaril), 25 mg t.i.d.; or hydroxizine (Vistaril, Atarax), 25 mg t.i.d. Try these medications in the sequence indicated. Each drug should be given long enough to be sure of its effectiveness, or lack thereof (a test period of at least 3 weeks). Avoid overmedication; do not give more than one major tranquilizer at the same time; if at all possible, start with relatively small doses and increase the dosage gradually.

For *chronic tension,* anxiety, or mild agitation: diazepam (Valium) 2 mg t.i.d., hydroxyzine (Vistaril, Atarax) 25 mg t.i.d., or doxepin (Sinequan) 25 mg b.i.d.

For *insomnia*: chloralhydrate (Noctec) 500 mg h.s.; or flurazepam (Dalmane) 15 mg h.s.

Recommendations for social and environmental management include the following.

Homecare, with adequate nursing help available as needed. Prevent admissions to hospital or other institutions whenever possible.

Structure *daily activities* according to a regimen that is consistent, predictable, and sufficiently diversified. A consistent repertoire of daily activities is essential in fostering the patient's sense of self-confidence and minimizing the risk of loss of control. The activity spectrum should provide diversions and stimulations in keeping with the patient's personal wishes and his remaining potentials. Avoid the extreme of excessive involvements and overstimulation, on the one hand, and that of social isolation and sensory deprivation, on the other, since each will exacerbate the symptomatology.

Recognize that attempts to alter longstanding character patterns are not only futile, but possibly harmful. The patient's behavior should be met with an attitude of *matter-of-fact acceptance.* Support must be given without being overbearing; helpful assistance should never be accompanied by undue efforts to correct him, or by pointing out to him (explicitly or tacitly) his deficits. The manifestations of anger, irritability, aggressive behavior, etc. may gradually get worse, as the dementia itself becomes worse, in time. It is helpful for persons having contact with the patient, especially those providing care, to remember that such negative emotions are not meant to be personally directed against them; they are, by and large, the manifestations of an illness: senile dementia.

Recognize his need to *maintain self-esteem*, and self-image of strength. The latter will require a certain amount of denial mechanisms on the part of the patient. This denial should be left intact, as long as it does not provide a serious risk to himself, others, or vital business matters. Interference with the denial mechanisms may lead to more serious and maladaptive defenses, such as paranoid projections.

The patient's *dependency* on others for providing him with basic support in the areas of memory and conceptual thinking, sets the stage for several possible undesirable developments. Since he has an obvious problem admitting "weakness" or dependency, he may react to increased dependency by becoming more controlling, angry, and defiant and insisting he can do without the help from others. If, for whatever reason, the supporting people in the environment happen to be absent or unresponsive, he will tend to feel lost, confused, and quite anxious. If the supporting persons try to point out that he was wrong, or try to correct him, he may react with anger; this can intensify to the point where he might feel that others "are against him."

The fact that he must rely on others for support in the area of *memory, abstract thought, and judgment* has the important implication that these persons, in order to be able to give such support, need to be well acquainted with the patient. This type of support cannot be expected, for example, from a nurse who has known the patient only briefly. Although this support needs to come from relatives and close acquaintances, the latter are advised not to get involved in manifestations that are the expression of psychopathology and matters that would require medical-psychiatric expertise.

While it is important to convey respect to the patient, and allow him to continue in roles in keeping with his self-image, it is also necessary to provide him with the *protection* that his condition requires. This protection can be given in tacit-implicit ways or in overt-direct ways. Tacit protection is called for when it is clear that the inherent demands of a situation would exceed the patient's capacities; e.g., tasks requiring the use of abstract thought, independent initiative, innovative problem-solving, or decisions involving complex issues with far-reaching consequences. Protective support can be given by letting others have the information available and provide this to the patient, in a matter-of-fact, casual (perhaps even surreptitious) manner. The patient may well accept such help and information, without openly acknowledging it as if he himself accomplished something important. If such tacit, subtle approaches of protecting the patient against the risks of his illness prove to be inadequate, a more direct, open approach is necessary. The element of firmness will then be essential. It is recommended that, if firm intervention is needed, this not be carried out by relatives, friends, or business associates, but by a physician, nurse, or other representative of the medical profession.

References

1. Goldstein, K.: Functional disturbances in brain damage. In: *American Handbook of Psychiatry*, edited by S. Arieti, vol. 1 chap. 39, Basic Books, New York, 1959. pp. 770–793.
2. Edwards, A. E., and Hart, G. M.: Hyperbaric oxygenation and the cognitive functioning of the aged. *J. Am. Geriatr. Soc. 22*:376–379, 1974.
3. Kral, V. A.: An overview of psychopharmacology of old age. *Psychopharmacol. Bull. 12*:51–52, 1976.
4. Branconnier, R. J., Cole, J. O., and Gardos, G.: ACTH 4–10 in the amelioration of neuropsychological symptomatology associated with senile organic brain syndrome. *Psychopharmacol. Bull. 14(1)*: 27–30, 1978.
5. Ban, T. A.: Vasodilators, stimulants, and anabolic agents in the treatment of geropsychiatric patients. In: *Psychopharmacology: A Generation of Progress*, edited by M. A. Lipton, A. Dimascio, and K. F. Killam, Raven Press, New York, 1978. pp. 1525–1533.
6. Hyams, D. E.: Cerebral function and drug therapy: the use of cerebral vasodilators, "vasorelaxants," "haemokinators" and "activators." In: *Textbook of Geriatric Medicine and Gerontology*, edited by J. C. Brocklehurst, ed. 2, Churchill Livingston, Edinburgh, 1978. pp. 670–711.
7. Rao, D. B., and Norris, J. R.: A double-blind investigation of hydergine in the treatment of cerebrovascular insufficiency in the elderly. *Johns Hopkins Med. J. 130*:317–324, 1972.
8. Ditch, M., Kelly, F. J. and Resnick, O.: An ergot preparation (hydergine) in the treatment of cerebrovascular disorders in the geriatric patient, double blind study. *J. Am. Geriatr. Soc. 19*:208–217, 1971.
9. Matejcek, M., Knor, K., Piguet, P. V., and Weil, C.: Electroencephalographic and clinical changes as correlated in geriatric patients treated three months with an ergot alkaloid preparation. *J. Am. Geriatr. Soc. 27(1)*:198–202, 1979.

10. Bazo, A. J.: An ergot alkaloid preparation (hydergine) versus papaverine in treating common complaints of the aged: double-blind study. *J. Am. Geriatr. Soc. 21*:63, 1973.
11. Smith, C. M.: Nicotinic acid therapy in old age. *J. Am. Geriatr. Soc. 11*:580, 1963.
12. Aderman, M., Giardina, W. J., and Koreniowski, S.: Effect of cyclandelate on perception, memory, and cognition in a group of geriatric subjects. *J. Am. Geriatr. Soc. 6*: 268–271, 1972.
13. Wright, I. S.: Comments on the use of anticoagulants in geriatric patients. *J. Am. Geriatr. Soc. 21*:1–3, 1973.
14. Ratner, J., Rosenberg, G., Kral, V. A., and Engelsmann, F.: Anticoagulant therapy for senile dementia. *J. Am. Geriatr. Soc. 20*:556, 1972.
15. Whanger, A. D., and Wang, H. S.: Vitamin B_{12} deficiency in normal aged and elderly psychiatric patients. In: *Normal Aging II*, edited by E. Palmore, Duke University Press, Durham, N. C., 1974. pp. 63–73.
16. Whanger, A. D.: Nutrition, diet, and exercise. In: *Handbook of Geriatric Psychiatry*, edited by E. W. Busse and D. Blazer, van Nostrand Reinhold Company, New York, 1979.
17. Jarvik, L. F., and Wilkins, J. N.: Aging, hormones and mental functioning. In: *Neuropsychopharmacology*, edited by P. Deniker, C. Radouco-Thomas, and A. Villeneuve, vol. 1, Pergamon Press, New York, 1978. pp. 49–57.

17

contact with the family

The structure and dynamics of the family unit depend on intrinsic factors (the characteristics of its individual members) and extrinsic factors (societal influences). In this chapter, our focus will be primarily on the first set of determinants.

THE DYNAMICS OF FAMILY CHANGE

The family, like other organisms, is not a static structure but a dynamic entity that continuously evolves. From a structural point of view, the relationships between family members can be described as horizontal (e.g., marital, between siblings) or vertical (e.g., parent-child). The family structure may be nuclear or extended. The former involves the smallest societal unit: husband-wife-child. The extended family includes members of more than two generations.[1, 2]

SOCIAL ROLES

From a functional point of view, family relationships can be described in terms of the roles of the individual members vis-à-vis each other. The role of one individual is complemented by the counter-role of one or more other family members, e.g., husband-wife, parent-child. If role and counter-role represent a good fit, the relationship tends to be harmonious. The concept of role is a social one; it refers to behavior carried out for and with others. It is clear that intrapsychic phenomena do not necessarily correspond to the social role: private thoughts and subjective feelings may or may not be in tune with one's social role. If they are in tune, there will be a state of relative harmony and absence of tension in the individual. If, however, social role and intrapsychic forces are in conflict, the former or the latter (or both) will feel the impact. Thus, a man may faithfully continue in various roles (husband, father, provider, disciplinarian) although inwardly he is aware of wishes incompatible with those roles. Chronic conflicts usually have a neurotic origin. In personality disorders, the conflict between social role obligations and intrapersonal tendencies typically does not last very long, because individual drives tend to win out over social responsibilities.

PHASES AND CHANGES

Phases of the Family

In the course of the years, the family undergoes modifications in structure and function, for example, when children are born, when they leave home, when the grandparents die, etc.[3, 4] The family passes through the following *phases*: preparental, parental, postparental, and the phase of the aging family (following retirement).[5] Thus, the relationships of the family members and the repertoire of roles change continuously. This may even happen within the span of a particular phase. During the parental phase, for example, the parents need to "grow up" along with their children. The behavior appropriate in the parent-infant relationship is very different from that between parent and teenager. The changing developmental tasks with which the child is confronted require concomitant, appropriate changes on the part of the parents.

Societal Alterations

The family may change, not only as the result of its own intrinsic developmental factors, but also due to broad *societal alterations* in the way the concept of family is viewed. In previous times (until the early 1900's), it was a common experience that one parent had died before the last child was grown up. Typically, the wife/mother would succumb to the risks attending pregnancy and childbirth. Medical progress has changed all that, so now-a-days the average marital couple still has many years together after their children have departed from home. The concept of the family as a basic societal unit has also been modified due to the changing role of contemporary woman, which has led to a reappraisal of many roles that were considered "traditional," or taken for granted. Society's impact on the family is further reflected by the increasing attention on children's rights. Finally, experimentations with alternative family organizations (e.g., solo-parents, multifamily living arrangements) have become more common and accepted.

Of special interest are the opportunities and constraints regarding living-together arrangements for old persons. Two major factors play a role in setting the stage for alternative arrangements. First, the number of old women exceeds that of old men, which has provoked some considerations with regard to polygyny as a possible solution.[6] Secondly, the economic facts of life may prompt older men and women, each of whom receives individual social security income, to co-habitate without formally legalizing this arrangement.

Belonging and Self-actualization

Experimentation with alternative types of family organization does not bewilder the thoughtful observer, since the basic themes are few and simple. They include the essential needs of *belonging and self-actuali-*

zation. Between these two motives, there is a natural tension. The sense of belonging evokes the image of the individual as being part of an interpersonal network within which he fits and finds shelter, as being a nodal point in a larger nexus that encompasses him. On the other hand, in the creative act of becoming a unique self, the individual stands out and stands alone. In becoming a person (a being that never was before, and never will return, a once-and-for-all kind of existence), the individual transcends the network he belongs to. Ideally, the tension between the two basic drives (to belong versus to stand out) is one of a healthy equilibrium. Thus, the sense of belonging would facilitate one's self-actualization and, conversely, the latter enables one to carve out a private niche of one's own in an alien world.

The motive of attaining a sense of belonging is reflected in the extended family organization. The emotional or spatial vicinity of three or more generations suggests ongoingness: the reassuring sense that one belongs to a family tree, whose survival does not depend on the fate of its individual branches. On the other hand, the drive toward self-actualization appears to correspond with the emphasis on the nuclear family unit. In this smaller type of family, it allegedly is easier to live a life that allows one "to be just yourself." The tension of having to subordinate (part of) oneself to the rules and roles of the extended family system may cause one to break away; the new, separate subsystem may be more free, but also more alienated. Conversely, the tensions inherent in the smaller nuclear family unit may prompt a search to join, or merge with, a larger, extended family.

In everyday life, we see both processes at work. It is now-a-days not uncommon for persons, who have reached middle age and fulfilled their obligations to their parents and children, to break away from it all and start a new life. The search is then for a new identity, to find out who one was all along, or to do what one always had wanted to. However, any breaking away from established ties (people and places) represents, per definition, a loss. The loss may be a calculated gamble to attain a long-term gain, like taking a few steps back to make a long jump forward.

Then, there are those who are more or less isolated or alienated, in search of a sense of belonging. The larger system which they eventually join may be the (extended) family group; but often, by way of mental processes of abstraction and generalization, this new, larger family system is a conceptual one: a belief, ideology, a group of people espousing a cause; etc. Considering the human life cycle in its entirety, it appears that the motive for a sense of belonging is relatively more prominent at either extreme of the continuum, i.e., in childhood and in old age.

ROLE REVERSAL AND FILIAL ROLE

Filial Maturity

It is often assumed that once the children are grown up and on their own, the relationship between them and their parents is pretty well finalized. In many instances, this is an oversimplification, because even between adult children and aging parents the relationship may continue to change. The very fact that the parents are aging is a major factor responsible for this. The adult children need to recognize that no longer can they look to their parents for the support they used to get. No longer are the parents strong or omnipotent, qualities ascribed to them by younger children. If the relationship between adult children and their parents has been mature, the role transition can be made without difficulties. The ability to relate to one's parents as a mature adult involves a genuine emancipation from them, and viewing them as persons in their own right, with their own unique identity. Such a mature, objective view cannot be clouded by remnants of conflict drifting over from the past. Such psychological changes, reflected in specific changes of role, are part of a developmental process which leads to *filial maturity*. The filial crisis of this stage occurs when one realizes that the aging parents are no longer the pillars of support they used to be, but that they themselves begin to need the support of their children.

Reversal of Roles

This transition involves, therefore, a *reversal of roles*, which to some individuals may cause considerable problems. The adult child does not assume a parental role to his own parents; rather, the filial role involves being depended upon and being dependable. The performance of the filial role leads to filial maturity which has characteristic gratifications of its own. The clarification of one's filial role and the delineation of one's obligations toward an aging parent may not come about, until after considerable upheaval.[7, 8]

> A 40-year-old man was hospitalized due to a stomach ulcer. He had been working under high pressure, one reason being that he had to support his aged mother who had been living in with him and his wife. Also, there had been chronic strife with his "fussy" wife. After 2 weeks in the hospital, the ulcer symptoms had improved and he returned home. Shortly thereafter, his wife packed her belongings, moved out, and announced her intentions to separate. This left the patient and his mother together at home, neither one feeling happy with the way things developed. The next happening was the hospitalization of the elderly mother, for ill-defined symptoms. While she was in the hospital, the wife returned and moved back in the home. Eventually, a living arrangement evolved with the aged mother residing in a rest home, and her son and his wife continuing to live together. Thus, in the course of a few months, these three people had tried out three types of living arrangements. First, the adult son removed himself from the home leaving his mother and his wife together. Then, the wife departed, leaving her

husband and his mother together. Finally, the mother went, leaving the home to her son and his wife. This last arrangement was arrived at by trial and error, causing undue hardship for all. What they had been trying to decide was an answer to the question: "Who is responsible for whom?"

Individuals who have remained immature, overly dependent, or neurotic frequently have problems in this area.[9, 10] The immature person has a strong need to depend on somebody who is strong and supportive. Thus, it may happen that the aging parent is not "permitted" to become more dependent on the adult child. Because the latter continues to regard his parent as (unrealistically) capable and self-reliant, the aging parent is subjected to multiple burdens: he has to play a role which he does not want and is not capable of.[11]

The source of the problem may also originate with the aging parent, for example, when he tenaciously adheres to an outdated set of roles or obsolete self-concept. Such a person may continue to see himself as head of the family, or as somebody who should have the final word in family decisions, being unaware that what once was an appropriate role, is no longer so. In most instances, the difficulties in the process of role reversal are due to psychological factors in both the aging parent and the adult child.

THE AGING FAMILY

A wide range of stresses affects the aging family (postretirement phase). Mentioned already was the potential stress inherent in reversal of roles between aging parents and their adult children. Other stressful factors are the effects of biological aging, retirement, economic deprivation, loss of spouse, loss of home, etc.[1, 5, 12, 13]

Three-Generation Relationships

Townsend[13] examined *three-generation relationships* in low income families and found that the social and family circumstances determined the capacity for adjustment and self-care in later life. For aged persons, especially women, the vertical family relationships become more meaningful than the horizontal ones. Non-family activities diminish; mates may pull apart with regard to their interests and activities. The first-generation woman is busy with her grandchildren and her daughters with whom she maintains frequent contact as a family helper. The sons visit the mother but usually come alone. The first-generation man is isolated from many friends through retirement, and from his wife by her relative independence. When a woman is ill or disabled, she tends to depend first on a daughter, then on close female relatives, and lastly on her husband. When the aged man is ill, the most common source of aid is his wife, then female relatives, and the daughter. Thus, the most isolated person was the first-generation man. When this isolation is complicated by loss of spouse or close friends and by changes in environment, the chances for survival are slim.

According to other authorities, the role of the older man in the multigenerational family is more significant.[14, 15] Compared with the maternal relationship, the paternal one would become more important in later years. The final task of becoming an adult may involve more of a coming to terms with "the old man" than with the mother. Undoubtedly, cultural factors and differences in socioeconomical status play a major role in determining the importance and significance of the aged man vis-à-vis the aged woman in the extended family.

Loss of Spouse

The reaction to the *loss of spouse* through death or illness depends among other things on predisposing factors, particularly lifelong character patterns.[10, 16] For example, the pseudoindependent person may be stripped of his facade, and overt manifestations of dependency may appear for the first time, much to the concern or dismay of children and friends. The stress factor of loss of spouse is illustrated by the fact that suicide rates are highest following divorce or separation, and next highest with widowhood. The rate of suicide after divorce (both for men and women) is about two and a half times greater than that of the general population. The risk of suicide is highest in the first year after the loss of spouse, but it remains higher than average for at least 5 years.[17, 18]

Women seem to adjust better to the loss of spouse than men do. There are several possible reasons for this. First, the loss of spouse often is a stress experienced by women at a younger age than in the case of men, when there is relatively still more potential and energy for coping available. In addition, women seem to prepare themselves for the possibility of widowhood by way of anticipatory rehearsal for the role of widow. Such a mental process is set in motion by the deaths of married men in the circle of friends, the loss of a woman's father, and the departure of her children. This anticipatory grief can be useful, and may represent adaptive coping.[19] The husband may react to loss of wife in several ways. He may remarry, for any number of reasons (e.g., a healthy sexual drive or strong dependency needs).[20] The family's involvement in this decision can precipitate another crisis. A less adaptive coping response to the loss of the wife is withdrawal from the family, while making demands indirectly by various complaints. The reaction to the loss of a spouse, on the part of the surviving marital partner, is not always easy to predict or understand, even in the light of life-long character patterns.

> A man, in his mid-70's, died after a long illness, of lung cancer. He had always been a strong, strong-willed person whose role as patriarch and ruler of the three-generational family was never disputed. In contrast to his dominance (maintained until his death), his wife

was "meek and mousy." Prior to his death, the man himself, as well as the three adult children, worried about "what would become of mother," if she should lose her pillar of strength. What did happen was somewhat of a surprise. Even on the very day of her husband's death, this presumably helpless woman took charge of all necessary arrangements. She turned out to have financial expertise, social leadership, and personal stamina that more than matched those of her late husband. It just so happened that, given his dominant personality, there could not have been "two skippers on the ship." It was her particular strength that, for so many years, she could stay in the background and accommodate him.

Loss of Home

Another crisis of the aging family is *loss of the home* or moving to a new environment. In younger years, moves are considered an expanding event but to the aged, a move is usually a constricting, isolating event. The same loss occurs when members of the family move away. Aged persons who are on the waiting list for a home for the aged undergo special types of stress, because of their status in limbo. Following admission to the home, anxiety usually decreases.[21]

CONFLICTS IN THE FAMILY

Family pathology comprises disorders of the family as a whole, and disturbed relationships between two or more individuals within the family. The former usually represent long-standing, habitual patterns, while the latter may be more acute and reactive in nature. Many varieties of disturbances occur in both of these categories, and some of the more common types will now be reviewed.

THE FAMILY AS A WHOLE

Pathology of the family as a whole refers to ingrained patterns, behavioral styles, and ways of doing things, of which the family members themselves are hardly aware.

Problems in Perceptiveness and Deficiencies in Communication

Among family members, these may have been present for decades. The aging parents, or other elderly relatives, may become the victim of such patterns. Insufficient perception and awareness of what is happening to the elderly family members may be due to denial, selective inattention, or rationalization. Accurate perception of age-related changes in the parents may be too threatening, as for example, in the case of an unmarried child, chronologically an adult but emotionally still dependent and childlike, who lives with an aging parent. Such a state of affairs may be a great burden on the aging parent who is forced to continue playing a role for which he or she is no longer suited. In other cases, selective inattention is expedient because it enables one to avoid confrontation with certain filial responsibilities, and some people do not want to be bothered. It is of interest that professional attempts to deal with such patterns of denial and disturbed communication in families with an aged, disabled member frequently are not successful.[8, 11]

Attraction of Neurotic Opposites

Marital partners normally are attracted to each other on the basis of differences in sex (gender), but similarities and a shared outlook in nonsexual matters. Of course, there are some apparent exceptions; for example, a man who is the silent, serious type may do well in marrying a vivacious, cheerful woman. Such complementarity does not contradict the general rule because this couple may share a common outlook, i.e., that seriousness and cheerfulness are neither good nor bad in themselves, but that their value is relative depending on factors in the situation. In the case of neurotic opposites, however, there is no true complementarity and stability because within the partners there exist specific neurotic conflicts. The conflict in one individual may be the reverse, or mirror image as it were, of that in the other. Typical of the conflict is that one part of it is beyond awareness. An example may clarify this.

Let us assume that a man has strong dependency needs which are kept unconscious for whatever reasons. What is outwardly manifest is excessive independency (a reaction formation). Such a man is likely to attract a dependent woman because role and counter-role form a good fit. This couple will get along reasonably well as long as the man's independent facade remains intact. If however, the reaction formation crumbles, due to aging or illness, the underlying dependency comes to the fore. Now there are two dependent partners in the relationship, a very unstable situation (See case on p. 128).

Other examples of such neurotic opposites are the following: one partner has cruel (sadistic) characteristics, the other is the suffering martyr (masochistic); one partner is chronically depressive and the other hypomanic (unduly optimistic and cheerful). In all these instances, we may find that the outwardly visible behavior has an invisible counterpart which is the opposite of the former. The masochist may be a sadist in disguise; the hypomanic defends himself against depressive feelings, etc.

Crisis-prone Family

For some families, stress and crisis is a way of life. The family members may complain about their burdens, e.g., the presence of elderly parents in their home, but in fact, it is precisely this stress that holds the family intact. There may be many reasons for this, only two of which will be mentioned. First, some families are close only during times of stress and crisis, because the only thing they are good at is the business of providing support. Secondly, some families may, secretly or unconsciously, welcome stressful circumstances because the external crises prevent them from having to face their inner conflicts. Thus, when relatives complain about the presence of aging parents in their home, it is wise to try to ascertain to what extent these relatives are *crisis-prone.* This can be done by taking a brief history of their past. If their past is a succession of crises or near-crises, then one should suspect that the external turmoil serves a defensive purpose.

Folie à deux (Shared Paranoid Disorder)

Few entities are more intriguing than *folie à deux*, the "psychosis of association," in which the same delusions are shared by two. Folie à deux in the aged is similar to folie à deux in the population as a whole, both with regard to incidence and nature of psychopathology. Among the factors common to folie à deux in patients of all ages are isolation and poverty, a very high proportion of blood relationships, particularly sister-sister combinations, a high level of dependency, and a high rate of persecutory delusions.[22, 23] (See Table 17.1).

The two theories most commonly presented to explain folie à deux suggest that the delusion is imposed on a weaker member by a stronger person or that two people simply become psychotic at the same time and one borrows the delusion from the other. Dependency is felt to be of importance in the development of the syndrome. It is probably more accurate to regard the need to preserve intimacy as the most important factor leading to a unitary delusional system. This view of the etiology of folie à deux would de-emphasize the role of contagion and emphasize the adaptive function of a unitary delusion, how both partners can project interpersonal and other frustrations outward while at the same time joining forces against a common enemy. If one of them assumes a dominant role in the relationship and the other a submissive role, then the chance for disagreement between them is further reduced and even greater closeness might result. Gralnick found persecutory delusions in nearly all cases in which relationships had been of extended duration.[22] Hostility was projected outward against a common enemy.

It must be kept in mind that folie à deux represents the extreme, at one end of the continuum. Along this continuum, we find instances of dyadic pathology of varying degrees. Thus, it is not unusual to encounter relationships between two relatives (either old-old or old-young) that are characterized by intense dependency as well as mutual exploitation. A fairly typical example is the situation of an aged, widowed, infirm parent, living together with an adult child who has one or more handicaps (e.g., mental retardation, alcoholism, physical disabilities). One can not help

Table 17.1

Psychosis by Association in Patients Aged 65 or Over, Reported in English Literature*

Case report		Patients involved				Characteristics of illness			
Date	Author	Relationship	Age	D or S**	Assoc. (yrs.)	Diagnosis	Nature of Delusions	Hallucinations	Type
1877	Lasegue and Falret	Mother and	66	S	28	Par. schiz.	Grandiose	?	FI
		daughter	28	D		Par. schiz.	Grandiose	?	
1888	Tuke	Husband and	70	?	26	Par. schiz.	P & A	?	FS
		wife	60	?		Par. schiz.	P & A	?	
1897	Elliot	Sister and	75	?	25	Par. schiz.	P & A	Aud.	FS
		sister	65	?		Par. schiz.	P & A	Aud.	
1917	Clark	Father and	68	D	life	Par. schiz.	P & A	?	FI
		son	?	S		?	P & A	?	
1934	Gotten	Father and	73	D	life	Par. schiz.	Religious	Yes	FC
		daughter	33	S		Par. schiz.	Rel. S & P	Yes	
1936	Grover	Sister and	65	D	46	Par. schiz.	P & A	Aud.	FC
		sister	67	S		Par. schiz.	P & A	?	
		Mother and	70	S	7	Par. schiz.	?	Aud.	FS
		daughter and	29	S		Par. schiz.	?	Aud.	
		daughter	26	D		Par. schiz.	?	Aud.	
1940	Postle	Mother and	81	D	25	Par. schiz.	P & A	None	FS
		daughter	48	S		Par. schiz.	P & A	?	
1942	Gralnick	Mother and	66	D	life	Par. schiz.	P	Yes	FC
		daughter	46	S		Par. schiz.	P	No	
		Twin sister and twin	66	D	life	Paranoia	P	No	FC
		sister	66	S		Paranoia	P	No	
1943	Kibzey	Father and	70	S	life	Par. schiz.	P & S	?	FC
		daughter and	33	S		Par. schiz.	P & S	Aud.	
		daughter	27	D		Par. schiz.	P & S	Aud.	
1949	Schmidt	Husband and	66	S	40	Simple schiz.	P & A	No	FI
		wife	63	D		Par. schiz.	P & A	Aud. & tactile	
1956	Dewhurst	Sister and	74	D	34	Sen. Par. Psy.	P & S	?	FS
		sister	64	S		Sen. Par. Psy.	P & S	Visual	
		Sister and	78	D	?	Senile Psy.	P & S	?	FS
		sister	71	S		Senile Psy.	P & S	Aud.	
		Mother and	80	D	42	Par. schiz.	P & A	Aud.	FI
		daughter	42	S		Par. schiz.	P & A	Aud.	
1963	Waltzer	Father and	72	D	17	Par. schiz.	P & A	?	FS
		mother and	37			Par. schiz.	P & A	?	
		9 children	4–15			Par. schiz. & emotional	P & A	Not stated	FS
1970	McNiel	Sister and	72	D-S	life	Par. schiz.	P & A	No	FS
		sister	77	S-D		Par. schiz.	P & A	No	

* See Ref. 23.

** D, dominant; P, persecutory; A, aggressive; S, sexual; FS, folie simultanée; FI, folie imposée; FC, folie communiquée; Aud., auditory.

but suspect that such a child was "selected" to stay at home, while the others were permitted to leave (Compare case example on p. 124).

CONFLICTS WITHIN THE FAMILY

Conflicts within the family may revolve around an aged parent, or develop between the aged husband and wife. Many of these maladaptive patterns are precipitated by the vicissitudes of the aging process, and are therefore relatively recent and acute.

Regressive Behavior

The aged person may react by becoming unduly helpless and turning to others in the family for assistance in almost all of his life activities. This *regressive* behavior may become an excessive burden on the other family members, not only because they provide so much support but also because the regressed person frequently feels angry and guilty about his child-like dependency. His dependency is often a hostile clinging, which is self-defeating, and it may become impossible to do anything that satisfies him. Depression may color the clinical picture, in which case the depressive symptoms may have the purpose of communicating to the other family members: "Look how miserable you make me feel."

In some instances, regressive behavior in one family member may be unconsciously encouraged by one or several other family members. To the latter, the burdens imposed by the regressive behavior of the former are the lesser of two evils. They are willing to pay a price, sometimes a very high one, to achieve an important gain. This gain often pertains to a power maneuver, e.g., the attempt to keep the other person (the helpless one) dependent, to keep him under control, or in line. Such power plays designed to keep another person attached to oneself are security operations (albeit maladaptive) to prevent the risk of object loss. The situation can get truly complicated if both marital partners are equally involved in such neurotic interactions, and if each one simultaneously is active instigator and passive recipient.

> A 63-year-old chronically disabled woman was referred for psychiatric consultation by a community agency. Her chief complaint was "I can't afford to pay for my medications anymore." She took 13 types of medication everyday. Especially significant was what her husband said during the interview. He considered himself almost as disabled as his wife. The medication count in his case came to seven. He stated that, if he no longer could take care of his wife, he would feel like killing himself. Underlying this neurotic interaction was the dual need in both partners, to be at once the helpless, passive recipient and the helpful, concerned caretaker. This pattern of vicarious dependency gratifications had begun after the children had left and sexual intimacies had stopped. The ensuing vacuum had been filled by regressive activities: i.e., hypochondriacal con-

cerns. Both partners needed each other for consensual validation of their new (regressive) identity. Only in the realm of physical symptoms could they still relate with each other. The maladaptive nature of the interaction is pointed up by the continuous escalation of medications, and increasing despair ("I'd rather kill myself if I can't take care of her anymore"). Management consisted in allowing them to view each other and themselves as physically sick; reducing the medications by 75 percent, enough to eliminate financial stress but not so much to cast doubt on the authenticity of their physical symptoms; and, introducing a set of caretakers, one for each partner. If the new caretaker had been one and the same for both partners, there would have been a risk of negative transferences, in the form of destructive sibling rivalry between husband and wife.[24]

Withdrawal

In the case of regression, interpersonal relationships have changed but they are not broken off. In *withdrawal* there is a moving away from other people, not primarily physical, but emotional. Withdrawal of this kind threatens to disrupt interpersonal relations, a fact of great importance since maintaining contacts with others is a crucial need for aging persons. The pattern of withdrawal may lead to isolation with its risks of self-absorption, hypochondriasis, disuse atrophy of social skills, or progressive loss of contact with reality.

Moving against Others

Regression and withdrawal represent flight responses (moving away from). It is also possible that the aging family member *moves against* others. This happens when he perceives them to be responsible for his plight (through projection). This pattern is usually associated with aggressive behavior, ideas of being neglected or maltreated, and angry accusations. Such a paranoid reaction is maladaptive because others in the family will respond with counterattack. The latter confirms the paranoid person's idea that his suspicions were correct after all.

Control of Others

Another type of aggressive reaction to stress is the attempt to *control* others. The individual may feel that others are capable of providing satisfaction, but he is uncertain that they are willing to provide it. The efforts to gain control are security and power operations manifested in several possible ways. One may manipulate others by trying to make them feel guilty, by flattery, by physical force, by depressive or self-destructive behavior. Or, one may attain a dominating position by making the other person dependent on oneself, by keeping him child-like, sick or incompetent. If this control is directed at a submissive person, there may be no conflict; most people, however, resent being manipulated and will respond with various countermaneuvers. As a result, family members may spend tremendous amounts of time and energy in this tug-of-war. The effects of such excessive security operations can be harmful not only to the aging person himself, but also to younger members of the family. A (rather tragic-comical) example of this is the following:

> A 50-year-old man was hospitalized because of recurrent depressions. He had been living with an uncle for the last 20 years. The circumstances which brought the patient and his uncle (then 62 years old) together were as follows. The aging uncle had no immediate family, but did have a big estate. The patient, then 30 years old, was asked by the uncle to live with him on his farm and to take care of him. As a reward, the uncle would, upon his death, leave the patient all his material possessions. The patient had figured that this was a winning proposition. He admitted having had the thought that his uncle, being sickly and all, would not live but a few more years, whereupon all his uncle's wealth would be his. But the uncle did not die at his appointed time. In his own mind, the patient had given him 5–10 years of additional life, when he had moved in with the uncle. When 10 years had passed, however, the uncle was still living, and the expenses incurred in providing medical and nursing care, inexorably nibbled away at the estate. Around this time the patient suffered his first depression. But he stayed on the farm with his uncle: since he already had invested 10 years of his life in this gamble, he felt that he could not afford to back out. During the next 10 years, the uncle continued to be alive, the estate continued to shrink, and the patient became more depressed.

Turning against Self

Instead of moving against others, a person may *turn against himself* and become depressed. This also involves a shift from primarily interpersonal to primarily intrapsychic pathology. In fact, the family may often be quite unaware that one of them is actually suffering from a depression. This is of great practical importance, in view of the fact that suicide is a serious risk of depression in elderly men.

The case example, described above, illustrates not only the attempt to control others, but also the turning of hostility against the self. The patient clearly had had death wishes toward his "beneficent" uncle. As the uncle overstayed his welcome, the intensity of the patient's death wishes increased proportionately. In this instance, it was difficult for the patient to face the death wishes, and realistically come to grips with them, because he had solemnly resolved to give his uncle the best of care.

Who Can Be the Sickest?

In some families we can observe a complex interaction involving regression, hypochondriasis, and competition. This transaction may be described by the phrase: "*Who can be the sickest*?" Characteristically, this involves two persons, for example, an aged marital couple, who have become progressively more dependent due to age-related loss of autonomy. They have begun to relate to each other in the manner of sibling rivalry, competing for the attention and support of a relative or parent figure, e.g., social workers.[24] The intervention needed here is to arrange adequate support for both partners individually, and to convey that support of one of them is not at the expense of the other. Only then will they feel secure enough to give up using physical symptoms in the service of competition and attention-getting.

> An aging couple was referred for psychiatric consultation, because of their constant bickering and arguing. Each had a number of chronic illnesses. The husband, now 83, used to be a mild-mannered, easy going man. But since the onset of arthritis and heart disease, which limited his activities and made him more dependent on his wife (76-years-old), his friendliness had been eclipsed by more and more irascibility. His wife, never having seen this side of him, had felt taken aback but tried to accommodate him. Her efforts along this line began to falter when her own health began to fail while her husband's regressive behavior (the irascibility) continued to worsen. At this point, a social caseworker had entered the scene, but the more she tried to help out, the more antagonism developed between her two clients. It was a baffling situation, because "both these people used to be so nice." Then, an exacerbation of the husband's heart disease required his hospitalization. During this time, both husband and wife reverted to their habitual friendliness. Following the husband's release from the hospital, the bickering began again, with a crescendo at each visit by the caseworker. Then the wife needed to be hospitalized, and again both were more peaceful during the separation. But once she was back home, the dissonance returned as well. And so it went, on and on, for some 2 years. Eventually it became clear that the hospitalizations were breathing spells for the two combatants. Both husband and wife showed regressive behavior which had a potentiating effect on each other; each had developed a strong transference toward the caseworker. They competed for attention by putting each other down and playing up their own symptoms. The caseworker, family physician, and psychiatrist reached a consensus that it would be best to place the couple together in a rest home, and provide each one with an individual caseworker. The security of the rest home and the reassuring knowledge of "having my own caseworker" acted in combination to decrease their anxiety, hypochondriacal games, and destructive sibling rivalry. A follow-up revealed that, once again, they had become the nice persons they used to be.

References

1. Bengston, V. L., Kasschau, P. L., and Ragan, P. K.: The impact of social structure on aging individuals. In: *Handbook of the Psychology of Aging*, edited by J. E. Birren and K. W. Schaie, vol. 2, chap. 15, van Nostrand Reinhold Company, New York, 1977. pp. 327–351.
2. Kerckhoff, A. C.: Nuclear and extended family relationships: normative and behavioral analysis. In: *Social Structure and the Family: Generational Relations*, edited by E. Shanas and G. Streib, Prentice-Hall, Englewood Cliffs, N.J., 1965.
3. Cohen, P., Dizenhuz, I. M., and Winget, C.: Family adaptation to terminal illness and death of a parent. *Social Casework*, 223–228, 1977.
4. Malinak, D. P., Hoyt, M. E., and Patterson, V.: Adults' reaction to the death of a parent: a preliminary study. *Am. J. Psychiatry 136:(9):*1152–1156, 1979.
5. Kerckhoff, A. C.: Husband-wife expectations and reactions to retirement. In: *Social Aspects of Aging*, edited by I. H. Simpson and J. C. McKinney, Duke University Press, Durham, N.C., 1966.
6. Kassel, V.: Polygyny after 60. *Geriatrics 21:*214–218, 1966.
7. Sheps, J.: New developments in family diagnosis in emotional disorders of old age. *Geriatrics 14:*433–449, 1959.
8. Savitsky, E., and Sharkey, H.: The geriatric patient and his family—study of family interaction in the aged. *J. Geriatr. Psychiatry 5:*1, 1972.
9. Birtchnell, J.: Recent parent death and mental illness. *Br. J. Psychiatry 116:*289–297, 1970.
10. Wahl, C. W.: The differential diagnosis of normal and neurotic grief following bereavement. *Psychosomatics 11:*104–106, 1970.
11. Miller, M. B., Bernstein H., and Sharkey, H.: Denial of parental illness and maintenance of familial homeostasis. *J. Am. Geriatr. Soc. 21:*278–285, 1973.
12. Pincus, L.: *Death and the Family*, Pantheon Books, New York, 1974.
13. Townsend, P.: *The Family Life of Old People*. Penguin Books, London, 1957.
14. Birren, J. E.: Life Review, reconciliation and termination. In: *The Psychology of Aging*, chap. 12, Prentice Hall, Inc., Englewood Cliffs, N. J., 1964.
15. Butler, R. N.: The life review: an interpretation of reminiscence in the aged. *Psychiatry 26:*109–114, 1963.
16. Vachon, M. L. S.: Grief and bereavement following the death of a spouse. *Can. Psychiatr. Assoc. J. 21:*35–44, 1976.
17. Payne, E. C.: Depression and suicide. In: *Modern Perspectives in the Psychiatry of Old Age*, edited by J. G. Howells, chap. 13, Brunner-Mazel, New York, 1975. pp. 290–312.
18. Bunch, J.: Recent bereavement and suicide. *J. Psychosom. Res. 163:*361, 1972.
19. Gerber, I., Rusalem, R., Hannon, N., Battin, D., and Arkin, A.: Anticipatory grief and aged widows and widowers. *J. Gerontol. 30:*225–229, 1975.
20. Cleveland, W. P., and Gianturco, D. T.: Remarriage probability after widowhood. *J. Gerontol. 31:*99–103, 1976.
21. Lieberman, M. A., Prock, V. N., and Tobin, S. S.: Psychological effects of institutionalization. *J. Gerontol. 23:*343, 1968.
22. Gralnick, A.: Folie à deux—the psychosis of association. *Psychiatr. Q. 16:*230–263, 1942.
23. McNiel, J., Verwoerdt, A., and Peak, D. T.: Folie à deux in the aged: reviewed and case report of a role reversal. *J. Am. Geriatr. Soc. 20:*316–323, 1972.
24. Laverty, R.: Reactivation of sibling rivalry in older people. *Social Work 7:*23–30, 1962.

18

environmental planning*

With advancing age, the capacity for homeostasis gradually declines; the range of adjustment and adaptation becomes smaller and narrower. This aspect of aging, the *decreased effectiveness of homeostasis*, deserves to be emphasized, because it implies an important principle: in environmental planning one should not primarily attempt to adjust the aged person to the demands of the environment, but adapt the environment to the needs and limitations of the aged person. When the environment (both in its physical and social aspects) has been adjusted to meet the needs of the aging individual, a state of equilibrium and health prevails. On the other hand, discrepancy between environmental stresses and capacity to cope with them leads to a state of disequilibrium and disease. For effective environmental planning, it is necessary to have a working knowledge of the specific needs and limitations resulting from the aging process.

PRINCIPLES AND PRACTICAL IMPLEMENTATION

Biological, age-related alterations occur in all of the organ systems. Changes in anatomical structure include decrease in size (atrophy), degeneration (e.g., arteriosclerosis), changes in the connective tissue (e.g., arthritis), etc. Associated with these are physiological changes which are of interest, from a practical point of view.

NEUROPSYCHOLOGICAL CHANGES

Impaired Vision

Complaints about *impaired vision* are extremely common and may be caused by cataracts, glaucoma, or macular degeneration. Cataract surgery can be performed regardless of age with few risks of complications. If macular degeneration is also present, however, the surgery will be less beneficial.[1] Generally, because of diminished visual acuity, there is need for greater illumination. In twilight and in the dark, visual impairment is especially prominent; hence, the frequent occurrence of confusion and the risk of accidents during nighttime.

* In collaboration with Alan D. Whanger, M.D.

Hearing Losses

Hearing losses, especially for high tones and sounds, increase with age. For this reason, an elderly person may comprehend the spoken words of a man but not those of a woman. It is important to speak slowly, enunciate clearly, and face the person to facilitate lip reading. A person who is continually unable to comprehend what others are saying frequently becomes suspicious. As with so many other prosthetic devices, the aged person frequently has problems in accepting a hearing aid and making effective use of it.

Mental Functions

The *brain* serves mental functions and neuropsychological capacities, such as thinking, perception, intelligence, memory, learning, and coordination of motor behavior. With aging, most of these functions show some decrement, but these changes are by no means uniform, and they vary from person to person. Individual personality factors and past life experiences have a significant influence on the final outcome.

Individualized Activity Programs. Life long practices and habits are not likely to change easily in the later years, and in planning *activity programs* for the aged, it is well to remember this. The program should be in keeping with the individual's habits and his potentials. The capacity for learning is not lost, although more time is needed to acquire new habits, ideas, or skills. An important principle is that functions which have been used regularly throughout life, and continue to be exercised in later years, tend to remain relatively more intact; not only intellectual functions, but also neuromuscular skills, exercise tolerance, sexual capabilities, social competence, etc.

Maintenance of General Intelligence. General *intelligence*, once it reaches its peak, may maintain this level in old age, especially if people continue to be active and if they suffer no deterioration due to excessive physical and neurological changes. Education fosters maintenance of intellectual ability; continued learning throughout life probably has a similar effect. Older people may compensate for a decline in intelligence by modifying their behavior or by adopting alternative responses (emphasis on accuracy rather than speed of performance). A high level of intelligence, a good education, and continuous practice in exercising the capacity to learn may help delay intellectual decline. Therefore, it is useful to develop continuing education programs for the aged. Some may want to complete high school or college education; others may want to pursue special interests and talents. Older citizens may be encouraged to participate actively in community affairs, especially organizations for and of the elderly themselves. Aged persons could be trained to function as "friendly visitors." The stimulation involved in such activities is likely to have a beneficial effect on overall intellectual alertness.

Loss of Speed in Function. General loss in *speed of function* affects many complex psychological processes. This slowing of response is largely related to altered brain function rather than the result of changes in the peripheral organs. The organization of behavior becomes progressively more difficult and accuracy is stressed above speed. The psychomotor skills involved in driving are also affected.[2] Healthy people in their 60's and 70's are more frequently involved in highway accidents than middle-aged persons, but they are safer drivers than teen-agers and many people in their 20's. Although reflexes are often slower, the elderly driver tends to exercise greater caution and better judgment than the younger driver.

Accident Prevention. This is an important aspect of environmental planning for the aged. The triad of loss of touch sensations in the feet, loss of visual and auditory acuity, and psychomotor slowness predisposes the aged person to disorientation in the dark, and falling becomes a hazard. To counteract the decrements in sensory acuity, it may be useful to magnify textural and visual contrasts and to intensify auditory cues from floors and surroundings. Accidents are the third most frequent cause of death among aged males, the fifth among aged females. For every fatal accident, there are many nonfatal but disabling accidents. Accidents are caused most frequently by cars hitting the aged pedestrian; by falls, the majority of which occur at home; and by burns.

MUSCULOSKELETAL CHANGES

Atrophic Changes

Atrophic changes in bone structure and stiffened joints may cause reduction in height, a stooped posture, as well as limitation in mobility. There is loss of muscular power and a decrease in the ability to perform rapid movements. Lack of activity aggravates these changes, and can lead to actual disability (e.g. the permanent contractions of joints of aged people who are bedridden). Although joints and ligaments become progressively stiffer, there is often a good preservation of motion. Changes in the muscular system make routine tasks more difficult and, more important, tend to impair the efficiency of such vital functions as breathing, urination, and defecation. Stiffening of the rib joints may also add to respiratory difficulties.

Skeletal Pain

Skeletal pain is a frequent complaint, and may be caused by osteoporosis, osteoarthritis, or less common conditions such as gout, rheumatoid arthritis, or bone metastases. Osteoporosis is a specifically age-related disabling condition which occurs much more frequently in women. There is need for additional research to establish the usefulness of estrogen replacement or other therapy in postmenopausal women, as a means to prevent the development of osteoporosis, or to treat it once it exists.

Hip Fractures

Hip fractures, due to falls, occur frequently and illustrate the interaction of multiple pathogenic factors. The fact that a fall causes the fracture, or that a spontaneous fracture causes the fall, illustrates the effect of aging on bone structure. The accident of the fall itself can be precipitated by many factors: sensory deficits and deficient psychomotor coordination, lack of adequate safety precautions and accident prevention, dizziness due to transient ischemic attacks, hypotensive episodes due to cardiac illness or drugs (antidepressants, antipsychotics), and so on. Once a hip fracture has occurred, many new complications may develop. The immobility in bed facilitates psychological regression, which again leads to more immobility and proneness to accident. Also, contractures may develop during the state of immobilization. Once a contracture exists, it is nearly impossible to correct it. Contractures develop under the same conditions as decubitus (pressure sores). They are prevented by not allowing the individual to remain immobilized in the same position, by encouraging as much activity as he is capable of, or by providing passive exercises, i.e., moving the individual's arms and legs for him. Prevention of contractures and decubitus is a major nursing problem in many aged institutionalized patients. Restoring and sustaining the ability to walk is the best protection. If the patient is confined to the bed or chair, it is necessary to change his position at regular intervals. Inspection of the skin may reveal the development of anemic areas, requiring meticulous hygiene and careful massage to promote local blood flow. Once the skin has broken down and a decubitus sore has developed, the wound tends to become larger and permanent. In short, a fall causing a hip fracture, which in turn produces physical immobilization, psychological regression, and possibly decubitus and contractures, can represent a milestone on the pathway toward senile regression.

NUTRITION

Atrophic Changes in Gastrointestinal Tract

Age-related changes that affect *eating habits* and *nutritional status* include loss of teeth and mandibular atrophy, atrophic changes in the tongue, tastebuds, and gastric glands, decreased gastrointestinal motility, decreased need for caloric intake, and so on. Changes in eating patterns include a decreased fluid intake, increased liking for sweets, and a preference for meals that are easy to fix and food that requires minimal chewing efforts. Associated with these, there is a greater risk of malnutrition, vitamin deficiencies, anemias, painful conditions in the mouth due to ill-fitting dentures, constipation, etc.[3] The loss of teeth is a serious narcissistic trauma and physical loss. The subsequent mandibular atrophy makes it difficult to fit dentures well. Because the latter tend to be painful, older persons often disregard or "lose" them.

Psychological Aspects

The *psychological aspects* of food and eating are also important. Food may symbolize affection or pleasure, security or strength. For many persons, eating is not only a matter of intake of calories, but also a social experience. Thus, people who live alone may begin to neglect their meals. Poor eating habits result in decreased physical and mental vigor, which, in turn, aggravates the poor eating syndrome. On the other hand, social isolation may create a constellation in which eating is the only pleasant experience in a bleak existence. When food replaces company, overeating or regressive food cravings may be the result.

Specific Regimes

In advising *specific regimes* of nutrition for various medical illnesses, it is useful to weigh the pros (of improving physical aspects of the illness) versus the cons (of depriving the patient of psychologically satisfying experiences). It is possible that any physical gains are outweighed by the development of emotional distress. A cardiac patient, for example, may be told to go on a low calorie, low fat, low cholesterol, low salt diet, and to stop smoking and drinking alcoholic beverages. His cardiac status may improve on this regime, but the patient may develop a depression that cripples him more than his heart disease did. The important point is to treat the whole patient; to evaluate physical and psychological aspects, to assess their relative importance and mutual effects on each other, and to treat both of them simultaneously.[4]

Since the psychological and social aspects of food and eating are so important, special booklets describing attractive and adequate menus for older people could be prepared and made available to community agencies for distribution. Such pamphlets could also be sent to the medical practitioners in the community. Perhaps even local restaurants and cafeterias might be interested along this line. Specific attention in the area of nutrition should be directed toward aged people who live alone or who require special diets due to illness. With regard to the institutionalized aged, it would be useful for a "geriatric dietitian" to have periodic consultation with managers of boarding homes, nursing homes, and other extended care facilities to discuss nutritional, psychological, and social aspects of meals.

ENVIRONMENTAL CHANGES

THE ELDERLY PERSON AND HIS FAMILY

Decision Making

The move to an institution (for example, a boarding home, nursing home, or mental hospital) usually is the final outcome of a long and difficult series of events. When the elderly person has been living at home with relatives, some degree of psychological stress and friction is the rule rather than the exception.[5] Although these problems in the family are not necessarily abnormal, it is useful to be alert to their existence. The psychological stress may arise from several sources, for example, the children's inability to accept age changes in the parent, the family's frustration about their inability to cope with the physical or mental problems, irritation due to the lack of improvement in the elderly person, and guilt about increasingly strong wishes to be freed of the burden of caring for one's disabled parent. Usually, a mixture of these emotions and attitudes is present in family members. The aged parent himself may vacillate between a wish to be close to and dependent on his children, and feelings of guilt or resentment about this dependency. Such ambivalence, a mixture of positive and negative feelings, may have a significant effect on the *making of decisions*. Effective decision making, e.g., concerning a possible move to a boarding home, requires a clear comprehension of the issues at stake. When positive and negative attitudes both are present (ambivalence), it becomes more difficult to have an undistorted view of the overall situation. This is particularly true when one set of feelings is being suppressed. The suppressed thoughts and feelings, however, continue to exert influence. The opposing sets of attitudes lead to impaired decision-making or persistent doubts about decisions that have been made. A relative's guilt feelings, for example, may prompt him to interpret the move to the boarding home as a rejection. If the decision amounts to a postponement of effective action, this will only aggravate the problem.

Counseling

Timely *counseling* and *guidance* concerning the issues at stake, with clarification of interfering emotional factors and support in carrying out a rational plan, represents the best intervention in such situations. In determining what course of action is best, each case should be evaluated individually, with consideration of the following factors.

Patient: his disability for usual life activities; the extent to which he is harmful to himself or to others, or is a social nuisance.

Family: economical resources (financial resources, available space in the home, etc.), attitudes toward the aged family member (hostility, rejection, ambivalence, ratio of ill-will versus good-will).[6]

Community: availability of mental hospital, nursing homes, boarding homes, and various programs of service for the aged.

Only by taking these factors into consideration can one arrive at a plan satisfactory to the patient and his family. That the relatives need professional assistance in decisions involving placement of a psychiatrically ill aged family member may seem rather obvious. Yet, one gets the impression that such professional assistance is often not available; or if it is, that the relatives are not aware of it and do not seek it. In many instances, counseling or guidance, or the services of information and referral agencies, may actually be more useful to the family than to the patient himself. The presence in the home of an aged person with psychiatrical illness is a stressful burden on the entire family, and may even precipitate psychopathology in the other family members.

MOVING TO A BOARDING OR NURSING HOME

Traumatic Effects

Whenever feasible, it is good practice to enlist the cooperation of the aged person himself. He should not, as a rule, be moved to a boarding home without his prior knowledge and approval. He should not be "taken for a ride." Ideally, the transfer to an institution or chronic care facility involves a consensus between the aged individual, the significant family members, and at least a third party (social worker, physician, the operator of the boarding or nursing home). A move should not be carried out suddenly, without due preparation, because this may lead to a "transplantation shock" in the aged person.[7, 8] In preparing him, one could arrange a series of preliminary visits to the boarding home prior to the move. When the move takes place, the individual should be encouraged to take some of his (most personal) possessions with him.

The *traumatic effects* of environmental changes on the aged person are generally well known. Essentially, a relocation can amount to a dislocation.

> A 74-year-old man had lived alone for years in a dilapidated shack. Holes in the walls permitted wind, rain, and cold to come in. Rats were visitors during all seasons. The man lived in filth and constant danger of being burned (he used a wood stove to prepare meals). For years, the social service department had tried to improve the habitat of this recluse, but in vain. None of the suggested changes and the material assistance were accepted. Finally, a solution seemed to present itself. A well-to-do farmer nearby had a cabin and offered it to the hermit. The cabin was a fine little building, with conveniences, such as plumbing and electricity. The old man was persuaded to make the move, and a long-standing problem (which had been a concern throughout the small community) appeared to have been solved in a humane fashion. A few days after the move, however, the social worker received an urgent call from the farmer in whose cabin the old man was now living. Upon her arrival, the social worker found the man in a state of acute confusion; he was lying in his bed, with the evidence of fecal incontinence all around him. (Neither disorientation nor fecal incontinence had been a problem before then.) The significance of this episode lies in the fact that, to the old man, "home" was the old

shack where he had lived for decades. It was there that he felt he belonged, not in the nice, new cabin. But those around him felt exactly the other way around. What mattered in the end was that the physical relocation became a psychological dislocation. In the unfamiliar environment, the old man lost his grip on the world, and this loss of control was reflected in the function of his sphincters: they, too, lost their grip. The loss of sphincter control was part of a general loss of control.

Preparing for Change

Such outward reactions to unfamiliar environments can be prevented by allowing the older person to make the change in a more *gradual* way. A comparison can be made with the mechanisms of immunity. A foreign element introduced into the organism elicits different reactions depending on quantitative factors. A large, all-at-once amount of an alien substance (virus, toxin, etc.) may overwhelm the organism's defense mechanisms. A smaller amount, however, stimulates some kind of defense or resistance. Repeated administration of small amounts can build up a solid immunity against the invasion of large amounts of alien elements. What is true on the physiological level applies also to the mental apparatus and the psychological level.

THE CONCEPT OF A HOME

Some psychological and interpersonal aspects of the boarding or nursing home deserve further discussion, with special emphasis on the concept of "home." We will define a home as a place where one belongs and where one has one's belongings; to feel at home is to belong. And, usually, a home is a place where a family lives. How does this apply to such facilities as a rest home, boarding home, nursing home, or even the chronic geriatric wards in mental hospitals?

Promoting a Sense of Belonging

First, in as much as the home is a *place of belonging*, it is our goal to promote in the elderly person residing in the institution a sense of belonging, and to make him feel "at home." Efforts in this direction include the following:

Private Space. The amount and type of *space* allocated to the elderly resident should be in keeping with the need for privacy and the principle of "territoriality." The latter involves the delineation of a space, which the person can regard as "my own." The boundaries of this space can be compared to what, on a psychological level, is the ego boundary. It is that space around me, in the center of which I myself am located, extending from me onto its boundaries. Everything within the perimeter of that space is felt to be my own, while the space beyond it is felt to be that of the "other." My private space can be invested, filled as it were, with my psychic energy or interest. The concept of *privacy* includes the sense of private ownership and the opportunity to be on my own, and to have visual privacy. Without being shielded from the eyes of others, there is a loss of personal dignity.

There are several ways to allocate space in such a way that the above requirements are met. Boundaries between the respective spaces belonging to the various residents are no problem when there is a one-person-per-room situation. With two persons in one room, a curtain in the middle can be a boundary that also ensures visual privacy. On wards with several patients, it is useful (but not easy) to arrange beds, chairs, nightstands, etc. in clusters and configurations that suggest and delineate individual life spaces.

Personal Belongings. Within the boundaries of this private space, the person is to have subspaces for his *personal belongings.* The location and characteristics of these spaces (e.g., individualized color schemes, type of furniture, pictures, plants, etc.) may facilitate in the aged person an experience of recognition that this is "my own," of remembering that "this belonging of mine is here, and that one belongs over there."[9]

> A 67-year old woman belonged to that category of patients designated as "having grown old in the institution." It was no longer possible to determine whether her intellectual and emotional deficiencies were the long-term consequences of simple schizophrenia or the manifestations of mental retardation (a differential diagnosis which is not always easy to make). The patient shared her room with three other elderly females. Her only furniture was a bed and a nightstand. Generally, she seemed mildly content and never displayed much emotion. During the routine ward rounds, we discovered that she was using the lower compartment of her nightstand as a crib for a doll. The crib was a primitive thing, consisting of pieces and remnants of towels. The doll had been assigned a permanent berth in this make-believe crib. When we expressed our pleasure at the sight of this touching scene, the patient responded with a smile. In fact, the only times she would smile at all were in connection with the doll. The doll in the nightstand represented a transitional object, which the patient treated as she herself wished to be taken care of (vicarious gratification). Also, the nightstand (something "out there") had become a part of herself. The boundaries of herself (her ego, her body image) had extended so as to incorporate that dark, intimate enclosure with its precious contents. Whether or not this is the acting out of a pregnancy fantasy is a matter of speculation. This same patient would regularly feed a patient in the bed across from her, who was blind.

Closeness or Distance. People differ greatly with regard to the amount of personal space, and the *distance* or *closeness* to the other (their neighbor) which they consider optimal. Part of the sense of belonging is the feeling of being part of a neighborhood. Some persons like (or don't mind) being close up against each other; others need to have a good bit of distance between themselves and their neighbor. Some of these differences are socioculturally determined; at other times, they are manifestations of specific psychopathology. Chronic patients on the wards of mental hospitals tend to distribute themselves in characteristic patterns across the ward space: most seem to feel crowded, and try to maintain maximum distance so that they are evenly distributed across the ward space. At the other extreme are those patients in search of closeness, physical touch, or togetherness. Such a patient may get in bed with another one, or is always following another patient around.[10] Although the final outcomes of chronic schizophrenia and senile dementia have much in common, it is our impression that one of the differences is that the chronic schizophrenic retains his distance, while senile patients often reach out for contact, as if starved for a personal touch. This reaching out for physical touch is also emotionally touching: it has a basic quality of urgency conveying the wish, "Be with me." This physical reaching out has it corollary in the verbal question often asked: "When can I go home?" If one then asks where home is, one is surprised to discover that the patient has no idea where his home is. Or, he may talk about a home he once had in the remote past. One can't help but feel that the question "When can I go home" is a primitive, concrete way of expressing something more abstract, like: "This place is not like home—I wish I could be at home—or feel at home—Is there anything you can do to make me feel at home here?" (see also p. 251.)

> An elderly male patient on the geriatric ward always had a small travel bag containing his belongings placed right in the center of his bed. The patient, who was profoundly confused, never was able to give a verbal explanation of his behavior. When asked about it, he just smiled. For that matter, he never tried to pick up his bag and leave. Yet, his actions signalled that he was "ready to go home."

Communal Space. Part of the concept of neighborhood is *communal space* where I can be in touch with others. This being-in-touch is not first of all physical, but represents contacts involving the experiences of seeing, hearing, and sharing things. This communal space ideally should contain activity centers that provide opportunities for a wide spectrum of human interests.

Dimension of Time. It is also necessary to pay attention to the *dimension of time.* The sense of time comes about as one moves through space. In the same manner that allocated space is to be made private and personal and filled with my belongings, so time should be filled with activities that are meaningful. The experience of the flow of time is an essential ingredient of optimal mental functioning. When time ceases to flow, a state of stagnation and timelessness results. This will exert a powerful regressive pull upon the patient. When he succumbs to it, he will be sliding into a state of regression, autistic withdrawal, or irreversible senility.[11]

Transference Phenomena

Now what about the home as a "place where a family lives?" Obviously it is not possible to replicate family life in the usual sense of the word. Upon entering the home, however, the elderly person takes with him characteristic attitudes and ways of relating to others. To a large extent, these feelings and attitudes are derived from past life experiences, including those which the individual had with his parents, siblings, and children. These feelings, expectations, attitudes, ways of looking at the world and others, are transferred from one situation to another. Thus, emotions, ideas, and expectations may be detached from the people in one situation, and transferred and attached onto persons in the new situation. This phenomenon of *transference* is universal in human relations.

When, in an institutional setting, transference phenomena occur, they will vary depending on the type of home and the personality of the resident. Since a boarding home is a home with an operator (manager, director) who is in charge, the operator may be seen as a parental figure and the other residents as siblings. This may happen regardless of any age differences. Thus, an elderly resident may (unconsciously) view a home manager 30 years his junior as a maternal figure; he may begin to relate to her in ways similar to the relationship he once had with his real mother. The concept of transference is not only of theoretical interest, but frequently there are important practical implications. This is especially true when negative feelings (hostility, guilt, envy) are being transferred. An individual who, at one time, had a troublesome relationship with his real mother, may (again, unconsciously) expect the same kind of difficulties with a rest home operator. If one is alert to the possibility of such transference distortions and tries to understand their underlying meaning, one is in a better position to tolerate unusual difficult behavior and to find the proper means to handle the real problem. In this connection, special attention may be needed for the home operator as well as the resident or patient. Possibly helpful would be information-exchange sessions specifically aimed at consulting with the supervisory staff of boarding homes, nursing homes, and other long-term care facilities.

THE SPECTRUM OF COMPREHENSIVE SERVICES

Comprehensive services are based on the recognition that a person's condition is determined by physical, psychological, interpersonal, cultural, economical, and environmental factors. Because these factors interact in a complex manner, comprehensive services must be flexible. To implement comprehensiveness as well as individualization of services, rigidity in organization should be avoided. A person with an economical catastrophe should receive assistance just as quickly as a patient with a serious illness. Aged persons in need should receive appropriate help without having to go through unnecessary "channels." To attain comprehensiveness, flexibility, and speediness of services, two sets of community resources are needed: a central agency that gathers and distributes information, and a spectrum of service facilities and programs concerned with medical care, health maintenance, economic and vocational assistance, etc.

THE INFORMATION AND REFERRAL AGENCY

The central facility that collects and distributes information relevant to aging is essentially an information and referral service.[12] Its basic functions include the following:

Information

The information and referral service aims at distribution of pertinent information. It needs to make itself highly visible and well known to the community, especially the aged. This can be done with the aid of local news media and by distributing special brochures and pamphlets. Efforts must be made to inform aged persons how to take advantage of community resources, and find their way through "the system."

Evaluation and Planning

This includes periodic review of existing services, and the conceptualization and initiation of new services. In these efforts, the central facility (or the information and referral service) can make specific contributions in terms of organizing meetings on the local level and disseminating pertinent information regarding policies and programs on the higher levels (regional, state, and federal). The planning and implementation of local developments are facilitated when they are attuned to, and fit in with, larger trends and currents. Program development is a "construction job" involving two phases of activity that differ with regard to their direction. The first, that of building from below upward, requires local initiative (in our case, it would be optimal to include a representative cross-section of the elderly population). The second phase is the process of building, from above downard; this involves governmental initiative. Both types of processes are essential for program development. The risk to be avoided is that "the twain never shall meet" and that the two components of program development fail to interlock with each other.[13, 14]

Facilitation and Coordination

The objective here is to initiate appropriate channels of contact and communication between important local services and facilities. For example, the moving of aged persons from their home to a boarding home, nursing home, general hospital, or mental hospital (and subsequent moves between these places) usually is not well regulated. This is largely due to lack of coordination between these institutions. What needs to be avoided in the development of multiple programs and services is that every one begins to assume that the problems will be solved by somebody else. With increasing numbers of service programs, the amount of buck passing can increase in geometrical terms. The elderly patient is passed from one agency (facility, program) to the next, that is, from pillar to post. The danger in a community network of multiple programs is that the staff of the respective agencies begins to believe that they have solved the problem by referring the patient elsewhere. In fact, they only solved their own problem, i.e., they got rid of the patient. Meanwhile, the patient himself falls down in the gaps of the network. Eventually, the patient may show up again at the initial agency. He has made the rounds, and gone from all the pillars to all the posts. When he returns to the starting point (the initial agency), it would be part of the pattern of self-deception to view his return as a "readmission." To the contrary, the patient is not readmitted for a recurrence of his problem or illness, but he returns because his problem never was ameliorated in the first place.[15, 16]

Central Clearinghouse

To reduce the frequency of such unfortunate malfunctions, the central facility (information and referral service) might explore the use of a special system of data collection and retrieval. This would involve a kind of central registry on elderly persons who, at any point, have entered the network of community service programs. The information to be recorded would include routine identifying data, data pertaining to the presenting problems (type, severity, causation), data on proposed problem solving or treatment plan, and follow-up data. The appropriate agency records the data and transmits them to the information and referral facility for data storage and further processing. The latter involves, among other things, the transmission of data to agencies (facilities, programs) that are nodal points in the network of services. The transmission and distribution of data could be routinized or automated so that relatively little additional expenditures of time and money are required. The objective is to have pertinent agencies share available information on elderly clients who have "entered the system," and to keep this information up to date. Such a clearinghouse or registry would prevent unnecessary expenditures of professional effort (e.g., repetitive history taking), the pitfalls of the patient's falling between the slats, and so on. It would also provide a valuable repository of data for research activities. The automation of data collection, retrieval, and distribution could be done by means of computers.

The advantages of data sharing need to be weighed against the disadvantages: the risks of loss of privacy and of confidentiality. The constraints of interagency data sharing are set by ethical principles and legal guidelines aimed at the protection of individual privacy and privileged information.

Case Detection

Case detection involves special efforts aimed at locating aged persons who have problems. Such individual case identification is facilitated by periodic local publicity about the existence of an information and referral service. It also requires the active interest and participation of key people in the community, such as physicians, the clergy, social caseworkers, department of public health, etc.

An example of such a survey, and an instrument used in it, is the Older Americans Resources and Services (OARS) Survey.[17] Other services can be added, depending on specific local needs and conditions. Thus, if an information and referral service is located in the outpatient clinic of a hospital, certain medical services may be incorporated into the basic structure. Be that as it may, there should be clear channels of communication with all other agencies and services relevant to the aged. Actual physical proximity to other facilities is desirable from a practical point of view.

COMPREHENSIVE SERVICES AND COMMUNITY CARE

Diagnostic Centers

Diagnostic centers or "Well-Aging Clinics" can be located in the outpatient clinic of a general hospital, in local departments of public health or social service, or they could be associated with a day care center or high rise apartment building for the aged. Timely detection of disease in the aged is always a problem. All too often patients come to medical attention at a relatively advanced stage of their illness. The assessment center would place primary emphasis on health maintenance since anxiety is not an optimal motivator. Some individuals avoid physicians for fear that a serious condition will be diagnosed, that hospitalization or surgery will be recommended, etc. A "Well-Aging Clinic" could take initiative in getting aged persons regularly to the clinic for routine checkups. Attention should be given to the problems of transportation to the clinic. Some aged persons have trouble driving; others have no car, or live far away. Transportation can be organized by community groups, churches, department of social services, senior citizens groups, etc. Perhaps there is merit in the idea of using buses (of the school bus variety) for transporting aged persons to such facilities as diagnostic centers, hospital clinics, day care centers, etc. The transportation expenses need to be solved by the community as a whole.[18, 19]

Extended Care Facilities

These include nursing homes and the geriatric units of mental hospitals.[20] Some general hospitals have facilities for chronically ill patients. Relatively large homes for the aged may have the capability to develop an adjoining infirmary. It is difficult to make generalizing statements about which type of facility is most desirable. The answer depends frequently on local conditions. This caution in generalizing also applies to the statement frequently heard now-a-days that "elderly patients in a mental institution should return to the community as soon as possible." Indiscriminate application of such generalizations facilitates the pattern of "passing the buck" from one institution to another, or from the institution to the community. Again, the patient is passed from pillar to post. Frequently, such moves only represent administrative (pseudo) solutions, and the aged patient is the victim of the resulting confusion. Mutual collaboration between local institutions concerning each other's goals and methods would prevent much of this confusion.[21] (See Scheme 18.1).

> The drive to "get patients back into the community" may result in good or bad consequences. An example of a good result is the case of a 73-year-old man who had spent more than 40 years in a mental hospital. Having existed in almost total isolation from the rest of the world, he was unfamiliar with modern society. Reportedly, he had never seen an airplane except on TV. Through the steady effort for 2 years of one caseworker, this man was prepared for living on the outside. The two of them made frequent, regular trips into the community so that the patient could discover what life on the outside was all about and prepare himself for the transition to a rest home.

The success of such efforts depends on a multitude of factors: the patient's assets, the availability of health care personnel with both mature judgment and a sense of commitment, the quality of available boarding homes, etc.[22–24] There is no question that the operators of many boarding homes are quite capable and responsible, and they provide a living environment superior to that of the mental hospital. On the other hand, some boarding homes are inadequate, certainly when compared with the renovated geropsychiatric facilities that have begun to emerge in some mental hospitals.[20]

Home Care Programs

Home care programs developed by local hospitals, the public health department, etc. are aimed at keeping selected patients at home, thus preventing the need for more expensive hospitalization. The home care team consists of a physician, a visiting nurse, and other therapists (physical therapy, dietitian, social worker, etc.). Such programs can be

SCHEME 1.*

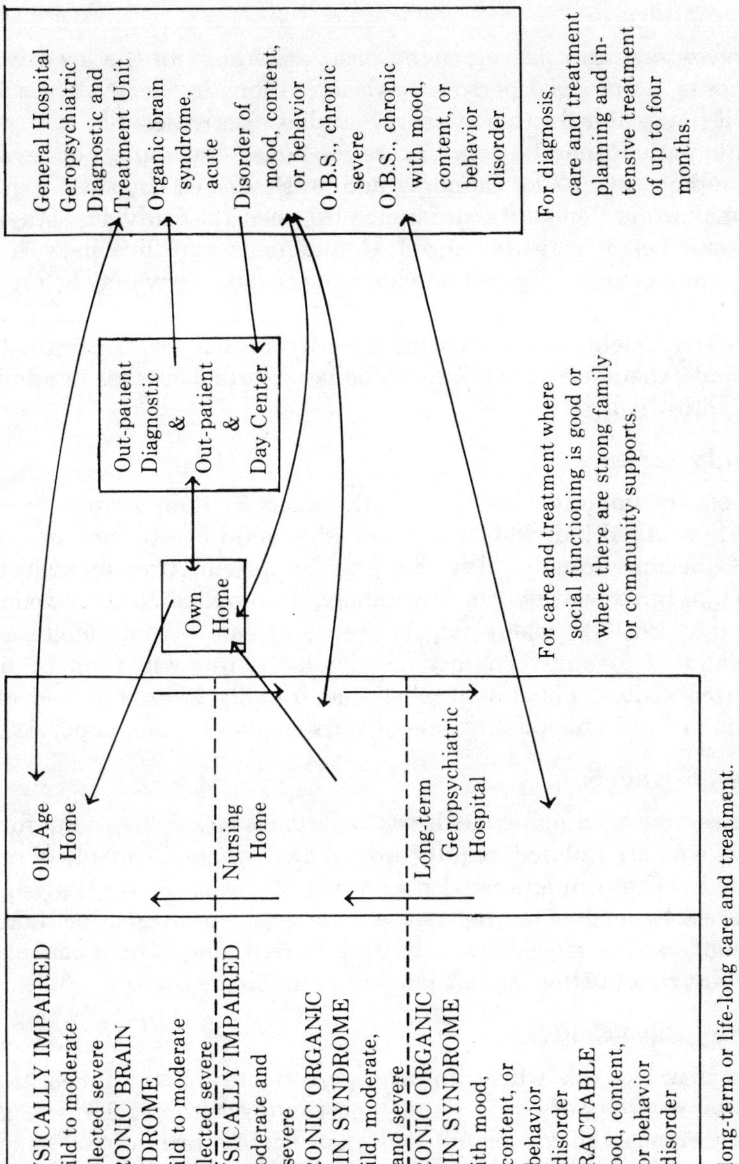

* Reprinted from Goldfarb[21] by permission of Brunner-Mazel.

combined with other services such as meals-on-wheels, friendly visitors, etc. Again, this points up the need for a central agency that can coordinate the various services and determine which package of services is indicated. The cooperation of the family members is essential in implementing home care programs.[25]

Homemakers

Homemakers can provide some basic assistance to the aged in their own home. Some aged persons have limitations in specific areas which make it impossible for them to carry out basic activities. For example, an arthritic patient may be able to care for himself at home, but unable to go shopping, to do the laundry, and wash dishes. In such a case, a homemaker may make the difference between the individual staying at home and being institutionalized. Companions may live in with older persons or a couple, or spend only part of the day. They may be recruited from the aged person's relatives, neighbors, etc. The companion may receive free lodging and some compensation for her services in the home. The total expenditures are likely to be less than in the case of admission to an institution.

Friendly Visitors

These are volunteers who visit the aged in their homes or in the institution. Aged individuals in reasonably good health may be encouraged to become friendly visitors themselves. Some friendly visitors can get caught up, unwittingly or unwillingly, in complicated family conflicts. They may rush in where angels fear to tread. When caught in the quicksand of a family conflict, a friendly visitor will soon become a frustrated visitor. This risk implies that friendly visitors should receive preliminary training for this type of work, or work under supervision.

Meals-on-wheels

The service of bringing meals to the home is especially useful for aged persons who are isolated, require special diets or are incapable of preparing meals. These programs also aim at preventing or breaking up any vicious circles leading to progressive undereating or overeating. Likewise, homemakers, friendly visitors, visiting nurses, and others can play an important role in altering deficient eating habits.

The Day Care Center

A facility like this where an aged person can remain during the day may offer a variety of services and opportunities. Group activities, games, hobbies, etc. can be carried out with the help of a recreational expert, or independently. Associated with the center may be a physician, psychologist, or social worker who could provide counseling and guidance, or conduct group therapy sessions. Limited medical-geriatric services may be offered as well. In planning a day care center, attention should be given to the types of services needed in view of the local conditions in the community. Ideally, there should be enough space around the center to make gardening possible, to keep pets on the premises, to go outside for walks on the grounds, etc. Recreational activities (e.g., music, films, discussion groups) can be organized by interested volunteers or by recreational therapists.[26]

Mental Health Services

Mental health services can be made available through the local mental health clinic, a nearby hospital, the out-patient clinic of a general hospital, the day care center, etc. These services are important in view of the frequent emotional disorders associated with physical illness, social isolation, or other deprivation. Effective mental health services can be offered only by a team of professionally trained individuals; the psychiatrist, the psychiatric nurse practitioner, and the psychiatric social worker represent the core of such a team. The community mental health programs would aim at methods of identifying and treating acute situational problems; counseling and guidance with regard to such problems as retirement, social role change, altered family relationships and leisure time activities, assistance to families caring for disabled or emotionally disturbed aged relatives, consultation with other community agencies, e.g., with regard to release planning for institutionalized aged patients, and organizing educational experiences for other professionals about normal and geropsychiatric aspects of aging.

Other Services

Other services and programs included in a comprehensive spectrum are protective services, legal aid, vocational projects, sheltered workshop, continuing education, foster grandparents program, etc.[27]

References

1. Eckstein, D.: Common symptoms and complaints of the elderly. *J. Am. Geriatr. Soc. 21*:440–443, 1973.
2. Gianturco, D. T., Ramm, D., and Erwin, C. W.: The elderly driver and ex-driver. In: *Normal Aging, II*, edited by E. Palmore, Duke University Press, Durham, N. C., 1974. pp. 173–179.
3. Whanger, A. D.: Vitamins and vigor at 65 plus. *Postgrad. Med. 53*(2):167–172, 1973.
4. Whanger, A. D.: Nutrition, diet, and exercise. In: *Handbook of Geriatric Psychiatry*, edited by E. W. Busse and D. Blazer, Van Nostrand Reinhold Company, New York. 1979.
5. La Barre, M. B., Jessner, L., and Ussery, L.: The significance of grandmothers in the psychopathology of children. *Am. J. Orthopsychiatry 30*:175–185, 1960.
6. Grauer, H., Betts, D., and Birnbom, F.: Welfare emotions and family therapy in geriatrics. *J. Am. Geriatr. Soc. 21*:21–24, 1973.
7. Aldrich, C. K., and Mendkoff, E.: Relocation of the aged and disabled: A mortality study. *J. Am. Geriatr. Soc. 11*:185–194, 1963.
8. Lieberman, M. A.: Relationship of mortality rates to entrance to a home for the aged. *Geriatrics 16*:575–579, 1961.
9. Peterson, R. F., Knapp, T. J., Rosen, J. C., and Pither, B. F.: The effects of furniture arrangement on behavior of geriatric patients. *Behav. Ther. 8*(3):464–4677, 1977.
10. Harris, H., Lipman, A., and Slater, R.: Architectural design: the spatial location and interaction of old people. *Gerontology 23*(5):390–400, 1977.
11. Carp, F. M.: Effects of the living environment on activity and use of time. *International J. Aging Hum. Dev. 9*(1):75–91, 1978.
12. *Guidelines for an Information and Counseling Service for Older Persons.* Center for

the Study of Aging and Human Development, Duke University, Durham, N. C., 1970.
13. Shanas, E.: Factors affecting care of the patient: Clients, government policy, role of the family and social attitudes. *J. Am. Geriatr. Soc. 21*:394–397, 1973.
14. *Psychosocial Needs of the Aged: Selected Papers*, edited by I. M. Burnside and R. H. Davis, Ethel Percy Andrus Gerontology Center, Los Angeles, 1973.
15. Friedman, J. H.: Misassignment of geriatric patients to a State mental hospital. *J. Am. Geriatr. Soc. 19*:172, 1971.
16. State Policy and the Long Term Mentally Ill: *A Shuffle to Despair*. City of New York Commission on State-City Relations, 1972.
17. Maddox, G. L., ed.: *Multidimensional Functional Assessment: The OARS Methodology. A Manual*, ed. 2, Duke University Center for the Study of Aging and Human Development, Durham, N. C. 1978.
18. Robinson, R. A.: The assessment center. In: *Modern Perspectives in the Psychiatry of Old Age*, edited by J. G. Howels, chap. 18, Brunner-Mazel, New York, 1975. pp. 379–396.
19. Barney, J. L.: *The Well-Being Report: A Look at Supportive Services for the Elderly*, Institute of Gerontology, Ann Arbor, Michigan, 1975.
20. Whanger, A. D., and Busse, E. W.: Care in hospital. Chapter 21. In: *Modern Perspectives in the Psychiatry of Old Age*, edited by J. G. Howells, chap. 21, Brunner-Mazel, New York, 1975. pp. 450–485.
21. Goldfarb, A. I.: Integrated services. In: *Modern Perspectives in the Psychiatry of Old Age*. edited by J. G. Howels, chap. 26 Brunner-Mazel, New York, 1975. pp. 540–569.
22. Gladue, J. R.: The role of the physician in the nursing home: past, present, and future. *J. Am. Geriatr. Soc. 21*:444–449, 1973.
23. Gutman, G., and Herbert, C. P.: Mortality rates among relocated extended-care patients. *J. Gerontol. 31*(3):352–357, 1976.
24. Lawton, M. P., Patnaik, B., and Kleban, M. H.: The ecology of adaptation to a new environment. *Int. J. Aging Hum. Dev. 7*(1):15–26, 1976.
25. Risdorfer, E. N., Primanis, G., and Dozoretz, L.: Family care as a useful alternative to the long term hospital confinement of geropsychiatric patients. *J. Am. Geriatr. Soc. 19*:150, 1971.
26. McConald, R. D., Naulander, A., Halod, O., and Holcomb, N. S.: Description of a non-residential psychogeriatric day care facility. *Gerontologist 11*:322, 1971.
27. Beattie, W. M., Jr.: Aging and the social services. In: *Handbook of Aging and the Social Sciences*, edited by R. H. Binstock and E. Shanas, chap. 24, Van Nostrand Reynold Company, New York, 1976. pp. 619–642.

19

protective intervention*

PROTECTIVE SERVICES: LEGAL AND PSYCHIATRIC ASPECTS

LEGAL ASPECTS

The term "protective services" essentially could be used for any medical, psychiatric, or social treatment modality, but in the course of the years, it has acquired a specific meaning. Now-a-days, protective services pertain to those services required to protect an individual from abuse, neglect, safety hazards, mistreatment, or exploitation. They are undertaken with or on behalf of persons who are unable or unwilling to secure them for themselves, or who are without able and responsible persons acting in their behalf.

In keeping with the contemporary concerns about patients' rights, laws are now being enacted to protect specifically the rights of elderly individuals. A Reporting Law for Protection of the Elderly became effective in North Carolina in 1974,[1] and was broadened to include all persons over age 18 in 1975[2] and 1979.[3] The current law defines an adult in need of protective services (including the elderly, who are still the main population in need) as anyone over the age of 18 who is disabled due to a wide range of physical as well as mental conditions. Anyone who has reasonable cause to believe that a person is in need of protective services must report this to the county director of social services. The latter must make a prompt and thorough evaluation, which includes a visit to the person and consultation with individuals familiar with the case. After completing his evaluation, the director of social services indicates whether or not protective services are needed.

Evidence of Abuse or Neglect

The law defines protective services in terms of measures necessary to prevent abuse or neglect. These services include medical and mental health care, assistance in hygiene, food, clothing and shelter, protection from health and safety hazards, and protection from physical mistreatment and exploitation. *Abuse* includes the willful infliction of physical injury or mental anguish and the deprivation by a caretaker of essential

* In collaboration with Robert D. Miller, M.D., Ph.D.

services. A *neglected* elderly person is one who lives alone and is unable to provide for himself or is not receiving the services from his *caretaker*. The latter is defined as a person responsible for the care of the elderly person as a result of family relationship or who has assumed such responsibility for the care of the elderly person voluntarily or by contract. The 1979 revision of North Carolina Statutes also includes adults who are residents of state hospitals for the mentally ill or centers for the mentally retarded, are in the opinion of the professional staff mentally incompetent to give consent for medical treatment, and have no legally appointed guardian.[3] If an elderly person consents to protective services but his caretaker objects, the director of social services may petition the district court for an order enjoining the caretaker from interfering. This petition is required to allege facts showing that the elderly person needs protective services, that he has consented to receive them, and that the caretaker refuses them to be provided. The judge may issue an order to enjoin the caretaker from interference.

Right to Decide

The law gives the elderly person *the right to decide* whether he will consent to protective services. The county director of social services has the legal responsibility to provide indicated protective services if the elderly person consents. If the latter does not consent, services may not be provided unless the director of social services determines that the elderly person lacks capacity to consent, in which case he may seek authority from the court to provide protective services under the procedures prescribed by the reporting law. If the elderly person consents but later withdraws his consent, the services must be terminated unless the director secures court authority to provide protective services on the grounds that the elderly person lacks the capacity to consent.

Lack of Consent Capacity

If an elderly person is abused or neglected and *lacks the capacity to consent,* the director can petition the court for an order authorizing protective services. The law requires that the district court has a hearing within 14 days after the petition is filed if sufficiently specific facts are alleged. The elderly person must receive at least 5 days' notice of the hearing. He has the right to be present and the right to counsel at the hearing. If the court finds that the elderly person needs protective services but lacks capacity to consent, the judge may order that the services be provided, and designate an individual or organization to be responsible for the welfare of the elderly person and to have the right to consent to protective services in his behalf.

If the elderly person does not require protective services, but is not capable of making decisions necessary to ensure his own welfare, such as consenting to medical or psychiatric treatment or making a reasonable disposition of his property, it may be necessary to petition the court for a legal guardian to be appointed. In addition to the full guardianship procedures available in all states, which are lengthy and complex, North Carolina also allows for a limited guardianship procedure presided by the clerk of court. This process provides for a guardian to be appointed for a specific purpose only, such as medical treatment or disposition of property.[4] Due process is well protected by the requirement for a comprehensive evaluation by a physician, a psychologist, and a social worker, but the decision can be made immediately in emergency situations. A previous law permitting the director of a state mental hospital to certify an in-patient to be incompetent without a hearing was repealed by the 1979 North Carolina legislature. The current set of statutes allows protection for the elderly person (for whom most of these procedures take place), and flexibility to permit a guardian to assist in making only necessary decisions, and only after a full evaluation and due process hearing at which the elderly person is guaranteed counsel.

A third avenue to provide protection to the elderly in North Carolina is that of commitment to a state hospital for the mentally ill or to a center for the mentally retarded. An elderly person at risk due to a mental disability may sign himself into such facilities voluntarily as long as he is competent to understand what he is doing. If he is not, or if he needs treatment but is unwilling to accept it, involuntary commitment may be employed provided that the following two conditions are met. First, the person (the law applies equally to all ages) must be mentally ill, mentally retarded, or inebriate; and second, he must be dangerous to himself or to others (dangerous to others in the case of mentally retarded persons). Mentally ill is defined statutorily as an illness which so lessens the person's capacity to use self-control, judgment, and discretion in the conduct of his affairs and social relations as to make it necessary or advisable for him to be under treatment, care, supervision, guidance, or control.[5] *Dangerousness to self* has recently been redefined to include, besides suicidal and self-mutilating behavior, actions indicating that the person would be unable, without care and the continued supervision of others, to exercise self-control, judgment, and discretion in the conduct of his affairs and social relations, or to satisfy his needs for food, clothing and shelter, protection, and safety, so that serious physical debilitation would ensue without treatment. *Dangerous to others* is defined as inflicting, or threatening to inflict, serious bodily harm on another, or acting in such a way as to create a substantial risk of such harm to another.[6] In the next section, the terms dangerous to self and dangerous to others will be discussed in a somewhat broader context; the legal definitions discussed above should be kept in mind, as involuntary commitment may be a viable alternative if other efforts to provide protective services fail.

A fourth area of interaction between the legal and the treatment services for the elderly is that of the provision of structured living environments for persons unable to live by themselves or with families. With the present trend towards deinstitutionalization and treatment of the mentally disabled (including a growing number of elderly) in the community, the concept of a group home, providing a family-like environment for a small number of disabled persons under the direct supervision of trained "houseparents," has become increasingly important. Unfortunately, in many cases there is community resistance to the placement of group homes in their neighborhoods. Efforts have been made through local and state zoning ordinances, as well as private covenants associated with wills and property transfers, to exclude group homes from residential areas, thus defeating the whole purpose of attempting to place disabled persons in an environment as nearly "normal" as possible.

A number of recent legal decisions have begun to define the principle that group homes cannot be excluded from residentially zoned areas *a priori*, and that they should be treated as single-family dwellings for zoning purposes.[6] These issues will continue to arise as long as there is no consistent federal and state policy concerning the rights of disabled persons to experience living conditions as normal as possible, and will have continuing impact on the provision of services to the elderly who suffer from a mental or physical disability.

PSYCHIATRIC ASPECTS

From the above, it has become clear that the central issue may not be the contents or substance of the protective services to be rendered, but the *manner* in which this is done. This implies the existence of any number of factors in the situation which function as obstacles and barriers. The successful implementation of a program of protective services depends on effectively removing these obstacles, by way of skillful and effective *intervention*. Under the heading of protective intervention, our concern here is with the following questions:

What kinds of conditions in old people would cause us to depart from our usual methods of making services available?

In what way do these methods differ from the usual ones?

Are there specific conditions which require the use of certain new techniques of making services available?

CONDITIONS REQUIRING MODIFICATION IN METHOD

Sooner or later anyone who has been working with elderly individuals in need of assistance discovers that certain problems arise in the implementation of a particular plan. There may be clear awareness that a problem exists, that a service is needed, and various services may be indeed available. But yet, obstacles begin to develop, and somehow one finds oneself unable to implement a program of action. There may be two reasons for this. First, the difficulty may rest with the clinician or practitioner himself. He may have arrived at an inaccurate evaluation of the client's problem, the service required, or both. It is also possible that, although correct with regard to the diagnosis and treatment plan, one is incapable of effective implementation due to inadequate training, or special problems such as "blind spots," personal idiosyncrasies, and sensitivities. A second set of obstacles are those presented by the client or his family who, for whatever reasons, resist efforts aimed at alleviating their distress. A review of these obstacles is presented, with brief mention of some psychiatric conditions in which they may occur.

DANGER TO SELF (PATTERNS OF SELF-DESTRUCTIVENESS)

Involuntary or Passive

a. inability to care for self (infirmity and disability);
b. inability to use available resources (physical isolation);
c. denial of illness or disability;
d. poor judgment;
e. faulty living habits;
f. regressive behavior;
g. accident proneness.

Voluntary or Active

a. refusal of assistance;
b. extreme social isolation;
c. suicidal tendencies.

DANGER TO OTHERS

Involuntary or Passive

a. being excessive burden on family;
b. social nuisance (exposing self, wandering, incontinence, etc.).

Voluntary

a. combativeness (including homicide);
b. geriatric delinquency;
c. malicious gossip.

MIXED (DANGER TO SELF AND OTHERS)

Pathological family dynamics, mutual suffering or cruelty, mutual destructiveness, etc.

DANGER TO SELF

This category refers to self-destructiveness in general. The various patterns can be relatively involuntary and unintentional, or they can be more or less voluntary, deliberate and willful.

Involuntary Patterns of Self-destructiveness

Inability to care for self may be due to physical or psychological infirmity and involve varying degrees of disability for basic daily living activities (eating, locomotion, personal hygiene, etc.). Serious problems may develop if there is lack of adequate assistance from family or neighbors. This category occurs frequently and calls for protective services in the sense of making routine supportive care available.

Inability to make use of available resources may be due to physical isolation, for example, an aged person who lives alone, far from neighbors, and has no means of transportation. This, too, is not an uncommon situation and does not necessarily create unusual obstacles, as long as the prospective recipient is cooperative.

In the following categories however, the obstacles are harder to overcome because the impediments are related to the individual's behavior and personality instead of external contingencies.

Denial of illness, disability, or need for assistance: In these cases, the aged person communicates, explicitly through verbal statements or implicitly through actions, his disagreement with, or resistance to, the opinion of others stating he needs assistance. The individual may deny the fact that he is sick or disabled; or, while acknowledging the illness and disability, he may deny its seriousness or the necessity to do anything about it. Patients with severe physical illness (e.g., cardiac illness or cancer) frequently deny the existence of their illness, or that the illness has serious implications. In manic patients, there may be an elated mood and grandiose behavior involving denial of underlying problems. The patient with organic brain syndrome may be unaware of many of his problems because he has lost the capacity to comprehend the real significance of what is happening to him.

Poor judgment is a manifestation of many psychiatric disorders. Inasmuch as good judgment is a function of intact ego functioning, the extent of poor judgment reflects impaired ego functioning. When good judgment is lost, the individual becomes accordingly more helpless and is at the mercy of forces over which he has no control. Such a person cannot protect himself adequately; also, he may inadvertently cause problems for others (e.g., a senile person who squanders his savings). Judgment is affected most severely in psychotic reactions, and in organic brain syndrome.

Faulty living habits involve behavioral patterns, which in the long run become deleterious to physical or psychological health, e.g., poor eating habits, alcoholism and other addictions, poor personal hygiene, etc. Such faulty living habits occur in many conditions, especially schizophrenia, organic brain syndrome, mental retardation, and certain personality disorders.

Regressive behavior includes phenomena related to loss of mastery and control, resulting in deterioration of the personal milieu, of personal hygiene, neuromuscular capacities, and sphincter control.

Deterioration of the personal *milieu* is a common complaint. Usually, these complaints are not made by these old people themselves, but by relatives, neighbors, case workers, etc. There are several ways in which such problems may develop and manifest themselves. The milieu in which a person lives, the space he calls his own, is a territorial extension of the self. The maintenance of a life space requires the expenditure of energy; when the energy required to create and maintain order is unavailable, the life space becomes a microslum. An imbalance between intake and output may result in congested clutter. Diminished ability to rid the personal milieu of excess or waste materials produces conditions of hoarding and filth. Typically, the elderly individual himself is not fully aware of the extent of decay, and this may present a problem in persuading him to accept protective services (e.g., home help).

Deterioration of personal hygiene frequently co-exists with the decay of the personal milieu. The old person becomes neglectful in bathing, grooming, and personal appearance; clothes are not cleaned or repaired, and the same old clothes may be worn constantly. Sometimes, idiosyncratic combinations are fashioned (one dress on top of another; special items such as a hat, a cane, briefcase, may become a permanent fixture of the appearance). There may be some last attempt to control the regressive drift. The individual may retreat into one room of the house, relinquishing control over the rest of his lifespace. Some individuals, oblivious to the disarray around them, become proportionately more concerned (sometimes obsessed) with personal cleanliness. A variant of the principle of sweeping dirt under the rug can be seen in some elderly women whose efforts consist of applying more and more make-up on their face. Isolated phenomena of an obsessive-compulsive nature further include increased preoccupation with housecleaning; with the purity of food, water, and utensils; etc.

> One elderly male had developed the compulsive habit of washing his walking cane every day.

The concerns about dirt may acquire phobic qualities; the patient becomes afraid of specific types of dirt, especially contamination of food. Various community agencies may get involved because the elderly person begins to call on them, complaining about the dangers he thinks he is exposed to, and asking for help.

Accident proneness may occur on the basis of unconscious guilt, or it may be due to sensory and motor deficits. The latter are more commonly found among the aged; impaired vision and hearing combined with motor weakness and poor coordination predispose individuals to accidents.

Voluntary Self-destructiveness

Behavior patterns of this type would appear to occur less frequently than involuntary self-destruction. When it does occur, it presents greater problems in management; this is so because the tendency toward self-destruction is no longer a simple drift with the individual being a helpless victim, but the tendency involves an active urge. Or again, it may manifest itself as an active resistance against any therapeutic intervention. Involuntary commitment to a hospital is frequently the only effective response to this behavior. We will mention three forms in which such self-destructiveness may be manifested.

Refusal of medical care sometimes occurs in aged persons who suffer from a treatable illness but who believe that any treatment is useless. They may feel that life is over for them, preferring to be left alone to die in peace, or they may fear the discomfort and expenses associated with medical care and hospitalization. The patient with a severe depression feels that he does not deserve to get well. The paranoid patient may refuse help because he is suspicious that others try to frame him, trick him, or gang up on him.

Extreme social isolation, as seen in the aged recluse, usually indicates serious psychopathology. These withdrawn individuals often are quite suspicious of others, and possibly paranoid. Since their isolation signifies a thorough insulation, it is difficult to reach out toward them; the withdrawn person misinterprets a stretched-out hand as a move with hostile intent.

Suicide is the clearest example of active self-destructiveness. It occurs most frequently in elderly males. Suicide prevention is a crucial aspect of protective intervention and one should be especially alert to the danger of suicide in aging white men.

DANGER TO OTHERS

Involuntary

Involuntary dangers and stresses to others refer to situations in which the aged individual by virtue of his specific age-related impairments, causes undue burdens on others. Neither the aged person himself, nor his family contribute to the problem by way of deliberate intent. Instead, the problem has come about from without, gradually encroaching on the patient and his family so that they tend to feel they are helpless victims of external circumstances or forces beyond their control. The aged person may be an excessive burden on his family in terms of depleting the family's economical and financial resources, or exhausting their physical and psychological reserves. The family may continue in their attempts to care for the aged family member because of a sense of duty and loyalty, or because they do not know where to turn for help. An aged person becomes a source of social nuisance when he is mentally so impaired that he continuously wanders away, exposes himself, is incontinent, is very boisterous, hoards a multitude of senseless items, etc.

Voluntary

Voluntary stresses or active threats posed by an aged individual may acquire the characteristic of deliberateness. Such an element of active initiative that is seemingly intentful occurs in conditions involving "geriatric delinquency."[8, 9]

Combativeness can reach the point of serious physical attack on others. A patient suffering from paranoid schizophrenic delusions, or a brain-damaged patient with impaired grasp of reality may feel that his relative or the fellow in the next bed is a mortal enemy, and then proceed to attack him. With suspicious, hostile or paranoid patients, one should try to solve the problem within a medical-psychiatric framework, rather than resorting to legal intervention. These patients are already inclined toward litigation, to begin with, and the use of legal interventions (police intervention, legal commitment, warrants, etc.) tends to solidify and petrify their combative stand; but these may be necessary as last resorts.

"Geriatric delinquency" includes, beside combativeness, behavior considered to be sexually deviant (e.g., making sexual advances to children, exhibitionism).[10]

One particular form of combativeness is not physical, but verbal, i.e., the *malicious gossip* which may occur in some paranoid or senile patients. Frequently this concerns relatives or neighbors, and the contents of the harmful rumors and gossip often has an erotic flavor.

MIXED SITUATIONS

An aged person and his spouse, or other family member, may be involved in pathological interactions in which all partners contribute to the destructive pattern. Usually what happens in such situations is that not only all the family members suffer subjectively, but also inflict suffering upon each other. These interactions may gather momentum in the manner of a vicious circle; and if outside intervention does not break up this vicious circle, the weakest link in the chain will give way, which may be the vulnerable aged family member. Such pathological family interaction can be seen, par excellence, in the relatively rare condition of *folie à deux* (shared paranoid disorder). (See p. 273.)

Two elderly sisters were legally committed to the mental hospital. This followed a lawsuit instituted by neighbors, charging that the sisters had made "unrestrained, vile, and untrue statements about them and that they were a public nuisance." On admission, the sisters were cooperative and friendly but insisted that their niece and nephew were after their property and that the niece, in fact, had destroyed it. They alluded to certain "whiskey people" who had antagonized them by throwing stones at them and placing dynamite in the basement. They complained that the neighbors ("whiskey people") had poisoned their chickens. Eventually the sisters boarded the windows and put up a fence. The difficulties came to a head by their shooting at the neighbor's clothespins.

DIFFERENCES IN APPROACH AND METHODS

In what way do the above conditions require a different methodology and approach? The traditional approach is usually based on the assumption that people who need help are willing, if not eager, to get it. This is the rational viewpoint and certainly would apply to most cases. But humans are not always rational, and some are never rational. Unfortunately these not-always-rational or always-irrational people often need help the most.

Rationality involves an element of freedom; conversely, the more irrational and the more impaired a person is, the more he has lost his freedom to act, and the more he is compelled to behave under the influence of impulses beyond his control. With this in mind, two principles can be formulated. First, the more a person is under the influence of irrational tendencies and the less rational control he has, the more he will be in need of a controlling agent or agency other than himself. Secondly, there are degrees of rational control and loss thereof, and the need for external controls will vary accordingly. This is not an either-or situation, in which control and reason are either present or absent, but a continuum of varying degrees.[11]

It is doubtful that among humans any really free and totally rational relations ever occur. In contacts with the aged there is ample opportunity to observe that freedom to choose as well as rational control of self and environment are significantly reduced. But usually, there seems to be no problem: the aged person "freely" accepts the inevitable, and the practitioner accordingly feels that no force or coercion needs to be used. But how often is it necessary to resort to some form of coercion, force, persuasion, limit setting, reinforcing of rules, suggestions, guiding, decision making, etc.? This is impossible to tell. There is no problem as long as the patient or client, more or less voluntarily, endows the professional worker with authority. In such a case there is a "fit" between the role of the client and the counter-role of the professional worker.

With increasing loss of rational control on the part of the client, there is increasing need for a substitute authority to step in and take over. This moving in of the external authority should take place on a graded scale—the amount and type of authority and control being attuned to the

Table 19.1

Degrees of freedom	Function and role characteristics: Clinician-practitioner	Function and role characteristics: Patient-client
Stage I		*CLIENT*
	a.—*information* no strings attached ("take it or leave it")	—"on his own"; free —no cooperation or relationship necessary
	b.—*counseling* no strings attached	—cooperative relationship
	c.—*guidance* more expectations regarding client; joint decisions	—more involved in collaboration, reciprocity; equal partners
Stage II		*PATIENT*
	a.—*suggestions & persuasion* active ("Do") and authoritative	—more passive, less on his own
	b.—*reinforcing rules & limit setting* more active ("Do"); also prohibiting ("Don't")	—beginning transfer of control and responsibility
	c.—*decision making, manipulation* commands & coercion	—increasing transfer of control and responsibility
	"Do this—or else"; "Don't do that—or else"	—freedom not yet totally lost because cooperation may remain
Stage III		
	a.—items a, b, c of Stage II, in greater quantity	—passive within the doctor-patient relationship
	b.—items a, b, c of Stage II, with additional backing (legal)	—totally passive, but usually no longer within doctor-patient relationship

specific needs and deficiencies of the individual. The schema above presents various degrees and techniques of taking over control and suggests three stages or types of relationships (see Table 19.1).

In Stage I, there may be no real relationship between practitioner and client at first (for example, when simple information is being given); or a relationship may just begin to develop. Either way, the client remains relatively free and "on his own" in this stage.

In Stage II, there is a definite relationship, in the course of which the client becomes less free, inasmuch as the professional worker assumes more and more control and authority. All this occurs within the setting of a structured relationship.

In Stage III, the relationship in terms of mutual cooperative action is beginning to be dissolved due to the increasing loss of autonomy and freedom on the part of the patient, and the concomitant increase of authority and control on the part of the clinician. Initially, or as long as the two participants agree on the transfer of authority, the structure of the professional relationship may still remain intact. When, however, this transfer becomes a matter of dispute, auxiliary reinforcements tend to be called into action, such as the family, the family physician, a consultant-specialist, the minister, or the court. By this time, the element of mutuality or reciprocity in the relationship has usually been considerably reduced because the client has become, so to say, an object that is being manipulated. In some cases, a skillful clinician-practitioner may call in auxiliary forces while still maintaining an intact relationship with his patient.

INDICATIONS FOR SPECIFIC TECHNIQUES

It is logical that the more authoritative, forceful, and controlling approaches are to be reserved for those conditions described above as being the most serious. Conversely, those conditions that are relatively mild and tractable require only a minimum of intervention and control. The *involuntary* patterns of danger to the self or others would require lesser amounts of authoritative intervention than patterns that are voluntary, active, self-initiated, or intentful. The reason is that a person caught in some involuntary pattern, has already abandoned control and lost his own authority. The outsider who steps in to take over is likely to be welcomed as a liberator, rather than seen as an intruder. Freedom, rather than being lost, is regained.

The question as to how much pressure, force, or persuasion to bring to bear on the intervention, depends also on the *severity* of the problem. For example, when a patient uses denial to avoid specific feelings about his being physically ill, then only Stage I type of intervention is indicated. If the patient acknowledges the existence of his illness, but denies the action implications (i.e., the need for medical help) then Stage II intervention is called for. And, if the patient denies the very fact of his illness, we would need to resort to Stage III. Likewise, poor judgment, faulty living habits, accident proneness may differ in terms of their seriousness.

Voluntary self-destructiveness and active, deliberate danger to others call for forceful application of external controls (Type III).

Family situations that involve pathological interactions and harmful vicious circles should, in principle, be approached with an attempt to reduce the pathological interaction by pulling the sparring partners apart. The clinical practitioner is, as it were, a referee who stops the boxing match when one fighter is getting too many blows. This may require Type II techniques appropriately "titrated" in strength and concentration so as to fit the occasion. The specific techniques should be employed with a degree of force or intensity that is just sufficient to have the desired effect.

Practical know-how and clinical skills are acquired through experience, and a thorough discussion of this falls beyond the scope of this review. It may be useful to keep in mind one last point. As clinicians and practitioners, we do have authority, whether we want it or not. This authority, inherent in the professional role, should be used with discrimination, not for its own sake but for protective intervention, and in a manner that is rational and well thought through. It should be dispensed in dosages sufficiently strong to have the desired effect. Legal means sometimes are necessary, but the court is to be reserved as a last resource.

References

1. *Protection of the Abused or Neglected Elderly Act*, Article 6 of General Statutes Chapter 108 (Social Services), Chapter 1378 of the 1974 North Carolina General Assembly.
2. *Protection of the Abused, Neglected, or Exploited Adult Act*, Article 4A of General Statutes, Chapter 108 (Social Services), North Carolina General Assembly, 1975.
3. *An Act to Amend General Statutes Chapter 108, Article 4A, Concerning Protective Services for Disabled Adults*, Chapter 1044 of the 1979 North Carolina General Assembly.
4. Turnbull, H. R.: Incompetency and Guardianship. In: *Law and the Mentally Handicapped*, ed. 2, Insitute of Government, The University of North Carolina, Chapel Hill, N. C., 1979.
5. *Admission of Patients; General Provisions*, Article 3 of the General Statutes, chapt. 122-36; North Carolina General Assembly, 1977.
6. *An Act to Amend Article 5A of Chapter 122 to Change and Clarify the Dangerousness Standard for Involuntarily Committing a Person to a Mental Health Facility*, Chapter 915, North Carolina General Assembly, 1979.
7. Turnbull, H. R., and King, N. P., Group homes for the mentally handicapped, zoning, and other considerations in community residence for the mentally handicapped. In: *Law and the Mentally Handicapped*, edited by H. R. Turnbull, ed. 2, Institute of Government, The University of North Carolina, Chapel Hill, N. C., 1979.
8. Hays, D. S., and Wisotsky, M.: The aged offender: a review of the literature and two current studies from the New York State Division of Parole. *J. Am. Geriatr. Soc.* 17(11):1064–1073, 1969.
9. Wolk, R. L., Rustin, S. L., and Scotti, J.: The geriatric delinquent. *J. Am. Geriatr. Soc.* 11:653–659, 1963.
10. Wilson, J. G.: Signs of sexual aberration in old men. *J. Am. Geriatr. Soc.* 4:1105–1107, 1956.
11. Regan, J. J.: Protective services for the elderly: commitment, guardianship, and alternatives. *William and Mary Law Review* 13:569–622, 1972.

20 work and retirement

ENGAGEMENT AND DISENGAGEMENT

PERSONAL AND INTERPERSONAL ASPECTS

Senescence is characterized by a reduction in physical activities and social interaction, and a constriction of life space. Some withdrawal from life activities by the aged is probably a normal developmental process of the later years. The change from striving to withdrawing has been described as disengagement.[1] The theory of disengagement proposes that there is a mutual withdrawal between the aging person and others in the social system. The equilibrium that existed in middle life between the individual and society now evolves into a new equilibrium characterized by greater distance. The depth and extent of a person's engagement can be estimated by the degree of potential disruption that would follow his sudden death. However, the death of someone who has an important symbolic engagement with his society (scientists, artists, political leaders, etc.), can result in simultaneous loss and gain because the survivors can rally around the symbols he represented, thereby reaffirming their universal or timeless value.

The notion of disengagement is complicated by the tendency to equate activity and engagement on the one hand, and withdrawal (or passivity) and disengagement on the other hand. To avoid confusion between these concepts, it must be kept in mind that activity is a more encompassing concept than engagement. That is, the latter refers specifically to the social aspects, while the former includes any and all activities of the human organism. It appears there are several types of combinations of being (in)active and (dis)engaged, as indicated below: engaged + active, engaged + inactive, disengaged + active, disengaged + inactive.

Engaged and Active

This type would refer to those persons who are socially engaged, in an active manner. In this constellation, we would also expect active use of somatic and psychological functions.

Engaged and Inactive

This type is socially engaged, but in a passive, inactive way. The individual needs the closeness or company of others, but does not necessarily actively reach out for this, or make active contributions to the social interaction. An example would be persons who are introvert and reticent, or individuals who are regressed, but not withdrawn. In fact, in the case of regression, interpersonal closeness is intensified inasmuch as the regressed person has become more dependent; and it is this very closeness which eventually may become even stifling.

Disengaged and Active

This combination is illustrated by a "well-adjusted" hermit. Such a socially isolated person has few, if any, social contacts but may remain quite active in other respects.

Disengaged and Inactive

If a person is socially disengaged, and also passive or underactive with regard to the use of his somatic and psychological functions, his survival may be at risk. It would seem that, for the sake of survival of the organism, the disadvantage implied in social disengagement, needs to be compensated for by an actual increase of nonsocial activities. Hence, of the four possible combinations, this one appears to be most maladaptive and conducive to psychopathology. Examples include cases of isolation and introversion that progress to the point of autism, or withdrawal decompensating into a state of apathy.

It would seem, then, that there is no sound basis for any conflict between proponents of "activism" and "disengagement." Of course, the disengagement theory should not be used as a pretext to acquiesce in all of the aspects of loneliness and withdrawal. But for some individuals, the isolation which accompanies introspection may be more like a freely chosen "retreat" than an "exile." An emphasis on introspection and reminiscence does not necessarily preclude the need for optimal engagement in various activities. Introspection can serve as an active, if not manifestly expressive, effort to find oneself. The point is that the emphasis on one or the other should be a differential emphasis based upon knowledge of all relevant clinical data and the life style of the older person.

> The various features of disengagement versus engagement, and activity versus passivity are vividly illustrated by the example of a 65-year-old professional man who decided to embark on a journey into the self. His plan had been carefully thought through and involved a self-chosen retreat in the mountains for 1 year. During this time, he would have no contacts with other people, and concentrate his energies on writing down his thoughts and impressions as they emerged from day to day. Before beginning his solo venture, he discussed the plan with various physicians, including a psychia-

trist, and had a physical, psychological, and psychiatric checkup. The data indicated that he was in good physical and mental health and that his plan for the retreat was not a manifestation of psychopathology. During the 12 months of his retreat, he did exist in isolation, not only as far as people were concerned, but also in terms of having himself cut off from telecommunications (radio, TV, newspapers). The journey into the self produced a monumental volume of writings (illustrating a high degree of activity and productivity, as well as the ability to maintain contact with reality, under the stress of prolonged social isolation). Basically, there were two dimensions to the quality and contents of his thoughts as they were entrusted to paper, day after day. The first one was vertical, reaching back in time, toward the beginnings of his existence, and was essentially autobiographical. The second type of mental activity was horizontal and impressionistic, in response to momentary observations. While the autobiographical process involved a great deal of mental effort, e.g., concentration, memory, and logical thought, the second (horizontal) thought processes required less effort, were more playful, and frequently employed "free association." Significantly, the autobiographical, "in-depth" thoughts were more frequent during the first half of the retreat, while the other type was more dominant during the second portion. After successfully completing the entire 12 months period of retreat, he re-entered the human world, and re-engaged himself without difficulties. Medical and psychiatric examinations did not show significant differences between preretreat and postretreat data.

OLD AGE AS A CONSUMMATORY PHASE

Returning once more to the notion of "goal" in senescence, the final phase of human development: in view of so much decline, how can old age be called "the golden years?" Is this a deceptive euphemism or does the phrase contain an element of truth? Talcott Parsons suggests that, as a kind of counterpart to the basic instrumental emphasis of our culture, old age should come to be viewed as a consummatory phase.[2] It should be the period of "harvest" when the fruits of previous instrumental commitments are gathered in. The tendency has been to think of the enjoyments of youth as the prototypes of consummation (the pleasures of exhibiting physical prowess, of sexual gratification, etc.) and to think of old age as entailing a renunciation of the "best" things. In contrast, the last phase of life could be viewed as a reward for a life well lived. What is needed is a reward system offered by society, which makes it clear that for most persons it is good to be old. A reward system would need to be delicately tailored to be the highly differentiated and specific styles of life which it is to reward. In addition, there is a task for older people themselves to learn to interpret their own life situations in appropriate terms, and to view old age as an opportunity for the sheer enjoyment of the consummatory phase of life.

These notions lead us to the concept of leisure time activities. *Leisure* refers to "private time," the time one has for oneself and during which one is free to engage in private activities. The latter can be described in terms of hobby, recreation, or private work (in contrast to the occupational work role). Education toward leisure time activities would seem to be an essential part of retirement counseling, either pre- or postretirement. Certain programs can be developed to acquaint aging persons with a variety of recreational activities and to provide educational experiences in the area of their interest.[3–5]

PSYCHOPATHOLOGY OF WORK AND RETIREMENT

PERSONAL WORK AND VOCATIONAL WORK

Energy

Energy is the capacity for doing work. The human organism is an open system which is capable of producing free energy. In the most general sense of the word, the human being is at work, from the moment of conception until death. In any system undergoing sensecence, there is a steady decrease in the energy yields of that system. As energy production decreases, there is a negative change in the rate at which utilizable energy is produced. Power can be defined as work per unit of time. Senescence may be conceptualized as a decline in free energy production with time.[6, 7]

The transfer and application of energy onto specific functions produce various types of work activities. During the early developmental phases (e.g., "autonomy," "initiative," "industry"), energy is transferred (cathected) into basic neuromuscular and psychomotor skills; and, later on, energy is used for the acquisition of highly specific, individual skills which prepare the individual for vocational work. Thus, vocational work patterns and skills are among the last to appear, developmentally speaking; and, later on in life, they will be among the first to disappear. The latter event corresponds, to some extent, with the social phenomenon of retirement.

Vocational Work Role and Private Work

Being-at-work, then, includes the vocational work role and the private work patterns. The *vocational work role* (occupational work) involves the following properties: expenditure of energy, financial remuneration, production of goods and services, social interaction, and social status.

Private work refers to other forms of energy expenditure, such as leisure activities, sports, hobbies, etc. Leisure and hobby activities do not necessarily have properties of vocational work, with the exception of expenditure of energy. Both types of work have also in common that they play a role in the economy of the mind: they pose challenges for mastery, offer satisfactions, or may become involved in psychological conflict. *Retirement* signifies the end of the vocational work role thus leaving the individual with the opportunity for private work only. Retirement, therefore, is a transition that involves both a loss and a gain. What is lost is the occupational work role; what is gained is the opportunity for private work.[8–10]

Any period of change and transition in life may lead to psychological difficulties. In the case of retirement, these can usually be traced back to specific psychological problems that existed earlier in life. In other words, the psychological aspects of retirement depend on the psychology of work; and conversely, the *psychopathology of work* tends to become the *psychopathology of retirement.*

INDIVIDUAL PATTERNS

The optimal expenditure of energy and the very exercise of bodily and mental functions are usually enjoyable experiences. This "functional pleasure" also applies to the exercise of skills in work and productivity, and can make work an enjoyable necessity.[11, 12] *Functional pleasure* in work activities may decline due to loss of energy, or due to loss of specific work activities, e.g., retirement. In the case of retirement, that quantum of energy invested in occupational work is freed, as it were, and will seek new outlets. This state of affairs is basically similar to a grief reaction. The loss of the work role usually represents a significant loss, because into our occupation, we have invested much of our time, interest, and energy.[9, 13, 14] A successful resolution of the grief reaction may be more difficult or become impossible due to the interference of specific emotional factors and attitudes, for example, ambivalence. Thus, ambivalent and conflictual attitudes toward work that existed during the working years may, at the time of retirement, interfere with the resolution of the loss and become obstacles in the process of role transition. In such cases, the individual may have considerable difficulty in directing his available energy toward new activities, or using it to reactivate old interests and hobbies.

We shall now briefly review some patterns and constellations encountered in individuals whose work was *in the service of conflict.* Of course, some people never appear really to invest any interest or energy at all in their work. Some lack basic drive or talent; others, during their formative years, did not invest the time or energy needed to develop skills. People who never learned or developed skills will have a steady but colorless work career at best, and an erratic career at worst. Since work has not meant very much to them, neither will retirement.

Lonely, Inwardly Isolated Person

The *lonely, inwardly isolated* person tends to view the world as a cold, inhospitable place. Work serves defensively as a way to avoid close contact with others and to build his own personal bastion of strength from which he can deal safely at a distance with other people. Upon retirement such a person will again face the original conflict, and thus become more lonely. The longstanding interpersonal conflicts that work has been taking care of for almost a lifetime, now come out in the open.

> A man in his late 60's, who had been a "sea captain," had always preferred to be alone at sea, pitting his own strength against the elements. When he was about to retire, he divorced his wife and went to a small town which was "a village that is dying." The dying village was an outward representation of his inner sense of isolation.

Attempt to Regain a "Lost Paradise"

Other individuals used work to *regain a "lost paradise."* They may have a vague memory of some idyllic state in their early life which they attempt to regain through hard work. Their aim is to earn their place in the sun, and in some instances, within the shortest time possible. There may be wishes or fantasies of retiring very early in life. Sooner or later, such people become aware that the lost paradise cannot be regained in reality. Feeling that their activities proved to be futile, they are overtaken by nostalgic depression and a sense of having "missed the boat."

> A 48-year-old man who had been a driving, hard-working business executive, had climbed to the top in the firm where he was employed. As his circumstances improved, his wife became more interested in material comforts which in turn made it necessary for him to work even harder. When, at the age of 41, he had reached the peak of his career, he and his wife went separate ways. By this time, he had accumulated sufficient wealth that he could afford to retire. Soon, however, he was hospitalized for a nervous breakdown. Against the advice of his doctors, he married the nurse who had cared for him during his emotional illness. The couple moved to a sunny climate, bought a ranch, and settled down in what promised to be a happy existence. Instead, there were frequent quarrels during which he experienced chest pains which turned out to be angina. In addition, his depression returned. By age 48, this man had gone through two marriages, seven years of retirement, and a series of depressions. He continued to be materially wealthy, but he was vexed by the problem that his life was basically empty, and that he had pursued something in life that turned out to be a mirage.

Overly Independent Person

A third type is the *overly independent* person. Such an individual may be excessively self-reliant, because he cannot accept dependency gratifications. Perhaps he perceives his dependency wishes to be so strong that he is afraid to give in to them or he was taught in his younger years that dependency was tantamount to weakness and rewarded for presenting a facade of strength. When such a person retires, he may find it difficult to alter his lifelong pattern. Since his self-esteem depends on a self-image of activity and independence, there is a tendency to remain overly active.

> A man in his mid-50's had opened his own restaurant. His one and only concern was to serve others. He slaved from the early morning to the late evening to provide the best for his customers, completely neglecting his own welfare. In spite of these considerable personal sacrifices, the restaurant did not do well. Yet, he would buy his wife expensive gifts. In short, it was all important for him to have a self-image of being generous and self-reliant. Finally, he began to suffer from chest pains. His wife called in a physician but the patient ignored the warnings, continued his excessive pace, and soon collapsed due to a myocardial infarct.

Perfectionists

Again another group comprises the *perfectionists*, those who pay more attention to the detail than the overall pattern. The compulsive or perfectionistic person works in order to do things right; at the right time, in the right place, etc. It is more important how he does it, than what he does. He works, usually with great energy, as long as he can do it the right way. When, however, the details can no longer be attended to, or when perfection cannot be attained, he tends to feel at a loss and his productivity may come to a halt. In senescence, there may occur a critical decline in the energy required to live up to his high standards. Feelings of helplessness, shame, and a sense of inadequacy may be the result.

> A 60-year-old man had, over a period of 3 years, gradually become unable to do any productive work. He spent his time drinking and making unrealistic plans to get back in business. In the past he had been in the realty business but had never been really successful, due to his tendency to be overly precise and presenting his clients with so many pros and cons that he hardly ever closed a deal. Becoming increasingly aware of his lack of success, he began to enroll in a number of business courses, to improve his skills and knowledge. However, he failed these courses, and then he withdrew from work altogether.

Aggressive and Competitive Individuals

Some people have, for a lifetime, struggled with extremely *aggressive* and *competitive* feelings. Important in this particular psychological constellation is the fact that these impulses exist primarily on the fantasy level, and that the capacity to channel them through socially acceptable outlets is somehow lacking. Consequently, there is a kind of accumulation of these competitive drives with a resulting proliferation of them in fantasy life. Since such persons never learn to distinguish clearly between hostility and normal self-assertion, they become overly fearful of asserting themselves. Every time success comes within their reach, they shrink back; success may connote to them that it was at someone else's expense that they succeeded. Their life is a succession of "near successes," or actual failures; their work career will be substandard. The end of the work career may be perceived as a final failure or defeat which provokes guilt and anger.

Personal Identity Problem

When a person has a problem in the area of *personal identity*, he may be unable to decide which goals in life to pursue or which course of action to choose. As a way out, he may choose a career or occupation which will serve as an identity, a name tag as it were, or as a way of becoming "somebody." The danger inherent in the loss of the occupation is a feeling of anonymity or a sense of identity diffusion.

Needless to say, there are many overlaps among these personality constellations, and none of them exists in pure culture. Generally, most individuals appear to handle the transition from the work role into retirement reasonably well. The elements of anticipation, foresight, and preparation probably play an essential role in a successful transition and may have two important implications. First, foresight may lead to appropriate planning, well ahead of time, for the future event (e.g., financial and economic planning). Thus, retirement will not find the individual totally unprepared from the economic point of view. Of course, the existence of retirement provisions tends to facilitate effective planning. Secondly, the imaginative anticipation of a future event may evoke specific emotional feelings associated with the event. In the case of an anticipated loss, a person may experience anticipatory grief. This has psychological value because when the loss finally occurs, a certain amount of the grief work will have already been done. Conversely, if anticipatory grief is absent, the person will have to absorb the full impact of the loss all at once. Frequently, interference with preparation for retirement is due to denial mechanisms. In those instances where work functions in the service of psychological conflict, denial mechanisms and lack of foresight are relatively prominent.

References

1. Cummings, E., and Henry, W.: *Growing Old: The Process of Disengagement*. Basic Books, New York, 1961.
2. Parsons, T.: Old age as a consummatory phase. *The Gerontologist* 3(2):53, 1963.
3. Pfeiffer, E., and Davis, G. C.: The use of leisure time in middle life. In: *Normal Aging, II*, edited by E. Palmore, Duke University Press, Durham, N. C., 1974. pp. 232–243.

4. Buhler, C.: Meaningful life in the mature years. In: *Aging and Leisure*, edited by R. W. Kleemeier, Oxford University Press, New York, 1961. pp. 345–387.
5. Buhler, C.: Old age and fulfillment of life with considerations of the use of time in old age. *Acta Psychol. 19*:124–148, 1961.
6. Calloway, N. O.: A general theory of senescence. *J. Am. Geriatr. Soc. 12*:856, 1964.
7. Elias, M. F., and Elias, D. K.: Motivation and activity. In: *Handbook of the Psychology of Aging*, edited by J. E. Birren and K. W. Schaie, chap. 16, von Nostrand Reinhold Company, New York. pp. 357–383, 1977.
8. Dennis, W.: Creative productivity between the ages of 20 and 80 years. *J. Gerontol. 21*: 1–8, 1966.
9. Jaslow, P.: Employment, retirement and morale among older women. *J. Gerontol. 31*(2):212–217, 1976.
10. Choron, S. M.: Morale, careers and personal potentials. In: *Handbook of the Psychology of Aging*, edited by J. E. Birren and K. W. Schaie, chap. 28, von Nostrand and Reinhold Company, New York. pp. 672–691, 1977.
11. von Bertalanffy, L.: General system theory and psychiatry. In: *American Handbook of Psychiatry*, edited by S. Arieti, vol. 3, chap. 43, Basic Books, New York, 1966. pp. 705–721.
12. Hendrick, I.: Work and the pleasure principle. *Psychoanal. Q. 12*:311–330, 1943.
13. Cobb, S.: Physiologic changes in men whose jobs were abolished. *J. Psychosom. Res. 18*:245–258, 1974.
14. Glamser, F. D.: Determinants of a positive attitude toward retirement. *J. Gerontol. 31*: 104–107, 1976.

21

intimacy, loneliness, and sex in senescence

THE CONCEPT OF INTIMACY

Human development is a process of becoming that encompasses the entire life cycle. During each one of the developmental phases of the life cycle, the sense of intimacy (and its counterpart, loneliness) differs with regard to some basic dimensions, such as the type of partners, the nature of sharing, the objects that are shared, and the way in which intimacy is subjectively experienced.

Typical for the first year of life is the intimacy between child and mother. Because this relationship is so close, and the sharing involves feeding and nurturing, we speak of a symbiosis. Later on, the child may have intimacy with the father, and in this relationship the child wishes to share the father's strength. Through intimate relationships with peers, such as siblings and friends, the child learns to play. It is through play activities that the child masters many insecurities and challenges.

During adolescence, there usually are intimate friendships with peers. Through these close relationships, the adolescent learns much about himself. By the end of this developmental phase, the young person has a unique identity. Only then, after a personal sense of identity has been formed, intimacy with the opposite sex becomes possible.

When one becomes a parent oneself, the intimacy of the parent-child relationship is again experienced, but now one is on the other side of the fence, as it were. Still, many young, perceptive parents may sense a peculiar familiarity about it all. This familiarity is a direct carry-over from the intimacy one had long ago with one's own parents.

Thus, in the course of time, many types of intimacy evolve and the new forms build on previous ones, thereby including rather than replacing them. During the middle years of life, a person can have many intimate relationships: with one's parents, one's friends and co-workers, one's spouse, children, grandchildren, and so on. On the other hand, middle-aged individuals may be so involved in many activities and relationships, that they are too busy to take time out for moments of intimacy.

Old age brings inevitable losses. Each loss represents the disappearance of an intimate relationship, and increases the likelihood of loneliness. Thus, one of the main psychological tasks in old age is to accept the inevitable losses and to learn to be more alone without feeling too lonely. The more an old person has become capable, through mental processes of abstraction and sublimation, of extending his interests to encompass phenomena that are not bound by time and space (e.g., art, science, religion, society, nature), the greater his psychic immunity against the risk of loneliness.

In the usual sense of the word, though, intimacy involves the contact with another person. Of course, we can be intimate with our own self: our body, our thoughts, feelings, and memories. In fact, this intimacy with oneself is enriching, and the self can be a source of creativity and a wealth of experiences. But the self being a "lonely fortress," the sense of intimacy is fulfilled most in the contact with another person. Now, what are some of the basic *qualities of intimacy* with another person, as for example between a man and a woman?

First, there is a *sense of belonging*, in terms of "I belong to you; you belong to me; we belong to each other." This implies a sense of fit and harmony. The fact that this or that experience is intimate means that I can fit it into my life, into what is already there, and harmonize it with my past, present, and future self. The sense of fit and harmony is perceived as something that could not be any other way. Thus, one person will say to the other, "We are made for each other"; or, they marvel that the forces of destiny directed their paths so as to meet each other, as if such a harmony of feelings could only be the work of a higher providence—"It had to be."

Second, there is the element of *familiarity*. One cannot be intimate with what is new or unfamiliar, strange or alien. In fact, the counterpart of intimacy is referred to as alienation. Thus, nothing that is new is intimate. And, everything intimate fits in with a previous experience. It follows that the mental process of recognition is essential. Now, recognition is repeated cognition, as is also true in the case of remembering (memory).

We can now add a third characteristic of intimacy: the fact that *repetition* is built into the experience. On the one hand, intimacy is experienced as repetition of a previous experience; on the other hand, one wishes it to be repeated in the future. Intimacy is not a brief encounter.

The idea that the past is repeated in the present, and the present in the future, points up the next characteristic, that of *sameness*, and permanence. Such notions as change and transience are alien to the experience of intimacy. Through sameness one attains a kind of transcendence, a transcending of time. There is a process of time binding, i.e., the tying together of past, present, and future into one cohesive perspective. But there also is an element of timelessness in this transcendence, as if one has risen above the flow of time. Such transcendence of time is a sort of eternity. In the experience of intimacy, we see this illustrated when one says to a loved one: "It is as if I have always known you" (transcending time backward into the past)—or "our love will last forever" (transcending time forward into the future). There is nothing new or strange about this timelessness. It is our unconscious that is timeless and knows nothing about clocks and calendars. Time, in the sense of objective calendar time, is learned over a period of years. A true appreciation of time and a mature time sense do not occur until early adolescence. The timelessness of intimacy corresponds to mental processes that can be traced back to the early origins of our existence, and that continue to be present in the deeper, unconscious layers of the mind.

Finally, the activity of intimacy is *sharing*. What may be shared is something material and external (possessions, money, etc.), or time and space (as in a home), or the phenomenon called "each other." In sharing each other, the I and the you create the we. The we encompasses something bigger than I and you added together by way of simple arithmetic. In the language of systems theory, the system as a whole (we) is larger, greater, more than the sum of its parts (I + you). As people sometimes describe love, "It's bigger than me." Christian doctrine, systems theory, and psychoanalysis converge at this point: the religious emphasis on love corresponds to the above mentioned principle of systems theory as well as to the psychoanalytic principle of sublimation. Sublimation refers to the mental process of becoming less self-centered and more selfless, of subordinating the wishes of the self to the interests of a larger entity. This larger entity that transcends the narrow self can be concretely human (the we, or a family), or this entity can be an abstraction (art, science, humanity, mankind).

It might be noted here that one measure of the success of one's life is the measure of one's *sublimations*. (The submerging of the self in the service of a higher cause is the religious theme of losing oneself in order to find it). Corresponding to sublimation, there is the simultaneous process of desexualization. By this we mean that one learns to transform sexual energy so that it can be used for selfless aims, for the higher things in life, as it were. In summary, sublimation involves an orientation away from the self toward a larger, transcendent phenomenon, and an orientation away from sexual pleasure toward nonsexual satisfaction and achievements. Ideally, the way intimacy would change, in the course of life, is along these same lines; that is, an increasing amount of sublimation (or love, if you wish). The outcome of this would be 2-fold: to belong intimately to something that is larger than I am, that transcends me and, in fact, will outlive me; and to transform sufficient amounts of sexual drive into nonsexual energy for the purpose of achieving something that lasts and endures.

THE CONCEPT OF SEXUALITY

In the broad sense of the word, sexuality refers to wishes, drives, and feelings that have a somatic-physiological origin and have the aim of attaining pleasure.

SOMATIC ORIGIN

Feelings or drives of a sexual nature originate from multiple sources in the body, such as the mouth and gastrointestinal tract, the sense organs, the skin, the muscles, and so on. In each case, the sexual drive or energy that originates from that organ system has a specific quality. At different stages of human development, different body parts or organs assume relative importance. For example, during the first year of life the dominant erogenous zones are the mouth, upper gastrointestinal tract, and the skin. Later, the lower intestinal tract, the neuromuscular system, and sense organs also become important. The emergence of a particular organ system as a significant source of pleasure (i.e., sexual stimulation and satisfaction) depends on processes of somatic and psychological maturation. For example, by age 5 or 6, parts of the genital organs begin to mature, and the strength of sensations originating from them increases significantly. Hence, this is called the phallic phase of development.

THE STRIVING FOR PLEASURE

The nature of sexual drives is the attainment of pleasure. In our present framework, pleasure is defined as the release of tension, or the removal of excitations originating in a particular organ system; and organ pleasure is defined as "sexual." When the organ system from which pleasurable excitations originate is the genital apparatus, we speak of genital-sexual wishes or satisfactions. The genital apparatus is relatively late in its maturation; other parts of the body, in the course of development, emerge sooner as an important source of sensations. For this reason, these nongenital sexual excitations are called *pregenital.* In this context, the term pregenital connotes something that happened before something else; the sexuality that precedes genital sex is called pregenital. But, there is a second reason for the term pregenital: the sexual feelings originating from within the genital system are stronger than those from other organ systems. We speak of the dominance or primacy of genital sexuality. In this context, pregenital refers to the quality of being a forerunner of genital sex; and, in that sense, pregenital is equivalent to being *subordinated* to genital sexuality. To put it differently, pregenital sex drives are like a prelude or foreplay vis-à-vis genital sexuality. In the case of normal adult sexuality, the former culminate in the latter.

The *primacy* of genital sexuality depends on the maturation of the genital apparatus as a result of hormonal, anatomical, and physiological factors. The dominance of the genital system comes into being during early adulthood (puberty) and lasts until some indefinite point in late life. Thus, genital sexuality is only one form of sexuality, albeit the dominant one. It appears last, developmentally speaking; and generally, what developed last is most likely to disappear first. That means pregenital sexuality not only precedes (antedates) genital sex, but also will outlast it.

Between *intimacy and sex*, there is no one-to-one relationship. One can have intimacy without sex, and sex without intimacy. Intimacy can be sexually neutral; and sex can be lonely. But often intimacy is sexual and sex is intimate. By the same token, sexual intimacy may involve genital sexuality (in terms of specific consummation), or pregenital sexuality. No statistics are known about this, but probably people spend considerably more time being together in sexual intimacy that is pregenital in nature.

SEX IN SENESCENCE

Research in sex in old age is a relatively recent phenomenon. Publications on adult sexuality began to appear in the late 19th century. Publications on adolescent and child sexuality appeared 20 to 30 years later (1920's), and those on sex in senescence again some 20–30 years later (1950's). This development may be related to several factors. First, social attitudes used to be characterized by the notion that older people are sexless, or at least that they should be. Second, the increase in the number of older people and the emergence of gerontology and geriatrics have focused attention on the problems of living in old age, including those of sex. Finally, although many older people live in conditions that are less favorable than those of other age groups, there have been positive changes, such as Social Security, Medicare, and improved retirement provisions. This has focused attention on old age as a phase with its own opportunities for leisure and recreation. As time goes on, more healthy individuals who are still vigorous and look forward to leisure, including the recreation of sex, will reach old age.[1–3]

THE EFFECTS OF AGING ON SEX

Sexual capacities and functions show definite age-related changes; in this respect, sex is not different from other biological and psychological functions that show a decline with increasing age.[4, 5] To the extent that we speak of "normal" aging phenomena, these age-related changes in sex can also be viewed as a normal process. In our research at Duke, we studied 254 men and woman, ranging from 60–94 years of age.[6, 7] Some of the relevant findings are presented below.

Sexual Activity

In the overall group, the incidence of sexual *activity* declined from a level of more than 50 percent during the early 60's, to a level of between 10 and 20 percent after age 80.

Sexual Interest

The incidence of sexual *interest* does not show an age-related decline: mild-to-moderate degrees of interest may persist into the 80's.

In general, the incidence of sexual interest is higher than that of activity, and this *discrepancy* is more prominent in men.

Marital Status

Marital status has little effect on the sexual activity and interest of aging men. Unmarried women have only a negligible amount of sexual intercourse, but about 20 percent of this group report sexual interest. The sexual activity and interest of men is greater than that of women, regardless of marital status.

The Influence of the Past

Living patterns of the earlier years set the stage for those of the later years. This also holds true for sexual behavior patterns. The sexual drives and activities of older people correlate with those of the younger years. Men and woman who used to enjoy sex when they were young are likely to still enjoy it when old. This finding disposes of the (superstitious) notion that one only has a limited amount of sexual energy, or that by keeping some in reserve one may have more sexual energy later on in life. Actually, the reverse is true: active and regular use of sexual capacities is likely to maintain them in old age. In this respect, sex is no different from other functional capacities (e.g., intelligence) that benefit from active and regular use.

Individual Variability

The final common path of human sexual behavior is under the influence of a great variety of factors, including biological endowment, developmental and age-related changes, psychodynamic forces, interpersonal relationships, and sociocultural factors. It is no surprise, therefore, to find a great deal of variability among aging individuals with regard to their sexual behavior. Some of these individual variations include the following:

Although, in general, elderly men are sexually more active than women, in the course of time the differences become smaller.

Among men surviving into the 80's and 90's, continued sexual activity is no great rarity; about one-fifth of these men are still sexually active.

Although sexual interest declines with age, about one-half of the subjects surviving into the 80's and 90's report they still have sexual interest of mild to moderate degree.

Unmarried men have about the same level of sexual activity and interest as married men. In fact, unmarried men report not infrequently a pattern of increasing activity and interest.

About one-fourth of the men, regardless of age, report an increase in the degree of activity or interest, over a period of time covering several years.

Increased Sexual Activity

Since sexual potency declines consistently beginning in the early adult years until well into old age, it follows that increased sexual activity in aging men is likely to be due to psychological or social factors (an exception, of course, would be increased sexual activity due to improved physical health).[8] Among such we may see the following.

Personality growth and emotional maturation, on the basis of general life experiences or due to psychotherapy, may result in a *lessening of earlier sexual inhibitions.*

Attempts to *compensate* for, or deny, the age-related decrease in potency (overcompensation, counterphobic behavior, denial) tend to increase sexual activity or even cause compulsive hypersexuality.

Certain emotional crises (depression, boredom, and monotony, a sense of existential meaninglessness, work pressures) may prompt a *quest for oblivion* by way of losing oneself in exciting experiences, including sex.

Success in one's life's work may bring about a sense of "having arrived." The reality of actually "having it made," combined with the increased self-esteem, makes it possible for one to take more time out for all sorts of enjoyable activities, including sex.

Economic success may enable one to create those settings conducive to increased sex, e.g., vacation trips with spouse or an extramarital relationship.

Changes in the family, e.g., when children begin to leave the home, may leave the middle-aged couple with more time and fewer responsibilities.

Many important factors pertain to the marital relationship. The *wife's menopause* may have a favorable effect when there no longer need to be concerns about the risk of unwanted pregnancies. But loss of the spouse's childbearing capacity may be felt as a loss by the man himself, in which case the wish to deny his own aging and to feel young again may lead to pseudohypersexuality or extramarital sex with younger partners.

THE EFFECTS OF SEX ON AGING

With regard to the influence of sexual activity on aging, there is some evidence from animal experiments suggesting that continued sexual activity may contribute to, or is associated with, longevity. In male rats, for example, regular mating improves their condition and increases longevity. It has been pointed out that married persons live longer than unmarried ones, but this does not prove the beneficial effects of continued sexual activity.[9] The Duke research data suggest that continued sexual activity may be a characteristic of vigorous individuals who may represent a *biological elite.* These aged people tend to be still married, even if quite old; to retain physical and psychological health, and to remain socially, as well as sexually, active. Continued sexual activity is a correlate of continued vigor.[10]

The notion of a life-prolonging or vigor-restoring benefit from sexual contact is very old, and encountered in several cultures. The alleged beneficial effect on old males from the proximity of a young woman is called gerocomy, or *Shunamitism,* a phrase derived from the story of King David (1 Kings 1:1–5). Reportedly, the famous 18th century Dutch physician Boerhaave advised the elderly mayor of Amsterdam to lie between two young girls to recover his strength and spirits. The influence allegedly responsible was the heat or breath of a young virgin, coitus being excluded as dangerous. The terms spirit and breath bring to mind the physiological processes of inspiration and their deeper figurative meaning: to inspire is to create life, to be inspired is to be creative.

Apart from any magical or superstitious elements, we wonder to what extent we see something like Shunamitism in settings where nursing care is given to geriatric patients. Often we are impressed by the enthusiasm of youthful nurses whose warmth restores the spirits of elderly patients. The close proximity and intimacy, expressed in so many ways (e.g., touch, voice, feeding), is an expression of sublimation, which means that the relationship has been desexualized and thus has become sexually neutral. The stimuli transmitted in such contact, far from having a sexual significance, have the much broader aim of restoration and of regenerating a sense of well being.

THE QUALITY OF SEXUAL EXPERIENCE IN LATER LIFE

It is important to keep in mind that the Duke project, from which the above data were obtained, studied groups of subjects at different points in time. Thus, the data reflect the "average profile" of specific groups rather than longitudinal changes in the sexual behavior of particular individuals. In addition, the nature of the research data is quantitative rather than qualitative. Research data involving quantifiable variables is "objective," in that it permits statistical validation and replication by other investigators. However, if sex in the postmature years (following middle age and covering as much as one-third of the life span) is to continue playing an important role, then its quality is a pertinent issue. The subjective quality of sexual experience is more relevant than the quantity. Our attempts to understand some of the qualitative aspects is facilitated by keeping in mind certain considerations.

Changing Patterns

Sexual behavior *changes continually* during the life span. The various phases of human development have their own psychosocial characteristics which are reflected in sexual behavior. Through the years the sexual drives change with regard to their physiological sources of origin, their purpose, and the human context in which the sexual needs are satisfied. The postmature years, those following middle age, may cover a period of 20–30 years, or about one-third of the lifespan. Pfeiffer and Davis[11] studied the determinants of sexual behavior in men and women aged 46–71 years. Their findings indicate that the sexual behavior in these individuals (between middle and old age) depends on multiple factors, including the level of sexual functioning in younger years, the age and sex of the subject, and the subjective and objective health ratings. The sexual behavior of men was influenced by a much greater number of variables than that of women. In the latter, the most important determinants are age, degree of past sexual enjoyment, and marital status. This again emphasizes the fact that for women the availability of a sexually capable and socially sanctioned partner is a crucial factor.[11, 12] This point has particular relevance to the multifaceted issue of widowhood. Because the life expectancy of women exceeds that of men, there is in later life, a discrepancy in the number of men and women. This problem has even prompted consideration of polygyny as a possible solution.[13]

New Ways of Intimacy

Because sex usually is no longer procreative, there may be more emphasis on its *recreative* aspects. In spite of the anatomical and functional decline of the genital apparatus, interest in sexual activity tends to persist.

Because of involution of the genital organs, there may be a shift of interest, away from traditional sex (sexual intercourse with orgasm), in the direction of other types of sexual activity, i.e., sexual drives and behavior that are not primarily aimed at discharging genital excitation through orgasm. These pregenital needs and activities include sexual excitations from many parts of the body and a great variety of stimuli (oral, touch, and temperature stimulation, etc.).

Predominance of Pregenital Drives

Such a relative *predominance of pregenital drives* in an older person cannot be simply compared with the sexual immaturity of children or adolescents. Old age is not a second childhood. A lifetime of experience makes the difference.

The aim of sexual activity may not be primarily orgastic release of sexual tension, but rather the developing or *maintaining of excitation.* In this context, sexual activity may also serve more general aims, e.g., the need for intimacy and warmth, or a sense of being alive.

PSYCHOPATHOLOGY AND SEXUAL PROBLEMS IN OLD AGE

Sexual problems may occur at any age, and old age is no exception. We do not know if the frequency of sexual problems in old age differs from that in other phases of life, or whether they are similar in nature. Sexual problems may begin with the aging process; they may ameliorate in old age; or, as a life-long problem they may be carried over into later years. Individuals with a background of life-long sexual adjustment or personality maturity tend to have few, if any, sexual problems in old age.

Pathological Responses to Involution

In these cases, sexual involution acts as a pathogenetic factor. Loss of any capacity, including sexual functions, gives rise to a grief reaction, to anxious concerns about disruptions in intimate relationships, and can be perceived as a narcissistic injury resulting in lower self-esteem. In men, sexual potency usually declines gradually, and this makes it possible to work through the grief little by little, and to accept the loss without severe emotional upsets. Sexual involution in women, the menopause, usually takes place at a more rapid rate than the climacteric in men. Consequently, in women the psychological reactions to the change of life are often stronger or more visible than the corresponding reactions in men. But the intensity of the grief reaction does not necessarily have a bearing on the final outcome. It is important to note that because women usually cope with involution problems at a younger age than men do, they may have greater adaptational capacity when they really need it.

To a large extent, sexual drives can be understood in terms of their role in human relationships. Eros tends to bring people together, and the loss of sexual capacity may lead to anxious concerns about possible disruptions of intimate relations (e.g., fear of loneliness). Also, the loss of an important function can be perceived as a narcissistic injury resulting in lower self-esteem. In order to maintain or restore self-esteem, several psychological techniques may be employed (denial, projection, regression, and withdrawal). Whether these mechanisms are adaptive or maladaptive depends mainly on the degree of the particular mechanism.

Denial. The individual who tries to *deny* his sexual decline may appear to be hypersexual. True hypersexuality, however, is very rare and usually it is "pseudo," in the sense of a hypersexual facade. Such persons may seek out a great number of sexual experiences or variations, and this activity has an urgent, compulsive quality. The person does not act his age, but behaves as a younger adult. Again, whether or not such behavior is normal (adaptive) depends on the degree of these traits. In fact, a certain amount of denial or compensation can be useful. Some ingredients of romanticism and role playing add spice to life. As long as fantasy and make-believe do not get to the point of actual self-deception, no problem exists. Along with romantic make-believe comes the search for beautification; and again, as long as the beautification measures are aesthetically appropriate, and consistent with the individual's age and life style, we are dealing with normal and adaptive behavior.

Possessiveness. Decline of sexual function may lead to fears concerning loss of love. Some persons are bothered by a nagging fear that they will lose their hold on the spouse. *Possessiveness,* the attempt to have a permanent hold on the other person, is based on insecurity or dependency. The possessive person suffers from jealousy, a pathological apprehension about the possibility of alienation of affection. (Clinically, pathological jealousy and suspiciousness may occur in involutional depressions, or in paranoid states.) The individual uses projection to find a scapegoat, often blaming the spouse for the trouble. What is ironic and tragic is that this becomes a self-fulfilling prophecy: suspiciousness alienates others, and the alienation then becomes proof of the original suspicion.

Retreating. When a person feels that, with regard to some important activity, he is less capable than he would like to be, he may protect himself by way of a *retreat.* He may retreat from those situations that provide opportunities for that particular activity. Such a protective retreat may also occur as a response to feelings of sexual inadequacy and manifest itself as a regression into hypochondriasis. The physical symptoms provide an alibi for the alleged inadequacy.

Withdrawal. Avoidance of sexual opportunities (because of the fear of failure) may lead to another risk, *viz., withdrawal* from the other person. After some time, a new relationship becomes solidified, with the two partners now being further away from each other. The fear of failure often is the result of an all-or-none view. If sex is viewed as an all-or-none business, without a place for intermediate sexual activities (sex short of orgasm through intercourse), then the options are limited. The husband, for example, may feel that to enjoy sex he is obliged to go all the way. Perhaps his wife feels likewise; more likely she does not. Of course, some women interpret any failure on the part of their husband as rejection. Instead of viewing sexual involution as a fact of life, they take it personally. Their sense of rejection or loneliness is not based on actual, but imagined, rejection.

Embarrassment and Shame. These are troublesome feelings that may originate in several ways. First, more people feel that aging does not enhance beauty, and that the aged body is less beautiful to see. Whereas in earlier years, looking at one partner's body was a source of sexual stimulation, this is no longer so. By the same token, being looked at by one's partner may evoke feelings of embarrassment or shame. No longer is the emphasis on showing and showing off, but more on the need to cover and have privacy, from one's own eyes and those of one's partner. The ideal of dignity has as its counterpart the risk of shame. Loss of face may be the result of acting inappropriately, i.e., not acting one's age. A third source of shame or guilt is related to the relative predominance of pregenital strivings. It is interesting that the experts may advise older persons to relax and not worry about guilt and inhibitions regarding sex. One gets the impression that older persons are being encouraged to enjoy the kind of sex that young people do, as if age made no difference at all.

Thus, a new (false) stereotype may develop, replacing the previous one of the sexlessness of old age. This new stereotype, that older persons can have sex lives comparable to younger persons, might be more damaging than the old one, because it tends to set a standard of behavior beyond the reach of the majority of old people. Such a development only would increase fears of failure and reinforce the view that anything short of heterosexual intercourse with orgasm is something to feel embarrassed about.

Identity Crisis. Personal identity is closely related to one's self-concept as a man or woman. Therefore, decline or loss of sexual functions may pose a threat to an individual's sense of identity, in particular sexual identity, i.e. being a man, being a woman. The resulting *identity crisis of late life* may be quite disruptive. Frequently, we find that earlier psychological problems (dating back to adolescence and childhood) are reactivated.

Sexual Symptoms as an Expression of Nonsexual Pathology

Ego, Superego, Object Relation Changes; Physical Illness. Sexual disturbances (sexual deviations, sexual acting out, etc.) may be due to *nonsexual age-related changes.* The latter include, for example, changes in the ego and superego, changes in object relations, physical illness, or iatrogenic factors. Decreased impulse control may result from age-related changes in the ego and superego. The importance of possible iatrogenic factors is illustrated by the case of a 60-year-old man, concerned about impotence, and being treated for depression. He reported that any time he would take imipramine, he had a "nearly uncontrollable urge to phone the little girls in the neighborhood and make sexual propositions to them" (see p. 162).

Organic Brain Damage. Patients with *organic brain damage* often present sexual problems of a specific nature. Because of the brain damage, there may be psychological impairments such as poor judgment and poor impulse control. Such elderly patients may show sexual behavior that is inappropriate with regard to time, place, and social context. Examples of such behavioral disturbances are exhibitionism, masturbation in public, pedophilia, and so on. Such behavioral manifestations of dementia may occur among geriatric patients in chronic care facilities. This can be upsetting to both the personnel and the other patients.

Sexual Acting Out. Geriatric patients in institutions may also present problems in terms of *sexual acting out.* What is acted out, through sexual behavior, can be a variety of impulses or psychological conflicts. For example, a patient may express hostile, defiant, or rebellious tendencies through provocative sexual acts. Another patient has discovered that exhibitionism is a guaranteed attention-getting device. Again, another type of patient seems to have learned, through some sort of conditioning, that the only opportunity to be touched by human hands is the forceful

restraint that follows his attack on somebody else, or being cleaned up after soiling himself. In the therapeutic management of these disturbances, it is helpful to have some understanding of the psychological problem that underlies the overt behavior. The knowledge that a patient's disturbed sexual behavior is a manifestation of his confusion, or is prompted by anger, loneliness, or boredom, enables us to see the disturbing behavior in the proper perspective, to maintain our professional attitude of detached concern, and to follow a plan of rational therapy that is aimed, not at the symptom, but at the cause.[14]

Eros versus Thanatos. Sexual preoccupations may cover up death anxiety. Thus, for example, delusions pertaining to sex, and life or death are not uncommon in aged patients close to death. Reference is made to some clinical case examples described earlier in this text: The 82-year-old schizophrenic woman (p. 82), the 71-year-old widow (p. 92), and the 85-year-old woman (p. 36). Some aged female patients complain of feeling "sex-starved." This may represent an instance of hypersexuality, where the emphasis on Eros is defensively used to cover up the approach of Thanatos. A corollary of this phenomenon might be found in the phrase "learning the facts of life." The facts of "life" are usually learned in early adolescence; what is overlooked, however, is that it is around this same time that the facts of death are fully discovered. Thus, the phrase "facts of life" is a euphemism, involving a certain element of denial of death.[8]

SEX AND CHRONIC ILLNESS

Many patients suffering from a variety of chronic *physical conditions* continue to have sexual interest, and maintain sexual activity. Chronic conditions such as heart disease, stroke, neurological diseases (e.g., multiple sclerosis, hemiparesis), and urogenital diseases interfere to some extent with sexual interest and activity. But this interference is not necessarily a total one. In the case of men, for example, who have had a coronary attack or a prostatectomy, approximately three-fourths are able to continue sexual activity.[15–19]

Certain problems, however, may arise in these situations, and these apply particularly to male patients. The disability resulting from the chronic illness may specifically interfere with the capacity to take sexual initiative and to perform in an active and sustained manner. It becomes, therefore, necessary for such patients (and their wives) to seek *new ways of sexual intimacy*. This requires, in both partners, open-mindedness and cooperation which in turn permit experimentation with new sexual techniques. An example of what might be a rather difficult readjustment is the change from an active mode to a less active or passive mode. Such a transition would be difficult for highly aggressive, independent, or self-assertive men.

The patient with a chronic illness (or the spouse) may come to feel that sex no longer has, or should have, a place in their life. For example, many women used to believe that a hysterectomy would signify the end of enjoyable sex. Or, a man may be convinced that prostate surgery will render him impotent. Unfortunately, such convictions may be self-fulfilling prophecies. Disfiguring and mutilative surgical procedures (mastectomy, colostomy, etc.) can be especially a problem for women. Women are generally more vulnerable to the trauma of disfigurement with the resulting loss of attractiveness, whereas men are more vulnerable to loss of power.

Reference

1. Greenblatt, R. B.: The psychogenic and endocrine aspects of sexual behavior. *J. Am. Geriatr. Soc. 22:*393–396, 1974.
2. Berezin, M.: Sex and old age: a further review of the literature. *J. Geriatr. Psychiatry 9:*189–209, 1976.
3. Butler, R. N., and Lewis, M. T.: *Sex after Sixty; A Guide for Men and Women in their Later Years.* Harper & Row, New York, 1976.
4. Kinsey, A. C., Pomeroy, W. B., and Martin, C. E.: *Sexual Behavior in the Human Male.* W. B. Saunders Company, Philadelphia, 1948.
5. Kinsey, A. C., Pomeroy, W. B., Martin, C. E., and Gebhard, P. H.: *Sexual Behavior in the Human Female.* W. B. Saunders Company, Philadelphia, 1953.
6. Verwoerdt, A., Pfeiffer, E., and Wang, H. S.: Sexual behavior in senescence. I. Changes in sexual activity and interest of aging men and women. *J. Geriatr. Psychiatry 2:*163–180, 1969.
7. Verwoerdt, A., Pfeiffer, E., and Wang, H. S.: Sexual behavior in senescence. II. Patterns of change in sexual activity and interest. *Geriatrics 24:*137–154, 1969.
8. Verwoerdt, A.: Normal psychology of the aging process, revisited, Discussion. *J. Geriatr. Psychiatry 9:*211–219, 1976.
9. Sheps, M. C.: Marriage and mortality. *Am. J. Public Health 51:*547–555, 1961.
10. Pfeiffer, E., Verwoerdt, A., and Wang, H. S.: The natural history of sexual behavior in a biologically advantaged group of aged individuals. *J. Gerontol. 24:*193–198, 1969.
11. Pfeiffer, E., and Davis, G. C.: Determinants of sexual behavior in middle and old age. *J. Am. Geriatr. Soc. 20:*151–158, 1972.
12. Christenson, C. V., and Gagnon, J. H.: Sexual behavior in a group of older women. *J. Gerontol. 20:*351–356, 1965.
13. Kassel, V.: Polygyny after 60. *Geriatrics 21:*214–218, 1966.
14. Wasow, M., and Loeb, M. B.: Sexuality in nursing homes. *J. Am. Geriatr. Soc. 27:*73–79, 1979.
15. Ford, A. B., and Orfirer, A. P.: Sexual behavior and the chronically ill patient. *Med. Aspects Human Sexuality 1:*51–61, 1967.
16. Hellerstein, H. K., and Friedman, E. H.: Sexual activity and the postcoronary patient. *Med. Aspects Human Sexuality 3:*70–96, 1969.
17. Finkle, A. L.: Sex after prostatectomy. *Med. Aspects Human Sexuality 2:*40–41, 1968.
18. Scheingold, L. D., and Wagner, N. N.: *Sound Sex and the Aging Heart; Sex in the Mid- and Later Years with Special Reference to Cardiac Problems.* Human Sciences Press, New York, 1974.
19. Herr, H. W.: Preservation of sexual potency in prostatic cancer patients after ^{125}I implantation. *J. Am. Geriatr. Soc. 27:*17–19, 1979.

22

training in gerontology and geropsychiatry

GEROPSYCHIATRY AS A DISCIPLINE

THE CONCEPT OF A DISCIPLINE

Concerning education in the various fields of aging, there is the question: "Who should teach what to whom?" The answer is related to the concept of discipline and specialty.[1–4] The term geriatrics usually denotes medical practice in the care of the aged which yet remains within the purview of a given medical or surgical specialty. Similarly, gerontologists tend to identify themselves primarily as biologists, psychologists, or sociologists who happen to be studying the aging process.[5] Since geriatrics is not clearly defined with regard to its position in medicine, the question has been raised if something can be gained from organizing geriatrics into a structured specialty.[6–9] The general impression is that the proponents and opponents are approximately equal in number, the proponents being more likely professionals with a clinical background (-iatry) than a basic science orientation (-ology). Those who are inclined to oppose geriatrics as a separate entity prefer to see it become an integral part of other disciplines and specialties. Those who favor the idea of a separate (sub) specialty frequently do so because of practical considerations, such as facilitation of professional identity; a higher degree of "visibility" in society, the opportunity to consolidate resources, and develop high-caliber clinical facilities.[9–11]

Cogent arguments are made either way, but few, if any, discussions are aimed at the question of what a discipline or specialty is, from a conceptual point of view. At the root of the issue is the very concept of "aging." Aging is a biological process; gerontology involves the study of time-related biological changes in living organisms. On this level, concepts such as aging, growth, development, change, becoming, etc. tend to become indistinguishable. Inasmuch as gerontology studies a time-related biological *process*, it would be only logical that it represents a specific dimension of various biological disciplines.

In the field of medicine, a discipline or specialty can be defined and conceptualized by way of two parameters: (1) the systematized study and accumulated knowledge with reference to clearly delineated interest areas and specific target phenomena; and (2) the type of professional activity directed toward these specific objects.

Target Phenomena

The *target phenomena*, or *interest area*, which provide a basis for a given medical discipline usually represent components of the human organism. Thus, the specialty of hematology is primarily aimed at cellular phenomena; cardiology, at a specific organ system; psychiatry, at the organism as a whole; and, public health, at the societal level. In some cases, the interest area pertains to a specific dimension of human life (e.g., industrial-occupational medicine; marital or family therapy).

The fact that there are no sharp boundaries in biology is reflected in the multiple interactions between disciplines. Thus, the boundary of a medical specialty is never static or absolute, but always semipermeable. Inasmuch as a medical specialty or discipline is only a nodal point in a larger framework, interdisciplinary contact is not a matter of choice, but a necessity. In the course of time, a body of scientific knowledge is accumulated with regard to the principal target of a discipline.

Methods of Practice

The second set of parameters pertains to the *methods of practice*, or *types of professional activity*, within a given discipline. These include:

Production of information, e.g., doing a physical examination, laboratory tests, making a diagnosis, basic research, clinical research.

Application of information, e.g., clinical treatment, cancer detection programs, community service programs, policy making.

Transmission of information, e.g., teaching, consultation, explaining a treatment plan to members of the therapeutic team, public relations.

Organization of information, e.g., the administration of research, training and clinical programs; recording, storing, and retrieving clinical data or research data; management of resources, talents, and personnel.

All medical professionals are involved in these four activities. Since the varying amounts of time and effort allocated to these activities add up to an infinite number of possibilities, no two professional career patterns will be the same.

GEROPSYCHIATRY: SCOPE AND PRACTICE

Geropsychiatry, the psychiatry of late life, encompasses the behavioral sciences, psychodynamic concepts, and psychiatric practice with reference to the aging personality and the mental disorders of late life.

Scope

In many respects, the senium is still a terra incognita. We need to know a great deal more about the psychosocial and intrapsychic processes involved in attaining a sense of integrity, the causes and mechanisms of its failure, the clinical expressions of such decompensation, and, most importantly, therapeutic modalities. An understanding of the final phase in human development can provide additional insights into earlier developmental periods and contribute toward a comprehensive theory of human behavior.

The focus of geropsychiatry is on the *process* of becoming old and the *outcome* of this process in specific individuals. The processes we are interested in studying are organic as well as psychodynamic in nature. The former pertain especially to the central nervous system; the latter, to the experience of loss, the vicissitudes of grief, and the various forms of decompensation that are the outcome of inadequate coping and restitution.

The psychopathology of senescence is either *specific* or *nonspecific* with regard to age.

Nonspecific Psychopathology. *Nonspecific psychopathology* is that which can be found among individuals of any age. When present in the senium, it may be a carry-over from earlier life phases. A schizophrenic, for example, who reaches the senium, is not suffering from specifically senescent pathology. From a process point of view, our interest is how aging can affect (in terms of amelioration, or further decompensation) these nonspecific disorders. Aging frequently has certain *pathoplastic* effects on psychopathology. Some schizophrenics, for example, show a lessening of psychotic symptoms with aging; on the other hand, certain involutional depressions gradually decompensate toward hypochondriasis or a paranoid position.

Aging as the Pathogenetic Factor. In psychopathology that is *specific* to senescence, aging is the *pathogenetic* factor. On the organic level, this usually involves age-related changes of the central nervous system (CNS). On the psychological level, the pathogenetic effects of aging include the awareness of, and need to cope with, the stress of physical, social, and economical losses, as well as the unique situation of facing the end of life. Specific psychopathological entities may develop depending on the various ways in which the involutional grief reactions decompensate. A depression may become chronic when ambivalence interferes with resolution of grief. Through withdrawal and distancing, hypochondriasis and self-absorption come about, reflecting a disturbance in intimacy as well as generativity. Persisting hypochondriasis leads to progressive decathexis of object relations and impoverishment of the self, predisposing to further decompensation. A variety of misanthropic depressions may occur at the end of the line, including bitter resignation, vindictive depressions, and depressive cynicism.

In some respects, the psychopathology of senescence may be intrinsically different from that of younger years. For example, it has been observed that the classical depressions with feelings of guilt are relatively rare in late life. But when we do encounter guilt feelings in elderly patients, they may have a special significance. When, for example, an elderly patient expresses guilt about past autoerotic activities (a fairly typical depressive symptom) the real issue may be a sense of hopelessness that so much opportunity for genuine intimacy has been irrevocably lost. It is more comfortable to feel guilt (and to imagine that one can correct things by doing penance) than to face the fact that one has missed the boat. Likewise, the nature of anxiety in aging persons is different. While in younger people, anxiety often is a danger signal in response to ego-alien impulses, in older people it pertains to fear of losing external supplies. In addition, anxiety will arise when, for whatever reasons, the older person's perspective changes from a sense of integrity in the direction of despair.

Geropsychiatric Practice

Clinical Aspects. Characteristics of the *physician-patient relationship* include problems of communication, transference, and countertransference. Communication with psychiatrically ill elderly persons may be difficult due to age-related CNS slowing, organic brain syndrome, or functional psychiatric disorders. In senile regression, for example, ideational phenomena dominated by primary process, frequently occur. The resulting thought disorder closely resembles that of schizophrenia.

When the older patient "lives in the past," the physician may not be recognized at all, or he may become one of the persons in the patient's past. By and large, elderly patients appear less able to distinguish the therapist as a real person from the therapist as a transference figure. Typically, transference phenomena are not interpreted or analyzed, in contrast to therapy with younger adults.

Countertransferences may present serious problems, too, such as gerophobic attitudes or unresolved fears of aging and death. Often, one may feel frustrated by his inability to modify life-long behavior patterns in aged patients and the need to accept limited treatment goals.

Many problems are related to the patient's dependency on other family members, and the multigenerational aspects of family conflict. The frequent need for *contact with relatives* makes it imperative for the geropsychiatrist to be skilled in the diagnosis of disturbed family interactions and in family therapy. Such approaches can be compared with those in child psychiatry. However, the nature of the transference, and of the identifications observed between the child patient and his parents, are the reverse of those observed between the child and the parent patient. The problems of role reversal that may develop in the aged parent and in the adult child are frequently sources of family pathology. The aged parent may be the one who clings to an obsolete role in the family; or, the child chronologically adult, but emotionally immature, may not permit his parent to become appropriately dependent. Without corrective intervention, such family pathology may be passed on from one generation to the next.

Geropsychiatric diagnosis always involves a complex formulation and never a simple descriptive term. The diagnostic formulation integrates multiple etiological factors (premorbid personality; past experience; current stresses; nature of coping behavior, etc.) in such a way that the disturbed mental functions can be understood as the outcome of the interaction of all these factors. In the etiology, organic, psychogenic, and social factors usually co-exist and their interaction leads to vicious circles which tax the patient's homeostatic capacity to the breaking point. Organic brain syndrome, for example, has been described in terms of a sociopsychosomatic syndrome.[12] The diagnostic formulation, at the same time, points the way toward the essentials of the treatment plan.

Geropsychiatric therapy is never a single treatment modality, but always a treatment program. The composition of a treatment program is determined by the significant elements making up the diagnostic formulation. By and large, an effective treatment program, which is an individualized package of specific treatment modalities, contains measures that are medical, psychotherapeutic, and social. Other measures, e.g., legal aid, financial assistance, are often included as well.

Another characteristic is that, while in younger age groups one tries to adjust the individual to the environment, in the case of geropsychiatric management, the environment needs to be adjusted to the patient. This principle follows from the age-related decline in homeostatic capacity. Therefore, environmental planning, protective services, and protective intervention are important aspects of geropsychiatric practice.

A major therapeutic goal is to assist the aged patient in actualizing his potential, to free him sufficiently from illness so that he will be able to attain specific goals: a sense of integrity, the maintenance of personal dignity, and the creative capacity to experience the last years as the consummation of life.

Complex as the diagnostic formulation and the treatment plan may be, the implementation of the latter is even more difficult. This touches on another facet of geropsychiatric work, i.e., providing leadership in planning and developing service programs for the elderly.

Interdisciplinary and Social Aspects. The lack of meaningful communication between researchers, practitioners, and planners has come into progressively sharper focus. Related to this is the realization that research findings must be translated, applied, and attuned to social issues and problems.[2, 13–16]

Social geropsychiatry involves cooperation with community agencies, consultation with nursing homes, environmental planning, and programs of releasing hospitalized patients into the community. It also includes retirement counseling. Since the psychopathology of retirement often reflects the psychopathology of work, the geropsychiatrist needs to be acquainted with the meaning of work, leisure, and recreation.

Research Aspects. Major areas where additional research is needed include: etiology and treatment of organic brain syndrome and senile dementia, the psychodynamics of coping with involutional losses, and the psychopathology of "despair," psychopharmacology and geriatric prosthetics, development of adequate service programs and optimal environments, ways and means to enhance the quality of life (e.g., marital and sexual; recreation).

TRAINEE CATEGORIES

TRAINEE CHARACTERISTICS

Trainee characteristics can be categorized according to the trainee's discipline, his principal type of professional activity (research, clinical work, teaching, administration), and his level of professionality (semi- or paraprofessional, masters level, graduate, postgraduate). Occupational groupings to which training activities can be directed would include:

Health and Medical Services

Health and medical services, e.g., clinical psychology, dietetics, dentistry, health education, nursing home management, nursing, nutrition, occupational therapy, medicine, surgery, podiatry, rehabilitation counseling, social work, and speech therapy.

Social Services

Social services, e.g., financial planning with older people, social casework, family counseling, intake services, and assisting in adjustment in institutions and hospital discharges, arranging for guardianships, organizing and administering home services, providing information, referral and placement services, conducting group programs for older persons, planning for community agencies.

Educational, Religious, and Recreational Services

Educational, religious, and recreational services, e.g., program planners, arts and crafts, vocational and avocational counselors, librarians, club leaders, senior activity centers, group workers, pastoral counseling.

Environmental Planning

Environmental planning, e.g., architecture, community organization, federal and state planning, institutional administration, and housing for older people.

Paraprofessional

To these may be added *paraprofessional* and *semiprofessional* personnel (e.g., hospital attendants, "friendly visitors").

Geropsychiatry can make contributions to the training of many of these professional service fields, as illustrated by the following examples. The rehabilitation counselor needs to know how psychological factors influence motivation, and how mental impairment affects performance. The nursing home manager can be more effective when he is aware of the high incidence of psychiatric symptomatology among nursing home residents, and has a working knowledge with regard to the implications for treatment programs and an optimal physical and social environment. The family counselor needs to be well informed about the psychopathology of senescence, and the possible effects of the presence of an aging person on other family members. Specialists in architecture and human engineering are better equipped to create optimal environments (retirement villages, recreation centers) when their basic expertise is supplemented by comprehension of the particular needs of elderly persons. Such complicated tasks as balancing the need for privacy against the risk of psychological withdrawal and social isolation, the need for stimulation and activity against the risk of undue passivity, the need for peer contact against the risk of alienation from younger people, can be more easily carried out if the persons assigned these tasks have had some appropriate exposure to information from relevant areas of aging.[17]

QUANTITATIVE ASPECTS

Personnel Shortage

On all levels, there is a *shortage of professional personnel* working with elderly patients, and the field of aging is not attracting enough scientists and practitioners.[7, 13, 18] Lack of adequate leadership is perceived to be critical in almost every area, in particular policy making, program planning, education, and bridging interdisciplinary gaps.[14, 19] There is a need to increase the skills of those already active in the field of aging.

An accurate assessment of the manpower shortage is not possible because most workers in the field of aging spend only part of their time with the aged while their basic professional identity remains rooted in other disciplines. This partial commitment to the fields of aging does not negate the need for a core group of professionals who spend *most* of their time in this area. Without a minimum number of such specialists, little effective training could take place in various branches of aging. Thus, generally speaking, two types of training activities are needed: (a) staff development and teacher training, productive of specialists with a major commitment both to education and to the field of aging; and (b) training of personnel whose work involves the rendering of services and care to aged patients.

Gerophobia

The lack of personnel is sometimes ascribed to gerontophobia, which is perceived by some authors as a serious problem.[26] It is often stated that students or physicians are not interested in working with elderly patients. A few authors, however, go beyond this by observing that the amount of interest generated by students depends on the extent to which they have opportunities to work closely with aged patients in a clinical setting, and on the caliber of such a geriatric facility.[4, 9, 10, 20]

There is reason to believe that gerophobia and the alleged lack of interest among students and physicians are manageable problems. Other subspecialties have their own prejudices to contend with (e.g., mental retardation, alcoholism). Furthermore, as long as most professionals in the field of aging are only part-time gerontologist, it would not be proper to place responsibility for lack of progress on outsiders. Although there is little question about the existence of gerontophobia, and lack of interest among students, these obstacles are not static impediments, but capable of dynamic transformation depending on our own efforts. Probably the best way to overcome lack of interest is to have excellent *geriatric facilities* which provide opportunities for clinical learning experiences. There is general agreement that there are not enough clinical facilities capable of providing optimal care and high-caliber training in geriatrics or geropsychiatry. Related to this the question to what extent elderly patients themselves would use geriatric facilities. It has been observed, however, that when geriatric facilities are available, offering high-caliber services, elderly individuals do make use of them.[21–23] This suggests that elderly patients themselves do not object to being identified as "geriatric."

METHODS OF TRAINING

DETERMINING FACTORS

Teaching methods depends on the training *objectives*, the curriculum *contents*, and on the *type and level of professionality* of the trainees. For example, the training may focus on clinical skills, on principles of research, or on teaching techniques. These objectives are further modified by the nature of the setting in which the trainee ultimately expects to work (e.g., academic, private practice, institutional). Teaching methods should be closely attuned to the subject matter to be taught. For example, it is not possible to master the science and art of psychotherapy without doing psychotherapy under close supervision. Nor can one learn to teach without the actual experience of instructing different types of students, or without proper feedback from an experienced teacher. Such a matching of course contents to practical experience is feasible, however, only in training programs of reasonable duration. It is a drawback of conferences, workshops, and short courses that they do not provide the time-consuming but crucial element of "experience."

Finally, methods of training are also determined by the type of professional to be trained and by the level of his education (e.g., physicians, clergymen, social workers, nurses, physical therapists, hospital aids, community volunteers). The differences in characteristics between these groups and levels require corresponding differences in focus and depth of content. The process of transmitting to others one's own knowledge requires that it be transformed into objective information that can be received and assimilated by others. The greater the "professional distance" between teacher and trainee, the greater are the potential difficulties in communication. It is then essential that the teacher has thoroughly understood, and clearly conceptualized for himself, what he is about to teach, and that he find the appropriate language for transmitting the information to his audience. One important advantage of relative closeness of the professional levels of teachers and trainees, is the opportunity of the former to serve as a professional role model for the latter.

SPECIFIC METHODS

Specific methods of teaching include conferences, workshops, or institutes, regular consultations, formal courses, and full-time professional training programs.

Conferences, Workshops, and Institutes

These are a popular means of disseminating information. This format usually involves a series of presentations by authorities in the field, the use of discussion groups, and panel discussions. The program may last from one to several days and usually has a fairly substantial attendance. The advantages of this approach are strategic (e.g., alerting a relatively large group of professionals to particular aspects of aging, creating enthusiasm); economical (e.g., little expenditure of time and money on the part of the participants), and social (e.g., the fringe benefits of conventioneering). The disadvantages include the risk of superficiality of the learning experience, and the difficulty in evaluating accurately the impact of the training effort. Institutes and workshops are most effective when participants are carefully selected, when the number of participants is small enough to permit group discussions, when the conference lasts long enough to allow for assimilation and integration of the information presented, and when the proceedings are later made available to the participants.

Consultation Programs

Consultation programs represent a format less clearly defined than other training programs. Consultation may take the form of problem-centered seminars or of individual and group supervision. The consultant, who may be of a different professional background than the consultee, usually functions in an advisory role and tends to avoid recommending personal solutions based on his own experiences.

Because of the relatively unstructured nature of the consultation process, special difficulties may arise, such as disillusionment when the consultees discover that the consultations do not answer all their questions. This points up the need for clearly defining the roles and expectations of consultant and consultees.

There is a variety of formats from which the consultant and consultees can select one that is suitable for their particular objectives. The components which can be used to put a consultation program together include the following.

Didactic presentations can be given by the consultant, usually at the beginning of the consultation session, in order to delineate the "subject matter for the day," to stimulate the audience for later discussion, or to set the stage for a case presentation.

Case presentations can be given by the consultees. They have a greater chance of being effective if a case summary is made available ahead of time to the participants, including the consultant. The case discussion involves two phases. During the first phase, the consultant essentially raises questions and stimulates the consultees toward greater intellectual effort. At the end of the first phase, there are numerous isolated bits of observation, but little closure. During the second phase, the consultant sees to it that the bits of information are integrated into a cohesive framework. This usually necessitates the providing of additional theoretical knowledge to the trainees which enables them to see the whole forest rather than the single trees.

Group discussions may be periodically scheduled to talk informally about topics about which the consultant has some expertise, for example, ward management techniques; the structure and function of the treatment team; contact with the patient's relatives; professional frustrations, etc.

Audiovisual presentations can be used as a teaching device in an ongoing consultation program (or any type of training program, for that matter). Some points to keep in mind, with regard to audiovisual (AV) presentations are the following. (1) Usually, the AV presentation is no better than the instructor who uses it; in fact, AV techniques simply represent a method by which an experienced instructor enhances his effectiveness in communication. (2) Most instructors prefer to use video tapes which they themselves produced. (3) No audiovisual presentation (film or videotape) should run uninterruptedly for more than 20–30 minutes, or the audience will get sleepy. (4) Technical perfection of both the audio and video aspects is an absolute must. (5) The preparation and utilization of audiovisual materials is expensive and time-consuming. This investment is justified if there is sustained utilization of the hardware and the software, in such a manner that teaching effectiveness is significantly enhanced.

Courses

Courses are usually offered as a part of a larger curriculum, such as continuing education programs, or as part of in-service training programs. Courses in geriatric subjects are not currently a regular feature of medical school curricula or residency training programs. Attempts are being made in several places and in several ways to tackle this problem.[4, 9, 18, 24, 25, 26] The general impression is, that lectures, reading assignments, and larger conferences are not effective in stimulating interest among students. On the other hand, when students have access to clinical work with elderly patients, this serves as an eye-opener. Thus, if a student is going to be interested in the field of aging, he is likely to do so by way of developing an interest in aged *persons.*

To go on with the medical student: although he may take certain courses in aging, these are not sufficient for geriatic clinical work later on. Rather, he should learn how the "being old" of his patient can cause age-related impairments; how these determine the patient's reactions to therapy; and how they influence the doctor-patient relationship. He should have the opportunity to apply this knowledge in clinical situations, under supervision and with opportunities to observe his instructor perform clinically with geriatric patients.

Similar considerations apply to other disciplines. In the area of occupational therapy, it is clear that elderly patients with mental disorders require therapeutic activities that are quite different from those for other age groups. In the field of nutrition, the need for specialized knowledge is underscored by the fact that many elderly patients have a host of peculiarities related to loss of teeth, diminution of the sense of taste and smell, altered gastrointestinal functioning, as well as many psychological, social, and economical factors. Thus, geriatric medicine, geriatric occupational therapy, and geriatric dietetics are sufficiently unique and complex so as to require special training experience organized by experts in these respective areas. The same applies to many other areas, such as geriatric dentistry, recreation, and social work.

Courses in medical and psychiatric aspects of aging have special relevance for persons already working with elderly patients. Among these groups, there is usually substantial interest in additional training opportunities. The largest number of persons engaged in the care of geriatric patients are probably the nursing aides and practical nurses in extended care facilities. These persons appear to receive little in the way of formal training in geriatric topics. For example, mental hospital aides usually receive a general course orienting them to work with psychiatric patients. Topics related to aging constitute only a small part of the curriculum. When these aides are placed on a geriatric unit, on-the-job training is expected to supplement their limited knowledge. It is questionable, however, if these circumstances foster an optimal degree of clinical know-how.

In-service training programs for this type of personnel are not without problems. First, there is the problem of finding staff with competence in specific content areas, as well as in teaching methods, who are willing to teach, and who have sufficient time. Second, additional personnel must be available to carry on with patient care while the trainees are in class. Third, mental hospital aides represent a heterogeneous group with regard to age, intelligence, and motivation. By and large, they are more interested in learning practical know-how than theoretical concepts.

A few comments on the *evaluation* of training programs may be in order here. Several methodological problems exist. (1) The accuracy and usefulness of the assessment data depend on determining the pretraining level of trainee knowledge and skills. (2) Knowledge and information can be more easily and accurately tested than the level of clinical skills. (3) Improved morale, self-confidence, and job satisfaction in the trainees, which can be a definite fringe benefit of training, are even more difficult to measure. These subjective phenomena may be evaluated on the basis of personal reports expressed by the trainees. (4) Occasionally, a paradoxical phenomenon occurs: some trainees seem to know less upon completion of training than at the start. One possible explanation is that these are individuals who, as a result of the training, have begun to ask themselves questions about phenomena previously taken for granted. The evaluation test catches them at a time when they have more questions than answers.

In-service training staffs tend to develop their own *course materials*: texts, reprints, bibliographies, edited lectures, illustrative clinical case write-ups, and so on. These materials can eventually be put together in the form of a compendium or manual. Once such course materials are available, they can facilitate extension of the training program to other institutions.

As mentioned above, audiovisual methods can add a unique dimension to educational programs. Closed-circuit television enables an audience to follow closely an actual interview and permits the instructor to make ongoing comments on the patient's behavior and the communication in the physician-patient relationship. Playback of previously recorded video tapes offers the advantage that, at any time, the videotape can be stopped to discuss specific behavioral phenomena, or to replay parts of particular importance. Another use of video tape materials is the development of a library of video tapes on such topics as psychopathology of senescence, techniques of interviewing, family dynamics, and intergenerational conflict. From the video tapes, instructional films can be made.

Formal Training Programs

Formal training programs in aging require full-time participation on the part of the trainee. They are usually oriented more toward training in research than in applied gerontology or geriatrics. This trend is not surprising because a professional orientation toward research in aging promises the rewards of prestige, and the intellectual detachment needed in scientific research may be preferable to the personal anxieties and professional frustrations with which the clinician has to come to grips. But this trend does suggest that, to recruit bright and well-motivated persons for clinical work with the aged, part-time research needs to be emphasized. In fact, diversification generally is wise: the investigator may get new hunches from clinical work, and the clinician may improve his professional effectiveness by participation in research.

Table 22.1 shows an example of areas of interest and topics to be considered for inclusion in the 2-year curriculum of a full-time Geropsychiatry Training Program. In this particular case, the trainees would be psychiatric residents at the 4th and 5th year level of training.[27]

Table 22.1
Example of Geropsychiatry Fellowship Curriculum

Geropsychiatry
- Psychodynamics of senescence (patterns of successful aging, coping with involutional losses)
- Psychopathology and psychiatric syndromes of senescence
- Psychotherapy (individual and group therapy, family therapy, etc.)
- Psychopharmacology and other somatic therapies
- Environmental planning (milieu therapy, reality orientation, etc.)
- Management and administration, e.g., of geropsychiatric in-patient unit

Geriatrics
- Geriatric mdicine and neurology
- Somatopsychology (changes in body image, psychological reactions to chronic illness and disability, etc.)
- Psychosomatic approach (the sick role, psychosocial factors in organic brain syndrome, rehabilitation techniques, management of hypochondriasis, etc.)

Psychosocial Gerontology
- The human life cycle
- Ecology of senescence, sociocultural determinants
- Social attitudes toward aging and mental illness
- Work and retirement (career patterns, psychopathology of work and retirement, leisure and recreation); retirement counseling
- Family dynamics and conflict
- Programs of care for the aged and chronically ill

Psychological Gerontology
- Age-related changes and measurement techniques of intelligence, perception, psychomotor skills, learning, and memory
- Neuropsychological deficits of senium (clinical and laboratory techniques)

Biological Gerontology
- Psychophysiology
- Neurophysiology (senescent electroencephalogram, cerebral blood flow studies)
- Neurochemistry and neuropharmacology
- Genetics and biology of aging

References

1. Lawton, A. H.: The role of medical education in gerontology. *J. Am. Geriatr. Soc. 17(1):* 230–234, 1969.
2. Lawton, A. H.: Continuing postgraduate medical education in geriatrics. *J. Am. Geriatr. Soc. 19(2):*97–101, 1971.
3. Sinex, F. M.: A view of training from within the medical school: attitudes, status, and structure (Symposium—The real world and the ivory tower). *The Gerontologist 14:* 538–542, 1974.
4. Bayne, J. R. D.: Geriatrics and gerontology in medical education. *J. Am. Geriatr. Soc. 22(5):*198–202, 1974.
5. Schaie, K. W.: Training of trainers to train trainers (Symposium—The real world and the ivory tower). *The Gerontologist 14:*533–535, 1974.
6. Beattie, W. M., Jr.: Gerontology curricula: multidisciplinary frameworks, interdisciplinary structures, and disciplinary depth (Symposium—The real world and the ivory tower). *The Gerontologist 14:*545–549, 1974.
7. Freeman, J. T.: A survey of geriatric education: catalogues of United States medical schools. *J. Am. Geriatr. Soc. 19(9):*746–762, 1971.
8. Goldman, R.: Geriatrics as a specialty—problems and prospects. *The Gerontologist 14:*468–471, 1974.
9. Libow, L. S.: A fellowship in geriatric medicine. *J. Am. Geriatr. Soc. 20(12):*580–584, 1972.
10. Arie, T.: Morale and the planning of psychogeriatric services. *Br. Med. J. 3:*166–170, 1971.
11. Weg, R. B.: A view from curricula for gerontology. (Symposium—The real world and the ivory tower). *The Gerontologist 14:*549–553, 1974.
12. Wang, H. S.: Organic brain syndrome. In: *Behavior and Adaptation in Late Life,* edited by E. W. Busse and E. Pfeiffer, chap. 13, Little, Brown and Company, Inc., Boston, 1969.
13. Wright, I. S.: A look into the future of geriatric medicine. *J. Am. Geriatr. Soc. 21(2):*55–57, 1973.
14. Elias, M. F.: Dialectics of professional training, education, and delivery of services to elderly persons (Introduction to the Symposium—The real world and the ivory tower). *The Gerontologist 14:*525–526, 1974.
15. Hickey, T., and Spinetta, J. J.: Bridging research and application (Symposium—The real world and the ivory tower). *The Gerontologist 14:*526–530, 1974.
16. Urban, H. B., and Watson, W.: Alternative approaches (Symposium—The real world and the ivory tower). *The Gerontologist 14:*530–533, 1974.
17. Verwoerdt, A.: Training in geriatric psychiatry. In: *Behavior and Adaptation in Late Life.* chap. 17, Little, Brown and Company, Boston, 1977.
18. Rao, D. B.: Fellowships in geriatric medicine. *J. Am. Geriatr. Soc. 21(4):*169–171, 1973.
19. Fauri, D. P.: Educating for gerontological leadership roles (Guest Editorial). *The Gerontologist 14:*466, 1974.
20. Libow, L. S., Viola, R. M., and Stein, M. F., Jr.: The extended care facility at Mount Sinai City Hospital Center, Elmhurst, New York: three-year experience. *J. Am. Geriatr. Soc. 16(10):*1164–1172, 1968.
21. Varner, R. V., and Clavert, W. R.: Psychiatric assessment of the aged: a differential model for diagnosis. *J. Am. Geriatr. Soc. 22(6):*273–277, 1974.
22. Feigenbaum, E. M.: Geriatric psychopathology—internal or external? *J. Am. Geriatr. Soc. 22(2):*49–55, 1974.
23. Furstenberg, F. F.: Should your hospital have an aging center? *Hosp. Pract.,* August 1963, 48–53.
24. Busse, E. W.: One medical school's approach to teaching problems of the aging. *J. Am. Geriatr. Soc. 17(3):*299–303, 1969.
25. Miller, M. B.: Restructuring medical education for management of the chronically ill aged. *J. Am. Geriatr. Soc. 22(11):*501–509, 1974.
26. Bunzel, J. H.: Recognition, relevance and deactivation of gerontophobia: theoretical essay. *J. Am. Geriatr. Soc. 21(2):*77–80, 1973.
27. Verwoerdt, A.: Careers in geropsychiatry. *Sandoz Monograph: Careers Directions,* vol. 5, No. 3, 1977, pp. 14–19.

23

the golden age

The term golden age suggests that old age is a period in life which has prestige, high value, or great satisfaction. Related to this is the optimistic belief that continued progress in medicine, science, and social conditions will eventually enable man to live the full length of his life span, "adding years to life and life to the years." Whether or not this utopian prospect will ever come about is a matter of speculation.

Or, maybe this view of old age as a golden age is a cover-up. Could it be an invention, or an unconscious expression of our own pessimistic, gerophobic attitudes? By creating the mirage of a golden age at the horizon of life, we may comfort ourselves and feel relieved from doing anything about the stark realities of old age. Then, the phrase would be a hypocritical euphemism and a form of self-deception.

Notions which younger people have about old age, e.g., gerophobia, must be in the nature of prejudice because they have not had first hand experience with being old. These prejudices are carried along by these people, through adult years, into old age. By this time, the prejudice boomerangs against its carrier: the old person has become what he used to be afraid of. Thus, preconceived, unfavorable notions about old age are self-defeating not only to the aged of today, but also to people who are still young but will be old someday.

Between the overly optimistic and overly pessimistic points of view, there may be a more realistic position.

The aging person does have a decline in physical functioning, and it is particularly these physical changes that underly our gerophobic tendencies. Nevertheless, it is important not to forget that many functions hold up reasonably well with aging, that aging is not synonymous with illness, that only a small minority of the aged (5 percent) is so disabled that they have to be institutionalized, that some of the chronic illnesses and disabilities occurring in old age may become more treatable in the nearby future, and so on. And it must be kept in mind that aging, physiologically and psychologically, is an individual matter: different organ systems in the same individual may age with different times of onset and at different rates of speed. Also, time of onset and tempo varies from one individual to another.

With regard to social aspects, there is, of course, little doubt that the aged are less involved and engaged than, say, middle-aged persons. Nevertheless, social functions appear to be relatively age-resistant, being interpersonal in nature and not quite as dependent on physical factors.

Most of the aged are not alone or do not feel lonely; most of them wish to retain some degree of independence and they seem to succeed reasonably well in this. Aging persons are as individual in their preference with regard to closeness versus distance to relatives as younger people are.

Retirement is not just the loss of one's occupational work role; it is also an opportunity for more private work. General progress in education in the younger years, and proper attention to preretirement planning will enable retired persons to make optimal use of their free time for recreation or even creative purposes.

Psychological capacities decline in effectiveness. There is a common notion that old people are more conservative and less flexible. By and large, productivity and creativity, following a peak in the 30's and 40's, decline gradually thereafter. Nevertheless, personality does not drastically change with aging. This does not mean that people do not change at all in the course of time, but in the midst of change, an individual's identity can remain the same. Rather than describing old people in terms of being rigid, conservative, or cautious, we should wonder about the totality of their life style. Certain functions are more apt to stand out in late life, such as historical perspective, wisdom, and judgment. The historical perspective that comes from accumulated life experiences involves also a perspective on one's own life. The life review is a creative mental process through which the aged person reflects on the meaning of his own life and sometimes life in general. Besides the subjective goal of recalling personal historical events, reminiscing can be useful for others by communicating historical and cultural values to members of younger generations. Productivity and creativity do not necessarily come to a standstill in late life, but their quality may change. Creative interests may have a different focus (e.g., interest in history, nature, etc.).

All of this has a familiar ring. Somehow it still lacks power of persuasion. The "nevertheless" element in all of the above considerations reminds me of a letter of recommendation which I had requested concerning somebody, many years ago. The respondent's letter started off with, "I have known Dr. X for 8 years. Nevertheless, I can recommend him very highly." I am also reminded of what a well-known geriatrician said after almost a lifetime of work in the field of aging, "Old age *is* a depression."

There are innumerable ways of being happy or miserable. In fact, it is hard to know what happiness is; it is ephemeral and evanescent. In order to see it, one needs to have astigmatic vision, because by directly focusing at happiness, it seems to disappear. The pursuit of happiness is probably a self-defeating method. Happiness is also elusive, because at the very moment of experiencing it, I become aware of its transience.

Be that as it may, there seem to be three principal ways of happiness. First, one can be happy in anticipation of something. Implicit in this happiness is the hope, trust, or certainty that the happy prospect will become reality. This happiness has a temporal quality of the "not yet." Second, there is the pleasure of actual gratification and the joy of attainment in the present. This is the happiness of the "now," a transient moment between the "not yet" and the "no longer." Third, there is the happy contentment of having had pleasure and happiness and knowing and remembering it. The temporal quality is that of "no longer," but the past experience can be retained as mental images and memories and they can be recalled at will.

Each of the three modes of happiness has its own specific risk of misery. The happiness of the hopeful anticipation may shift toward anxiety, i.e., doubt about the probability of the hoped-for prospect. The happiness of the actual satisfaction in the here and now may be mixed with a nostalgic awareness of the transient nature of pleasure and its evanescence. The happiness of contentment and fulfillment may be replaced by depression or despair, when the person believes that his past was empty and that it is now too late to do anything about it.

> A 75-year-old man, for example, stated that "Since I was 15 years old, when I got started on my own, I have had 100 hours of happiness." Over a 60-year period, that comes to approximately 2 minutes of happiness per week.

People in general differ in regard to their preference for these modes of happiness. Eager anticipation is more typical for young people. Involvement in the present is more characteristic for the middle years. And ideally, late life is the time for a sense of completeness: the certainty that was once a promise has been fulfilled. The retrospective access through one's memories to the shares of happiness may result in a sense of gratitude. All of this may add up to a perspective in old age which could be a strong counterforce against cynicism or despair.

> The key is the attainment of a sense of a fulfillment. A young patient, 20 years of age, who was on a path toward schizophrenia, once said during an interview, "I wish that I were old." At first, I did not quite understand his point. He did not sound depressed, or tired, but one thing was beyond a doubt: the depth of his anxiety. Facing the openness of his future terrified him. What his statement implied was something to the effect of, "I wish that I were old. Then I would have completed all the living ahead of me; then I could at least say that all the experiences of a lifetime would be unalienably mine. Nobody could take them away. Nobody could touch me. I would have made it to the other side, without dying before my time."

Anxiety in younger years often reflects fears of missing out on life's opportunities, or dying before one's time. Having lived a full life places one beyond anxiety, in a sphere of serenity.

Related to the concept of fulfillment is the idea of coming home. The theme of "home" or "going home" is a leitmotiv in old age. The senile patient goes back home, to where he was born. The religious person looks forward to going home in a very different sense. A pervasive nostalgia is all around. But regardless of what home and where, aren't we also talking about being at home with myself, a special sense of belonging between me and myself? Being at one with myself is not a place, but an inner quality of being.

Up to this point, we have evaded the most difficult question, viz, what about people whose lives were empty? Are they victims to be abandoned to despair? Erikson defines integrity as the acceptance of life and the people in it, as something that had to be and that, by necessity, permitted no substitution; and as the acceptance of one's life and what happened in it, as one's own responsibility. Something that has to be "by necessity" is in accordance with the laws of determinism, fate, or Necessity (Ananke). On the other hand, my responsibility is based on freedom and choice. The transcendence of fate and the transformation of Necessity into Providence is ultimately possible only because of the sovereignty of the self. Man creates his own world, makes his own history, and is his own historian. History is not mechanical copying of facts, but selective choosing of relevant events. And who is the one to decide what is relevant? What judge is there to go to? Even the choice of a judge would be my decision. In the end, there is no one else to go to for the final answers except oneself.

CONCLUDING REMARKS

The emphasis in this last chapter has been on finding the positive elements and accounting for the goal in the golden age. Those of us who are in regular contact with the aged do not have to be convinced of the need of presenting the aged themselves with a message of hope. If it should become a habit to bring them messages of decline and depression, we would soon be without an audience, if not without work. On the other hand, it is equally difficult to hand out false reassurances and to deceive our aged clients and ourselves with Pollyannish pronouncements. All of this, far from being philosophical, is an urgently practical matter.

The various points presented above as positive elements have to be thought of as goals and ideals. Few people reach all of their goals and few reach any one goal as completely as they had wished. Goals and ideals are guideposts; they point the way. Old people vary greatly with regard to the progress they have made toward the end goals. It is safe to say that the overall situation of the aged nowadays, in spite of many recent improvements, is still not conducive toward assisting the aged to attain their goals. We hope improvements will continue to occur so that many ideals will be more closely approximated.

Apart from any and all such improvements, we must keep in mind that the golden values of the golden age do not come without work, conflict, and struggle. The value of gold lies precisely in the fact that it is rare and that one has to work hard at getting it. Finding it makes all the hardships worthwhile; knowing there is indeed gold present makes it possible to continue working with confidence.

index